W9-BGG-730

Management of Stroke:
A Practical Guide for the Prevention, Evaluation, and Treatment of Stroke

Third Edition

Harold P. Adams, Jr, MD
Professor and Director
Division of Cerebrovascular Diseases
Department of Neurology
University of Iowa College of Medicine

Gregory J. del Zoppo, MD
Associate Professor
Department of Molecular and Experimental Medicine
The Scripps Research Institute
Division of Hematology/Medical Oncology
Scripps Clinic and Research Foundation
La Jolla, California

Rüdiger von Kummer, MD
Professor of Radiology and Neuroradiology
Department of Neuroradiology
Technical University
Dresden, Germany

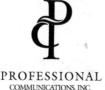

PROFESSIONAL
COMMUNICATIONS, INC.

Copyright 2006
Harold P. Adams, Jr, MD, Gregory J. del Zoppo, MD,
Rüdiger von Kummer, MD

Professional Communications, Inc.

A Medical Publishing Company

Marketing Office:
400 Center Bay Drive
West Islip, NY 11795
(t) 631/661-2852
(f) 631/661-2167

Editorial Office:
PO Box 10
Caddo, OK 74729-0010
(t) 580/367-9838
(f) 580/367-9989

All rights reserved. No part of this publication may be reproduced or transmitted in any form or by any means, electronic or mechanical, including photocopy, recording, or any other information storage and retrieval system, without the prior agreement and written permission of the publisher.

For orders only, please call
1-800-337-9838
or visit our website at
www.pcibooks.com

ISBN: 1-932610-16-2

Printed in the United States of America

DISCLAIMER
The opinions expressed in this publication reflect those of the authors. However, the authors make no warranty regarding the contents of the publication. The protocols described herein are general and may not apply to a specific patient. Any product mentioned in this publication should be taken in accordance with the prescribing information provided by the manufacturer.

This text is printed on recycled paper.

DEDICATION

We thank Leah, Nancy, and Hella
for their love and support.

ACKNOWLEDGMENT

The authors thank Ms. Kimberly Aggson for her assistance in preparing this book.

TABLE OF CONTENTS

Introduction **1**

Organization of Stroke Services **2**

General Measures to Prevent Stroke **3**

Diagnosis and Evaluation of Patients With Suspected Stroke **4**

Imaging of the Brain and Blood Vessels in Stroke **5**

Emergency Medical Management of Stroke **6**

General Management After Admission to the Hospital **7**

Treatment of Hemorrhagic Stroke **8**

Acute Treatment of Ischemic Stroke: Blood Supply to the Brain **9**

Acute Treatment of Ischemic Stroke: Neuroprotection **10**

Prevention of Ischemic Stroke or Recurrent Ischemic Stroke **11**

Rehabilitation After Stroke **12**

Index **13**

TABLES

Table 1.1   Levels of Evidence and Recommendations Used for Guidelines in Management of Patients With Cerebrovascular Disease................16

Table 2.1   "Brain Attack": Public Educational Program About the Common Symptoms of Stroke.............22

Table 2.2   Differences Between Stroke (Brain Attack) and Myocardial Infarction (Heart Attack).............22

Table 2.3   Information to be Obtained in the Field by Emergency Medical Services.................25

Table 2.4   Members of the Acute Stroke–Care Team.............26

Table 2.5   Components of a Stroke Unit................28

Table 3.1   Factors Associated With an Increased Risk of Stroke.................34

Table 3.2   Cardiac Causes of Embolization to the Brain.......36

Table 3.3   Atherosclerotic Causes of Ischemic Stroke...........37

Table 3.4   Nonatherosclerotic Vasculopathies Causing Ischemic Stroke.......................38

Table 3.5   Hematologic or Coagulation Disorders Leading to Ischemic Stroke....................40

Table 3.6   Leading Causes of Intracranial Hemorrhage.........42

Table 3.7   Definition and Treatment of Hypertension............45

Table 3.8   Trials of HMG-CoA Reductase Inhibitors in Lowering the Risk of Ischemic Stroke.................49

Table 3.9   Recommendations for Treatment of Hypercholesterolemia in Patients With Ischemic Stroke.......................50

Table 3.10 Rules of Thumb for the Diagnosis of Transient Ischemic Attack.....................58

Table 3.11 Symptoms of a TIA...............60

Table 3.12 Alternative Diagnosis: Transient Ischemic Attacks.....................60

Table 3.13 Key Questions When Evaluating and Treating a Patient With Suspected TIA or Ischemic Stroke.................61

vi

Table 3.14 Rules of Thumb in the Diagnosis of Warning
Leak of Subarachnoid Hemorrhage 62

Table 3.15 Differential Diagnosis: Minor
Subarachnoid Hemorrhage....................................63

Table 4.1 Differential Diagnosis of Stroke 70

Table 4.2 Historical Features of Ischemic or
Hemorrhagic Stroke 71

Table 4.3 Causes of Neurologic Worsening:
Patients With Stroke..72

Table 4.4 Territories of the Carotid and
Vertebrobasilar Circulations..................................73

Table 4.5 Signs of Ischemic Stroke in the Brain Stem
or Cerebellum...74

Table 4.6 Signs of Ischemic Stroke: Cerebral
Hemisphere 76

Table 4.7 Lacunar Syndromes...77

Table 4.8 Localizing Signs: Infarctions of Cerebral
Hemispheres...78

Table 4.9 Features Distinguishing Ischemic From
Hemorrhagic Stroke 80

Table 4.10 Symptoms and Signs of Hemorrhagic Stroke 82

Table 4.11 Symptoms and Signs of Subarachnoid
Hemorrhage..84

Table 4.12 National Institutes of Health Stroke Scale 85

Table 4.13 Hunt and Hess Scale: Subarachnoid
Hemorrhage..86

Table 4.14 Glascow Coma Scale...87

Table 4.15 Emergency Diagnostic Studies: Evaluation of
Patient With Suspected Stroke 88

Table 4.16 Special Diagnostic Tests of Coagulation to
Screen for Prothrombotic Cause of
Ischemic Stroke...97

Table 5.1 Imaging Techniques for Assessment of a
Patient With Suspected Stroke 104

Table 5.2   What Can Be Imaged in Patients With
Acute Stroke?..105

Table 5.3   Key Questions for Brain Imaging in
Patients With Stroke...106

Table 5.4   Recommendations for Performance of CT in
Patients With Suspected Stroke............................107

Table 5.5   How to Interpret a CT Scan in a Patient
With a Suspected Stroke......................................116

Table 5.6   Recommendations for the Use of Magnetic
Resonance Imaging in Patients With
Suspected Stroke...122

Table 5.7   Guide to Interpretation of Magnetic
Resonance Imaging Studies in Patients
With Suspected Stroke 123

Table 5.8   Magnetic Resonance Imaging Signals of
Blood Degradation Products 128

Table 5.9   Sequence of Vascular Imaging Tests:
Patients With Acute Stroke..................................130

Table 5.10 System for Stratification of Patients
With Acute Stroke: Initial Site of Occlusion
and Collateral Flow 141

Table 6.1   Components of General Emergency Treatment
of Patients With Acute Stroke 148

Table 6.2   Cardiac Abnormalities Associated With
Acute Stroke...151

Table 6.3   Issues Related to Emergency Management
of Arterial Hypertension Associated
With Stroke...153

Table 6.4   Approach to Elevated Blood Pressure in
Acute Ischemic Stroke 156

Table 6.5   Prevention and Treatment of Increased
Intracranial Pressure Following Stroke...............163

Table 7.1   Leading Causes of Neurologic Worsening
Following Acute Stroke..176

Table 7.2   Orders for Multidisciplinary Management
and Treatment of Acute Stroke:
First 24 Hours...178

Table 7.3   Complications of Stroke....................................180

Table 8.1   Intracranial Hemorrhage Associated With
             Medications That Affect Hemostasis 193

Table 8.2   Treatment of Coagulation Abnormalities
             Associated With Hemorrhagic Stroke.................196

Table 8.3   Management of Aneurysmal Subarachnoid
             Hemorrhage..205

Table 8.4   Treatment to Prevent Vasospasm and
             Ischemic Stroke After Aneurysmal
             Subarachnoid Hemorrhage...................................206

Table 9.1   Interventions to Restore or Improve Blood
             Flow to the Brain During Acute
             Ischemic Stroke..222

Table 9.2   Favorable Outcomes at 3 Months in
             Patients Treated <90 Minutes After Onset
             of Acute Ischemic Stroke 225

Table 9.3   Favorable Outcomes at 3 Months in
             Patients Treated 91 to 180 Minutes After
             Onset of Acute Ischemic Stroke...........................226

Table 9.4   Hemorrhagic Events Noted in Patients
             Treated in the European Cooperative Acute
             Stroke Study-I 228

Table 9.5   Mortality and Intracranial Hemorrhages in
             Patients Enrolled in the NINDS rt-PA Trial 229

Table 9.6   Community Experience: Emergency
             Administration of rt-PA in the Treatment
             of Acute Ischemic Stroke 231

Table 9.7   Regimen for Treatment With rt-PA:
             Acute Ischemic Stroke 236

Table 9.8   Results of Trial of Intra-arterial
             Prourokinase in the Treatment of Acute
             Ischemic Stroke..239

Table 9.9   Rates of Symptomatic Hemorrhage
             Trials of Emergency Anticoagulation:
             Acute Ischemic Stroke 242

Table 9.10 Favorable Outcomes: Trials of Emergency
             Anticoagulation in Acute Ischemic Stroke..........246

Table 9.11   Administration of Heparin Following
Acute Ischemic Stroke 249

Table 11.1   Therapies to Prevent Thromboembolic Stroke....280

Table 11.2   Cardiac Conditions Associated With the
Highest Risk for Thromboembolism...................284

Table 11.3   Desired Levels of Anticoagulation.....................285

Table 11.4   Potential Contraindications and Cautions
for Treatment of Patients Taking Oral
Anticoagulants...289

Table 11.5   Ranges of Effective Doses and Most
Common Adverse Experiences With
Antiplatelet Agents..292

Table 11.6   Factors That Predict an Increased Risk
of Perioperative Complications or
Contraindications for Carotid Endarterectomy ...301

Table 11.7   Leading Complications of
Carotid Endarterectomy 303

Table 11.8   Endovascular Procedures 305

FIGURES

Figure 4.1   Evaluation for Suspected Stroke 90

Figure 4.2   Emergent Evaluation for Hemorrhagic Stroke......92

Figure 4.3   Evaluation for Intracranial Hemorrhage 93

Figure 4.4   Emergent Evaluation for Acute
             Ischemic Stroke..96

Figure 4.5   Algorithm for Ordering TEE or TTE 98

Figure 5.1   Cerebral Hematoma 108

Figure 5.2   Subtle Subarachnoid Hemorrhage.......................110

Figure 5.3   Subdural Hematoma..112

Figure 5.4   Early Stages of Ischemic Infarction 113

Figure 5.5   Large Middle Cerebral Artery
             Territory Infarction...114

Figure 5.6   Watershed Infarctions..115

Figure 5.7   Old and Acute Ischemic Lesions..........................120

Figure 5.8   Carotid Dissections 124

Figure 5.9   Occlusion of Middle Cerebral Artery Trunk 125

Figure 5.10 Acute Hemorrhage Into the Precentral Gyrus.....126

Figure 5.11 Bilateral Subacute Cerebral Hematomas 129

Figure 5.12 Duplex Ultrasound of Right Internal
             Carotid Artery Stenosis 132

Figure 5.13 Magnetic Resonance Angiography in
             Venous Sinus Thrombosis Before and After
             Treatment With Heparin.......................................134

Figure 5.14 Computed Tomographic Angiography of
             a Carotid Artery Occlusion..................................136

Figure 5.15 3-D Reconstruction of Rotational Digital
             Subtraction Angiography in a Patient
             With Basilar Aneurysm 137

Figure 8.1   Digital Subtraction Angiography After
             Subarachnoid Hemorrhage and the Effect
             of Coil Embolization...208

Figure 9.1   Algorithm for Mandatory Baseline Assessment
              Prior to Treatment With rt-PA 234

Figure 9.2   Restoration of Cerebral Blood Flow in
              Progressing Stroke by Stenting the Internal
              Carotid Artery...256

Figure 11.1   Algorithm for Prevention of Stroke or
              Recurrent Stroke Based on Presumed Cause
              and Arterial Territory..282

1

Introduction

During the last third of the 20th century, both the frequency of and mortality due to stroke declined in the United States and many other industrialized societies. The drops probably were due, in part, to improved awareness and treatment of risk factors of accelerated atherosclerosis, stroke, and, in particular, hypertension. In addition, the prescription of stroke-prevention therapies to the highest-risk patients also had an effect. However, the decline has stopped.

The impact of stroke likely will grow during the first half of the 21st century. The rates of stroke likely will rise in both developed and developing countries. In the former, aging of the population and improved treatment of heart disease mean that the number of persons at the highest risk for stroke will increase. In developing societies, improved treatment of infectious diseases, changes in diet and lifestyle, and the extension of life expectancy mean that stroke will be a worldwide public health problem.[1] Currently, approximately 750,000 Americans will have a stroke every year and similar or higher rates are noted in many other parts of the world.[2-5] Stroke is the third most common cause of death in the United States and is the second most common etiology of death in the world.[4,6]

Stroke also is a leading cause of disability and long-term institutionalized care. It is second to Alzheimer's disease as a cause of dementia, and cerebrovascular disease also exacerbates the cognitive and behavioral consequences of degenerative dementia. Stroke is an expensive illness, costing the American economy more than $40 billion annually. Similar high costs are noted around the world. The costs are secondary to both health care expenses (including rehabilitation and long-term care) and losses in productivity. Thus effective prevention and treatment of stroke are important for:

- Patients and their families
- Local communities
- Health care providers (physicians, hospitals, rehabilitation services, long-term care providers)
- Insurance companies and other payers
- Social security and other disability programs
- Governments.

Several misconceptions exist about stroke. Stroke is not a cerebrovascular accident (CVA); it is a vascular event secondary to real diseases of blood vessels of the brain. There is a presumed reason or cause for every stroke. Stroke is not one illness but rather it includes several diseases that lead to occlusion of a vessel that deprives blood supply to an area of the brain or that predisposes to bleeding into or around the brain. While the incidence of stroke is highest among the elderly and advancing age is an important predictor of stroke, vascular events also are important causes of neurologic disease in children and young adults. Within most age groups, stroke occurs more frequently among men than women. The causes of stroke also differ between men and women. Still, stroke is a major public health problem in women. For example, among women younger than 45 years of age, stroke is much more common than myocardial infarction. Stroke kills approximately twice as many women as does carcinoma of the breast. Overall, approximately more American women than men die as the result of stroke.

The management of persons with cerebrovascular disease is multifaceted. In continues to evolve along with advances in diagnosis and treatment. Different aspects of management take priority at different stages of a person's life and not all people will need all aspects of treatment. In particular, the most cost-effective treatment is prevention. Currently, management options include the following:

- Primary or secondary prevention
  - Control of risk factors in large populations of healthy persons or high-risk asymptomatic or symptomatic persons
  - Evaluation and institution of therapies aimed at the probable cause of stroke
- Use of medical or surgical interventions to treat the highest-risk patients
- Emergency management of an acute stroke
  - Treatment of acute ischemic stroke
  - Treatment of acute hemorrhagic stroke
- Prevention or treatment of neurologic or medical complications of the stroke
- Rehabilitation to maximize recovery from stroke.

For too long, stroke was approached with a sense of nihilism by physicians and a sense of resignation by patients and their families. A positive attitude toward stroke is crucial. Patients with cerebrovascular disease should be considered to have an illness that can be treated successfully. The risk of stroke may be lessened. Lives may be saved. Disability may be avoided. Outcomes may be improved.

Parallel to improvements in management of cerebrovascular disease, the development of guidelines permits communication about the strength of clinical data and permits sharing information about these advances.[7-20] The recommendations contained in the guidelines are based on the levels of evidence from available data and the strength of the supporting information (**Table 1.1**). In some instances, when definitive data are not available, a recommendation may be based on the consensus of the members of the panel that author the guidelines. Differences exist

TABLE 1.1 — Levels of Evidence and Recommendations Used for Guidelines in Management of Patients With Cerebrovascular Disease

Class I	Conditions for which there is evidence for and/or general agreement that the procedure or treatment is useful and effective
Class II	Conditions for which there is conflicting evidence and/or a divergence of opinion about the usefulness/efficacy of a procedure or treatment
Class IIa	Weight of evidence or opinion is in favor of the procedure
Class IIb	Usefulness/efficacy is less well established by evidence or opinion
Class III	Conditions for which there is evidence and/or general agreement that the procedure or treatment is not useful/effective and in some cases may be harmful
Level of Evidence A	Data derived from multiple randomized clinical trials
Level of Evidence B	Data derived from a single randomized trial or nonrandomized trials
Level of Evidence C	Expert opinion or case studies

Sacco RL et al. *Stroke*. 2006;37:577-617.

among the recommendations contained in the several guidelines; these disparities should not be surprising and probably reflect interpretation of relevant data. The recommendations included in the most recent guidelines are incorporated in this text. While guidelines cannot provide definitive advice about all aspects of a complex disease such as stroke and physicians must continue to use judgment when treating the individual patient, the statements do provide benchmarks that help expedite diagnosis and treatment. In general, guidelines provide the following basic advice about components of management of stroke:

- Selection of the appropriate diagnostic studies to evaluate for stroke and its potential cause
- Administration of interventions that will improve outcomes from stroke or prevent stroke
- Details about when and how to prescribe effective therapies
- Avoidance of dangerous or ineffective therapies.

This text emphasizes the acute management (diagnosis and treatment) of patients with stroke. Information about prevention and rehabilitation also is included. The sequence of chapters is arranged in a presumed chronologic order for a hypothetical patient with cerebrovascular disease:

- Prevention by control of factors or conditions that predispose to stroke
- Emergency evaluation of a patient with suspected stroke
- Acute treatment aimed at lessening the neurologic consequences of stroke
- General management to prevent or control complications of stroke
- Prevention of recurrent stroke with medical or surgical therapies
- Rehabilitation to maximize recovery after stroke.

REFERENCES

1. Poungvarin N. Stroke in the developing world. *Lancet.* 1998;352(suppl 3):SIII19-SIII22.
2. American Heart Association. Heart disease and stroke statistics–2004 update. 2004.
3. Sudlow CL, Warlow CP. Comparing stroke incidence worldwide: what makes studies comparable? *Stroke.* 1996;27:550-558.
4. Bogousslavsky J, Aarli J, Kimura J; Board of Trustees, World Federation of Neurology. Stroke: time for a global campaign? *Cerebrovasc Dis.* 2003;16:111-113.
5. Asplund K. What MONICA told us about stroke. *Lancet Neurol.* 2005;4:64-68.
6. Bergen DC. The world-wide burden of neurologic disease. *Neurology.* 1996;47:21-25.
7. Adams HP Jr, Brott TG, Furlan AJ, et al. Guidelines for thrombolytic therapy for acute stroke: a supplement to the guidelines for the management of patients with acute ischemic stroke. A statement for healthcare professionals from a Special Writing Group of the Stroke Council, American Heart Association. *Stroke.* 1996;27:1711-1718.
8. Adams HP Jr, Adams RJ, Brott T, et al. Guidelines for the early management of patients with ischemic stroke. A scientific statement from the Stroke Council of the American Stroke Association. *Stroke.* 2003;34:1056-1083.
9. Adams H, Adams R, del Zoppo G, Goldstein LB; Stroke Council of the American Heart Association; American Stroke Association. Guidelines for the early management of patients with ischemic stroke: 2005 guidelines update: a scientific statement from the Stroke Council of the American Heart Association/American Stroke Association. *Stroke.* 2005;36:916-923.
10. Demaerschalk BM. Evidence-based clinical practice education in cerebrovascular disease. *Stroke.* 2004;35:392-396.
11. Mayberg MR, Batjer HH, Dacey R, et al. Guidelines for the management of aneurysmal subarachnoid hemorrhage. A statement for healthcare professionals from a special writing group of the Stroke Council, American Heart Association. *Circulation.* 1994;90:2592-2605.
12. Broderick JP, Adams HP Jr, Barsan W, et al. Guidelines for the management of spontaneous intracerebral hemorrhage: a statement for healthcare professionals from a special writing group of the Stroke Council, American Heart Association. *Stroke.* 1999;30:905-915.
13. Albers GW, Amarenco P, Easton JD, Sacco RL, Teal P. Antithrombotic and thrombolytic therapy for ischemic stroke: the Seventh ACCP Conference on Antithrombotic and Thombolytic Therapy. *Chest.* 2004;126:483S-512S.
14. Albers GW, Hart RG, Lutsep HL, Newell DW, Sacco RL. AHA Scientific Statement. Supplement to the guidelines for the management of transient ischemic attacks: a statement from the Ad Hoc Committee on Guidelines for the Management of Transient Ischemic Attacks, Stroke Council, American Heart Association. *Stroke.* 1999;30:2502-2511.
15. Hacke W, Kaste M, Olsen TS, Orgogozo JM, Bogousslavsky J. European Stroke Initiative: recommendations for stroke management. Organisation of stroke care. *J Neurol.* 2000;247:732-748.

16. Asia Pacific Consensus Forum on Stroke Management. *Stroke.* 1998;29:1730-1736.

17. Hack W, Kaste M, Bogousslavsky J, et al; European Stroke Initiative Executive Committee and the EUSI Writing Committee. European Stroke Initiative Recommendations for Stroke Management-update 2003. *Cerebrovasc Dis.* 2003;16:311-337.

18. Albucher JF, Martel P, Mas JL. Clinical practice guidelines: diagnosis and immediate management of transient ischemic attacks in adults. *Cerebrovasc Dis.* 2005;20:220-225.

19. EEC Committee, EEC Subcommittees, ECC Task Forces; and Authors of Final Evidence Evaluation Worksheets 2005 International Consensus on Cardiopulmonary Resuscitation and Emergency Cardiovascular Care With Treatment Recommendations Conference. 2005 American Heart Association guidelines for cardiopulmonary resuscitation and emergency cardiovascular care. Part 9: adult stroke. *Circulation.* 2005;112(suppl):IV-111–IV-120.

20. Sacco RL, Adams R, Albers G, et al; American Heart Association; American Stroke Association Council on Stroke; Council on Cardiovascular Radiology and Intervention; American Academy of Neurology. Guidelines for prevention of stroke in patients with ischemic stroke or transient ischemic attack: a statement for healthcare professionals from the American Heart Association/American Stroke Association Council on Stroke: co-sponsored by the Council on Cardiovascular Radiology and Intervention: the American Academy of Neurology affirms the value of this guideline. *Stroke.* 2006;37:577-617.

2

Organization of Stroke Services

A successful approach to management of patients with acute stroke involves the collaboration of the public and all medical services.

Public Education and Response

Members of the public should recognize the importance of the symptoms of stroke and the best response to the illness.[1,2] Unfortunately, most people do not know the presentations of stroke and some of the highest-risk groups (ie, the elderly) are among those with the least knowledge about stroke.[3-6] The public should learn the most common symptoms of stroke (**Table 2.1**). Public educational campaigns are needed to emphasize the symptoms of stroke.[7,8] These programs for stroke (brain attack) are modeled on those used to convey information about heart attack. However, unlike heart attack, which primarily presents with severe chest pain, the heterogenous symptoms of stroke often do not include pain or headache (**Table 2.2**). Awareness of symptoms or clarity in thinking may be impaired because of the acute brain illness, and a person may not recognize that a stroke is occurring. Thus besides the high-risk person himself/herself, family members, friends, neighbors, and coworkers should be knowledgeable about the symptoms and signs of stroke.

The public also should learn the correct response to a stroke — to seek medical attention immediately.[2,8,9] The message should be simple: the goal is to take the patient to the appropriate emergency department (ED)

TABLE 2.1 — "Brain Attack": Public Educational Program About the Common Symptoms of Stroke

• Sudden onset of symptoms
• Symptoms occur alone or in combination
• Weakness, clumsiness, heaviness or numbness:
  – One side of the body
  – May be restricted to arm and face
• Drooping of one side of the face
• Slurred speech or difficulty finding words
• Difficulty understanding others' speech
• Loss of or blurred vision in one or both eyes
• Dizziness (vertigo) or imbalance
• Unusually severe headache

TABLE 2.2 — Differences Between Stroke (Brain Attack) and Myocardial Infarction (Heart Attack)

• People respond more rapidly to severe pain:
  – Pain is prominent with heart attack
  – Pain often missing with brain attack
• Presentations of heart attack are relatively stereo-typed:
  – Severe, radiating chest pain
  – Dyspnea
  – Nausea
• Presentations of brain attack vary considerably (see **Table 2.1**)
• Public awareness:
  – Know importance of symptoms of heart attack
  – Do not recognize symptoms of brain attack
• Fear and anxiety may delay seeking medical attention with both
• Cognition and thinking:
  – Usually is normal in heart attack
  – May be abnormal or prominent in brain attack
  – Do not recognize signs of right hemisphere stroke because of the brain injury

as quickly as possible. The fastest method is to use emergency medical transportation. Patients should be encouraged to call the local emergency number (911 in most communities in the United States.) Alternatively, they may go directly to an ED, but the patient should not drive the vehicle. Patients should be advised not to contact their physician's office or answering services. They should not accept a scheduled outpatient visit. The worst response is to do nothing in the hope that the symptoms will resolve spontaneously. If the patient contacts a neighbor or relative for advice, the response should be to activate the emergency system.

Emergency Medical Services

While public educational programs are important, there is no reason to organize a public educational campaign if hospitals and physicians are not ready to react to an acute stroke. The health care system should respond quickly because of the relatively short window for successful treatment of stroke.[2,5,10,11] Any potential delay should be identified and tactics implemented to overcome the delay.[12,13] Local or regional plans should be developed to expedite treatment.[14-16] The plans should involve collaboration of physicians, hospitals, emergency medical services (EMSs), and ambulance systems. The support of third-party payers and government also is critical. For example, a coordinated regional stroke-care plan may involve bypassing hospitals that do not have the resources to provide emergency stroke care.[17] In the United States, the Joint Commission on Accreditation Healthcare Organizations has developed a system to certify primary stroke centers that would give modern emergency stroke treatment, including intravenous thrombolysis. Another approach is to develop stroke centers of excellence.[18] The development of regional stroke programs has been successful in increasing the number of patients with acute stroke who can be treated with effective therapies.[19] These systems can work in both rural and urban settings. Each community should address its hurdles to rapid treatment; potential strategies include helicopter transport of patients or telemedicine.[20-25]

Persons answering the telephone, including 911 calls, (EMS dispatchers, physicians' answering services, clinic receptionists, or hospital operators) should recognize the symptoms that reflect stroke and should expedite transport to the ED.[2] They should recommend that the patient go to the ED immediately or they should direct an ambulance or rescue squad to go to the patient's location. Some health maintenance organizations (HMOs) require notification prior to a patient's seeking emergency medical care.[26] Because delays must be avoided, these third-party payers should develop systems to avoid putting such barriers in the way of emergency treatment of stroke. The EMS system also should respond with alacrity.[2,27,28] Stroke should have the same high priority as does acute myocardial infarction.

Upon arrival at the patient's location, EMS personnel should survey the relevant medical history and perform a brief assessment.[29,30] Information about the time of onset of stroke is especially important (**Table 2.3**). Because relatives or observers may travel by private vehicle, their arrival at the ED may be delayed. Some patients may not be able to tell the time of onset of stroke or their neurologic condition may not permit elicitation of a clear history. Thus the EMS personnel should collect the key components of the history that may be needed during the emergency evaluation at the receiving hospital.

Life support should be given and an intravenous catheter should be inserted in order to administer emergency medications.[2] In the future, emergency treatment of the stroke may begin in the field, but to date, such

TABLE 2.3 — Information to Be Obtained in the Field by Emergency Medical Services

- Time and onset of neurological symptoms
- Determine nature of the neurological findings:
  - Weakness of arm or face
  - Slurring of speech or abnormal language
- Rate the score on the Glasgow Coma Scale:
  - Language
  - Eye movement
  - Motor responses
- History of recent illness, surgery, or trauma
- Recent use of medications, in particular anticoagulants

therapies have not been established as effective.[31] The paramedics also may obtain blood samples so that hematologic, biochemical, and coagulation tests may be performed upon arrival at the hospital. The patient should be transported to a hospital that has brain imaging tests and a stroke-responsive team available on a 24-hour-per-day, 7 day-per-week basis.[17,32-34] When ambulance personnel give advance warning that a patient with a stroke is being transported to the ED, this update should expedite mobilization of the appropriate resources at the hospital.

The hospital should have a predesignated acute stroke–care team to coordinate the initial evaluation and treatment. The team should include physicians, nurses, radiology staff, laboratory personnel, and pharmacists.[2,33] Each member of the team has specific duties during the acute period of evaluation and treatment (**Table 2.4**). The team should be mobilized when word is received about the impending arrival of the patient with a possible stroke. The components of the emergency evaluation are outlined in Chapter 4, *Diagnosis and Evaluation of Patients With Suspected Stroke* and in Chapter 5, *Imaging of the Brain and Blood Vessels in Stroke*. The initial treatment of

TABLE 2.4 — Members of the Acute Stroke–Care Team

Area of Expertise	Duties Performed

Physicians
Emergency medicine
Primary care
Neurology
Radiology
Neurosurgery
	• Assess history
	• Perform examinations:
	  – Physical
	  – Neurologic
	• Determine NIHSS score
	• Provide emergency medical care
	• Screen for treatment with rt-PA
	• Order and review diagnostic studies
	• Read CT scan
	• Treat stroke

Nurses	• Help in triage
	• Regularly assess vital signs
	• Assist in baseline evaluation:
	  – Obtain blood tests
	  – Pregnancy test
	• Assist with emergency care:
	  – Starting intravenous access
	  – Administer medications

Technicians	• Do laboratory work • Radiology • Do CT scan • Laboratory • Do electrocardiogram • Do chest x-ray (in some patients)
Pharmacist	• Prepare medications

Abbreviations: CT, computed tomography; NIHSS, National Institutes of Health Stroke Scale; rt-PA, recombinant tissue-type plasminogen activator.

patients is described in Chapter 6, *Emergency Medical Management of Stroke.*

Stroke Units

The care of patients after admission to the hospital is detailed in Chapter 7, *General Management After Admission to the Hospital.* A key component of modern stroke care is treatment in a specialized treatment facility commonly called a stroke unit.

In general, admission to an inpatient unit that specializes in treatment of patients with stroke is associated with an increased likelihood of a favorable outcome. Studies show that care in a facility dedicated to patients with stroke reduces the chances of dying and lessens both disability and the need for long-term institutionalized care (Level of Evidence A).[35-41] As such, treatment in a stroke unit is recommended in most stroke guidelines and statements[42,43] (Class I Recommendation). Overall, the success of stroke-unit treatment is as great at the potential benefit from emergency treatment of ischemic stroke with recombinant tissue plasminogen activator (rt-PA/alteplase).[44] The favorable effects can be detected as long as 10 years after the stroke. In addition, the potential benefits of stroke-unit care can be offered to a broad spectrum of patients, including those who are not eligible for treatment with rt-PA.[45]

The definition of a stroke unit usually includes a geographically defined facility within a hospital that focuses on the treatment of patients with acute stroke (**Table 2.5**). Physicians, nurses, and other professionals who have expertise in the treatment of patients with cerebrovascular disease staff these units. A stroke unit should have the capacity for cardiac monitoring and close neurologic observation. Invasive monitoring, such as continuous arterial pressure monitoring lines, also may be available. Stroke units usually do not repli-

TABLE 2.5 — Components of a Stroke Unit

- Geographically defined facility (4 to 8 beds):
  - Cardiac monitoring
  - Blood pressure monitoring
- Skilled personnel:
  - Physicians (most commonly neurologists)
  - Nurses
  - Rehabilitation specialists:
    - Physical therapy
    - Speech pathology
    - Occupational therapy
  - Discharge planners
- Stroke protocols – stroke-care maps:
  - Acute treatment
  - Monitoring for complications
  - Evaluation
  - Treatment to prevent recurrent stroke

cate an intensive care unit (ICU) because ventilators are not present. Fortunately, most patients do not require ventilatory assistance. However, a critically ill patient, such as a person who is comatose or who has bulbar paralysis, usually needs protection of the airway and ventilatory support. Such a person also needs extensive nursing care and should be admitted to an ICU.

Patients who need urgent surgical procedures, such as evacuation of a hematoma or clipping of an aneurysm, usually are admitted to an ICU after the cranial operation.[46-48] Seriously ill patients may be transferred from the ICU to a stroke unit when their condition improves. In this scenario, the stroke unit serves as a "step-down" unit.

Management in the stroke unit includes close observation to watch for neurologic worsening or responses to acute treatment. In addition, management includes measures to prevent or control acute or subacute medical and neurologic complications. Evaluation for the cause of stroke and starting therapies to prevent recurrent stroke are expedited. Finally, the initial aspects of poststroke rehabilitation and discharge planning can begin. The development of stroke protocols or care maps, which might include preprinted order forms, may help expedite all components of management.

The success of stroke-unit care probably reflects the involvement of all the professionals who expedite all components of acute care. While the initial expenses of treatment in a specialized stroke unit likely are greater than those in a general acute-care ward, the reductions in costs (ie, length of stay, reduction in chronic morbidity that requires long-term institutionalized care) should appeal to groups trying to reduce health care costs.

Once a patient's condition is stable, they may be moved from a stroke unit to a nonmonitored bed for subsequent care. There, management, including planning for discharge or transfer to a rehabilitation unit, is continued.

REFERENCES

1. Hill MD, Hachinski V. Stroke treatment: time is brain. *Lancet.* 1998;352(suppl 3):SIII10-SIII14.
2. EEC Committee, EEC Subcommittees, ECC Task Forces; and Authors of Final Evidence Evaluation Worksheets 2005 International Consensus on Cardiopulmonary Resuscitation and Emergency Cardiovascular Care With Treatment Recommendations Conference. 2005 American Heart Association guidelines for cardiopulmonary resuscitation and emergency cardiovascular care. Part 9: adult stroke. *Circulation.* 2005;112(suppl): IV-111–IV120.
3. Williams LS, Bruno A, Rouch D, Marriott DJ. Stroke patients' knowledge of stroke. Influence on time to presentation. *Stroke.* 1997;28:912-915.
4. Kothari R, Sauerbeck L, Jauch E, et al. Patients' awareness of stroke signs, symptoms, and risk factors. *Stroke.* 1997;28:1871-1875.
5. Kothari R, Jauch E, Broderick J, et al. Acute stroke: delays to presentation and emergency department evaluation. *Ann Emerg Med.* 1999;33:3-8.
6. Yoon SS, Byles J. Perceptions of stroke in the general public and patients with stroke: a qualitative study. *BMJ.* 2002;324:1065-1068.
7. Montaner J, Vidal C, Molina C, Alvarez-Sabin J. Selecting the target and the message for a stroke public education campaign: a local survey conducted by neurologists. *Eur J Epidemiol.* 2001;17:581-586.

8. Schneider AT, Pancioli AM, Khoury JC, et al. Trends in community knowledge of the warning signs and risk factors for stroke. *JAMA.* 2003;289:343-346.

9. Broderick JP. Logistics in acute stroke management. *Drugs.* 1997;54(suppl 3):109-116.

10. Brott T, Bogousslavsky J. Treatment of acute ischemic stroke. *N Engl J Med.* 2000;343:710-722.

11. Adams HP Jr. Treating ischemic stroke as an emergency. *Arch Neurol.* 1998;55:457-461.

12. Yu RF, San Jose MC, Manzanilla BM, Oris MY, Gan R. Sources and reasons for delays in the care of acute stroke patients. *J Neurol Sci.* 2002;199:49-54.

13. Wester P, Radberg J, Lundgren B, Peltonen M. Factors associated with delayed admission to hospital and in-hospital delays in acute stroke and TIA: a prospective, multicenter study. Seek-Medical-Attention-in-Time Study Group. *Stroke.* 1999;30:40-48.

14. Katzan IL, Graber TM, Furlan AJ, et al. Cuyahoga County Operation Stroke speed of emergency department evaluation and compliance with National Institutes of Neurological Disorders and Stroke time targets. *Stroke.* 2003;34:799-800.

15. Gil Nunez AC, Vivancos Mora J. Organization of medical care in acute stroke: importance of a good network. *Cerebrovasc Dis.* 2004;17(suppl 1):113-123.

16. Kennedy J, Ma C, Buchan AM. Organization of regional and local stroke resources: methods to expedite acute management of stroke. *Curr Neurol Neurosci Rep.* 2004;4:13-18.

17. Kidwell CS, Shephard T, Tonn S, et al. Establishment of primary stroke centers: a survey of physician attitudes and hospital resources. *Neurology.* 2003;60:1452-1456.

18. Willerson JT. Editor's commentary: centers of excellence. *Circulation.* 2003;107:1471-1472.

19. Scott PA, Temovsky CJ, Lawrence K, Gudaitis E, Lowell MJ. Analysis of Canadian population with potential geographic access to intravenous thrombolysis for acute ischemic stroke. *Stroke.* 1998;29:2304-2310.

20. Silbergleit R, Scott PA, Lowell MJ. Cost-effectiveness of helicopter transport of stroke patients for thrombolysis. *Acad Emerg Med.* 2003;10:966-972.

21. Thomas SH, Kociszewski C, Schwamm LH, Wedel SK. The evolving role of helicopter emergency medical services in the transfer of stroke patients to specialized centers. *Prehosp Emerg Care.* 2002;6:210-214.

22. Handschu R, Littmann R, Reulbach U, et al. Telemedicine in emergency evaluation of acute stroke: interrater agreement in remote video examination with a novel multimedia system. *Stroke.* 2003;34:2842-2846.

23. Wang S, Gross H, Lee SB, et al. Remote evaluation of acute ischemic stroke in rural community hospitals in Georgia. *Stroke.* 2004;35:1763-1768.

24. Wang S, Lee SB, Pardue C, et al. Remote evaluation of acute ischemic stroke: reliability of National Institutes of Health Stroke Scale via telestroke. *Stroke.* 2003;34:e188-e191.

25. Wiborg A, Widder B; Telemedicine in Stroke in Swabia Project. Teleneurology to improve stroke care in rural areas: The Telemedicine in Stroke in Swabia (TESS) Project. *Stroke.* 2003;34:2951-2956.

26. Neely KW, Norton RL. Survey of health maintenance organization instructions to members concerning emergency department and 911 use. *Ann Emerg Med.* 1999;34:19-24.

27. Crocco TJ, Kothari RU, Sayre MR, Liu T. A nationwide prehospital stroke survey. *Prehosp Emerg Care.* 1999;3:201-206.

28. Harbison J, Massey A, Barnett L, Hodge D, Ford GA. Rapid ambulance protocol for acute stroke. *Lancet.* 1999;353:1935.

29. Kothari R, Barsan W, Brott T, Broderick J, Ashbrock S. Frequency and accuracy of prehospital diagnosis of acute stroke. *Stroke.* 1995;26:937-941.

30. Kidwell CS, Starkman S, Eckstein M, Weems K, Saver JL. Identifying stroke in the field. Prospective validation of the Los Angeles prehospital stroke screen (LAPSS). *Stroke.* 2000;31:71-76.

31. Crocco T, Gullett T, Davis SM, et al. Feasibility of neuroprotective agent administration by prehospital personnel in an urban setting. *Stroke.* 2003;34:1918-1922.

32. Alberts MJ, Hademenos G, Latchaw RE, et al. Recommendations for the establishment of primary stroke centers. Brain Attack Coalition. *JAMA.* 2000;283:3102-3109.

33. Alberts MJ, Chaturvedi S, Graham G, et al. Acute stroke teams: results of a national survey. National Acute Stroke Team Group. *Stroke.* 1998;29:2318-2320.

34. Adams R, Acker J, Alberts M, et al. Recommendations for improving the quality of care through stroke centers and systems: an examination of stroke center identification options: multidisciplinary consensus recommendations from the Advisory Working Group on Stroke Center Identification Options of the American Stroke Association. *Stroke.* 2002;33:e1-e7.

35. Treib J, Grauer MT, Woessner R, Morgenthaler M. Treatment of stroke on an intensive stroke unit: a novel concept. *Intensive Care Med.* 2000;26:1598-1611.

36. Indredavik B, Bakke F, Solberg R, Rokseth R, Haaheim LL, Holme I. Benefit of a stroke unit: a randomized controlled trial. *Stroke.* 1991;22:1026-1031.

37. Indredavik B, Bakke F, Slordahl SA, Rokseth R, Haheim LL. Treatment in a combined acute and rehabilitation stroke unit: which aspects are most important? *Stroke.* 1999;30:917-923.

38. Indredavik B, Bakke F, Slordahl SA, Rokseth R, Haheim LL. Stroke unit treatment improves long-term quality of life: a randomized controlled trial. *Stroke.* 1998;29:895-899.

39. Indredavik B. Stroke units—the Norwegian experience. *Cerebrovasc Dis.* 2003;15(suppl 1):19-20.

40. Ronning OM, Guldvog B. Stroke units versus general medical wards, I: twelve- and eighteen-month survival: a randomized, controlled trial. *Stroke.* 1998;29:58-62.

41. Ronning OM, Guldvog B. Stroke unit versus general medical wards, II: neurological deficits and activities of daily living: a quasi-randomized controlled trial. *Stroke.* 1998;29:586-590.

42. Adams HP Jr, Adams RJ, Brott T, et al. Guidelines for the early management of patients with ischemic stroke. A scientific statement from the Stroke Council of the American Stroke Association. *Stroke.* 2003;34:1056-1083.

43. The European Ad Hoc Consensus Group. Optimizing intensive care in stroke. A European perspective. *Cerebrovasc Dis.* 1997;7:113-128.

2

44. Barnett HJ, Buchan AM. The imperative to develop dedicated stroke centers. *JAMA*. 2000;283:3125-3126.

45. Gilligan AK, Thrift AG, Sturm JW, Dewey HM, Macdonell RA, Donnan GA. Stroke units, tissue plasminogen activator, aspirin and neuroprotection: which stroke intervention could provide the greatest community benefit? *Cerebrovasc Dis*. 2005;20:239-244.

46. Mayberg MR, Batjer HH, Dacey R, et al. Guidelines for the management of aneurysmal subarachnoid hemorrhage. A statement for healthcare professionals from a special writing group of the Stroke Council, American Heart Association. *Circulation*. 1994;90:2592-2605.

47. Broderick JP, Adams HP, Jr, Barsan W, et al. Guidelines for the management of spontaneous intracerebral hemorrhage: a statement for healthcare professionals from a special writing group of the Stroke Council, American Heart Association. *Stroke*. 1999;30:905-915.

48. van Gijn J, Rinkel GJ. Subarachnoid haemorrhage: diagnosis, causes and management. *Brain*. 2001;124:249-278.

3

General Measures
to Prevent Stroke

Prevention is the most effective way to avoid death or suffering from stroke. Successful preventive strategies are cost-effective because they eliminate the expenses of acute hospital care, rehabilitation, and long-term institutionalized care. In addition, forestalling stroke also avoids the economic consequences of lost productivity and the consequences of disability. Although no measure to prevent stroke is uniformly successful, currently available interventions do lower the chances of a major, disabling, or fatal cerebrovascular event.

Prevention of stroke generally involves two different strategies. One consists of interventions that are applied to large segments of the population and includes health promotion and identification and treatment of common factors that increase the risk of either hemorrhagic or ischemic stroke (**Table 3.1**). The measures fall under the strategy of *primary prevention*. These interventions (eg, control of hypertension and stopping smoking) may have limited benefit for an individual patient, but their aggregate effects are substantial when looking at the impact on the health of a large population.[1-3]

The second approach involves the use of potentially more dangerous therapies given to smaller groups of persons judged to be at the highest risk. In some circumstances, these interventions are prescribed as a primary prevention strategy in high-risk asymptomatic people. *Secondary prevention* implies the use of treatments to prevent stroke or other ischemic vascular events in persons who already have had symptoms and includes

TABLE 3.1 — Factors Associated With an Increased Risk of Stroke	
Epidemiologic, Nonmodifiable Factors	
Age	Elderly > middle-aged or young adults > children
Sex	Men > women in most age groups
Race	African Americans > Asians or Hispanics > Whites
Geography	Asia > Europe or North America Eastern Europe > Western Europe Southeastern United States > other regions
Family	Stroke or heart disease in persons <60 years of age

Other potentially modifiable factors:*
- Diastolic or isolated systolic hypertension
- Diabetes mellitus, type 1 or type 2
- Hypercholesterolemia (hyperlipidemia)
- Elevated low-density lipoprotein (LDL) cholesterol
- Low high-density lipoprotein (HDL) cholesterol
- Hyperhomocysteinemia
- Smoking
- Alcohol abuse
- Drug abuse
- Use of oral contraceptives
- Pregnancy
- Migraine

* A combination of the potentially modifiable factors rapidly increases the risk.

treatment of a spectrum of people who have evidence of symptomatic atherosclerotic disease, such as:

- Myocardial infarction (MI)
- Angina pectoris
- Claudication
- Abdominal aortic aneurysm
- Amaurosis fugax
- Transient ischemic attack (TIA)
- Ischemic stroke.

In reality, the division into primary and secondary prevention is somewhat artificial because much of the management of patients in both groups basically is the same.

Risk Factors for Stroke

Because stroke encompasses a heterogenous group of vascular diseases, the conditions or factors that predispose to or increase the risk of a cerebrovascular event are diverse (**Table 3.2**, **Table 3.3**, **Table 3.4**, **Table 3.5**, and **Table 3.6**). The general categories of diseases that lead to ischemic stroke are:

- Large-artery atherosclerosis
- Small-artery occlusive disease (lacunes)
- Cardioembolic
- Nonatherosclerotic vasculopathies
- Disorders of coagulation.

Systems to categorize these vascular events have been used in both research and clinical settings.[4-6] While some conditions that lay the groundwork for ischemic stroke also may lead to brain hemorrhage, additional factors may promote bleeding. Conversely, other risk factors for ischemic stroke do not appear to predispose to intracranial hemorrhage.

Some factors that predispose to stroke are not modifiable. Advancing age is the single most important

TABLE 3.2 — Cardiac Causes of Embolization to the Brain

Atrial Fibrillation
- In particular, complicating structural diseases

Left Ventricular or Intraventricular Lesions
- Recent myocardial infarction, in particular anterior wall
- Ventricular aneurysm
- Akinetic segment after myocardial infarction
- Dilated cardiomyopathy
- Mural or intraventricular thrombus

Left Atrial, Intraatrial, or Interatrial Lesions
- Atrial septal aneurysm
- Atrial septal defect
- Patent foramen ovale
- Atrial turbulence
- Atrial thrombus
- Atrial appendage thrombus
- Myxoma

Valvular Lesions
- Congenital valvular abnormality
- Rheumatic stenosis of mitral valve
- Mitral valve prolapse
- Infective endocarditis
- Nonbacterial thrombotic (marantic) endocarditis
- Libman-Sacks endocarditis
- Mechanical or bioprosthetic valve, in particular mitral position
- Mitral annulus calcification
- Calcific aortic stenosis

Cardiac Procedures
- Cardiac catheterization
- Coronary artery bypass surgery
- Percutaneous transluminal coronary angioplasty
- Percutaneous transluminal valvuloplasty
- Intra-aortic balloon pump
- Cardiac transplantation

**TABLE 3.3 — Atherosclerotic Causes
of Ischemic Stroke**

- Aortic atherosclerosis ("shagbark" aorta)
- Extracranial large-artery atherosclerosis:
  – Origin of the internal carotid artery
  – Origin of the vertebral artery
  – Subclavian artery
- Intracranial large-artery atherosclerosis:
  – Distal portion (siphon) of the internal carotid artery
  – Proximal portion of the middle cerebral artery
  – Distal portion of the vertebral artery
  – Middle segment of the basilar artery
  – Disseminated atherosclerosis
- Fusiform (dolichoectatic) aneurysm:
  – Basilar artery
  – Internal carotid artery
- Small-artery disease (lipohyalinosis or microatheroma):
  – Penetrating arteries

predictor of a high risk for stroke.[7] Although stroke is much more common among elderly persons, it also is an important cause of neurologic disease in children and young adults with stroke.[8-12] Approximately 3% of ischemic strokes occur in people younger than the age of 45. The ratio of hemorrhagic stroke to ischemic stroke is higher in younger people than in the elderly.

In addition, the causes of stroke vary by age. Atherosclerotic disease and cardioembolism (particularly associated with atrial fibrillation [AF]) are the leading etiologies of ischemic stroke in the elderly, while the differential diagnosis is much broader in younger persons.[13] Similarly, cerebral amyloid angiopathy and chronic hypertension are leading causes of intracerebral hemorrhage in older persons, while vascular malformations, acute hypertensive crises, or aneurysms are more likely to explain bleeding in young adults.

TABLE 3.4 — Nonatherosclerotic Vasculopathies Causing Ischemic Stroke

Noninflammatory Causes	Inflammatory, Noninfectious Causes	Infectious Causes
• Arterial dissection (traumatic or nontraumatic)	• Polyarteritis nodosa	• Syphilis
• Post-traumatic vasospasm	• Wegener granulomatosis	• Herpes zoster (ophthalmic division of trigeminal nerve)
• Vasospasm, including migraine	• Churg-Strauss angiitis	• Cysticercosis
• Fibromuscular dysplasia	• Granulomatous angiitis (isolated CNS vasculitis)	• Acquired immunodeficiency syndrome (AIDS)
• Moyamoya disease and Moyamoya syndrome	• Systemic lupus erythematosus	• Bacterial meningitis
• Saccular aneurysm	• Rheumatoid arthritis	
• Amyloid (congophilic) angiopathy	• Scleroderma	
• Ehlers-Danlos syndrome, type IV	• Sjögren syndrome	
• Pseudoxanthoma elasticum	• Takayasu syndrome	
• Marfan syndrome	• Giant cell (temporal) arteritis	
• Homocystinuria	• Behçet disease	
• Fabry disease	• Ulcerative colitis and regional enteritis	
• CADASIL	• Sarcoidosis	
• Neoplastic angioendotheliosis (intravascular lymphoma)	• Relapsing polychondritis	
	• Drug-induced vasculitis	
	• Henoch-Schönlein purpura	

	• Association with radiation or neoplasia • Dermatomyositis–polymyositis • Cogan syndrome

Abbreviations: CADASIL, cerebral autosomal dominant arteriopathy with subcortical infarcts and leukoencephalopathy; CNS, central nervous system.

TABLE 3.5 — Hematologic or Coagulation Disorders Leading to Ischemic Stroke

- Polycythemia rubra vera
- Sickle cell disease
- Leukemia
- Essential thrombocytosis
- Thrombotic thrombocytopenia purpura
- Heparin-induced thrombocytopenia
- Antithrombin III deficiency
- Protein C or S deficiency
- Deficiency of factors V, VII, XII, or XIII
- Heparin cofactor II deficiency
- Dysfibrinogenemia
- Factor V Leiden
- Prothrombin gene mutation
- Antiphospholipid/anticardiolipin antibodies
- Nephrotic syndrome
- Malignancy
- Pregnancy
- Oral contraceptives
- Dehydration

The likelihood of stroke also differs between men and women.[14] In most age groups, the relative risk of either ischemic or hemorrhagic stroke is higher among men than in women. Atherosclerosis, trauma, and X-linked metabolic diseases are more common in men.[15] Women have strokes secondary to pregnancy, puerperium, oral contraceptive use, migraine, or saccular aneurysms.[16-18]

The frequency of stroke varies by geographic location and among different ethnic groups. Some of the differences among ethnic groups first reported in the United States also have been described in Canada and Europe. In the United States, stroke is of particular concern among African Americans.[19-21] The differences in rates between African Americans and other ethnic groups are most pronounced among younger persons. In addition, the severity of stroke and mortality are increased among African Americans. The cause of the high rate of stroke among African Americans has not been established, but some potential factors that might lead to a high risk are:

- Genetic predisposition, including sickle cell disease
- High prevalence of arterial hypertension
- Diet
- Economic or social factors
- Lack of access to health care.

At younger ages, a higher rate of stroke is found among Hispanic Americans than whites, but this association seems to disappear among older populations.[22,23] Some of the associated risk seems to be secondary to a high prevalence of diabetes mellitus in Hispanic Americans. Stroke is especially common in Asia, particularly in Japan and China. The sites of atherosclerosis also differ among ethnic groups. Intracranial atheromatous lesions are located in persons of Asian or African background, but the lesions are more common in extracranial sites among those of European ancestry.[24]

A family history of stroke or other ischemic vascular events, particularly when occurring at younger ages, portends an increased likelihood of stroke.[25] A number of factors, including a genetic predisposition to atherosclerosis, may explain the association. Amyloid angiopathy, saccular aneurysms, and vascular malformations are among the causes of hemorrhage that may occur in a familial clustering.[26] In addition, several inherited disorders of coagulation, including hemophilia, may lead to brain hemorrhage.[12,15,27] A family history of deep vein thrombosis, pulmonary embolism, MI, or spontaneous abortions may be associated with an inherited prothrombotic disorder.[28-31] Ischemic stroke also may be secondary to inherited vascular diseases such as cerebral autosomal dominant arteriopathy with subcortical infarcts and leukoencephalopathy

41

TABLE 3.6 — Leading Causes of Intracranial Hemorrhage

Trauma

Hypertension
- Chronic (Charcot-Bouchard aneurysm)
- Acute, severe (hypertensive crisis)
- Eclampsia

Aneurysm
- Saccular (berry)
- Intracranial arterial dissection
- Infective
- Neoplastic
- Traumatic
- Dolichoectatic (fusiform)

Vascular Malformation
- Arteriovenous malformation
- Telangiectasis
- Cavernous malformation
- Venous malformation

Amyloid Angiopathy

Vasculitis
- Isolated central nervous system vasculitis
- Multisystem vasculitis
- Drug-induced vasculitis
- Peripartum vasculopathy

Venous Thrombosis

Hemorrhagic Transformation of an Infarction

Neoplasm
- Glioblastoma multiforme
- Metastatic (lung, renal cell, thyroid, melanoma, choriocarcinoma)

Bleeding Diatheses
- Thrombocytopenia
- Leukemia
- Hemophilia A or B

Continued

3

> *Pharmacologic Agents or Drugs*
> - Thrombolytic agents
> - Anticoagulants
> - Antiplatelet aggregating agents
> - Cocaine
> - Amphetamines
> - Phenylpropanolamine

(CADASH) or Marfan syndrome. However, genetic diseases are a relatively uncommon cause of stroke in the population as a whole. In addition, shared diet, lifestyle, or environmental factors (eg, smoking) may explain some of the familial clustering of stroke.

Modifiable Risk Factors

The list of risk factors for hemorrhagic or ischemic stroke that may be modified or controlled is included in **Table 3.1**. Some of the interventions to prevent stroke are aimed primarily at slowing the course of atherosclerosis, preventing the fracture of atherosclerotic plaques, or stabilizing the arterial endothelium. Therapies are aimed at controlling those risk factors or conditions that promote development of advanced atherosclerotic lesions. Attention to these risk factors is critical when making decisions about the primary and secondary prevention of stroke. Some interventions involve changes in lifestyle — altering diet, losing weight, increasing exercise, and stopping smoking. Other interventions include medications to treat the medical conditions that are associated with accelerated atherosclerosis.

■ Hypertension

Arterial hypertension is the premier manageable risk factor for both hemorrhagic and ischemic stroke.[32-35] Regardless of age, diastolic arterial hypertension is associated with an increased chance of stroke. Among the elderly, isolated systolic hypertension also is correlated with an increased likelihood of stroke.[36,37] The association between arterial hypertension and stroke is much stronger than the relationship between high blood pressure and ischemic heart disease. Hemorrhage also complicates chronic hypertension and acute hypertensive crises, including eclampsia.

Improved and successful treatment of hypertension probably is one of the leading reasons for the decline in stroke during the last third of the 20th century. A number of antihypertensive agents are available (**Table 3.7**). The selection of medications is made on a case-by-case basis and involves consideration of other factors, such as concomitant diseases.[38] For example, an angiotensin-converting enzyme (ACE) inhibitor often is administered to help protect renal function in diabetic patients[3] (Class I Recommendation, Level of Evidence A). Conversely, patients with hypertension secondary to renal artery stenosis are not treated with an ACE inhibitor. In many cases, β-blockers or oral diuretic agents are prescribed initially. Patients with concomitant symptomatic heart disease often are administered either β-blockers or calcium channel blockers. There has been some decline in the enthusiasm for use of calcium channel blockers for treatment of hypertension to prevent stroke. The α-blockers do not seem to be as effective as other antihypertensive agents in lowering the risk of stroke among persons with hypertension.

There is evidence that some of the newer antihypertensive agents (ACE inhibitors or angiotensin receptor blockers [ARBs]) may have additional benefit in lowering the risk of vascular events among persons with hypertension.[39] These agents may stabilize the vascular endothelium, which in turn may lower the risk of acute thromboembolism. These medications usually are given in conjunction with other medications to prevent stroke and often are supplements to diuretics for treatment of elevated blood pressure. Several trials demonstrate the benefit of the medications in lowering

TABLE 3.7 — Definition and Treatment of Hypertension

Definition	
Optimal level of blood pressure	Systolic ≤120 mm Hg and diastolic ≤80 mm Hg
Normal level of blood pressure	Systolic ≤130 mm Hg and diastolic ≤90 mm Hg
Hypertension	Systolic >130 mm Hg or diastolic >90 mm Hg
Treatment	
Lifestyle	Lose weight, limit alcohol consumption, increase exercise, reduce sodium intake, maintain intake of potassium, calcium, and magnesium, stop smoking
Medications	Diuretics, β-blockers, calcium channel blockers, angiotensin-converting enzyme (ACE) inhibitors, angiotensin receptor blockers

the risk of stroke among patients with hypertension, including those who have had a previous stroke[40-46] (Level of Evidence A). These data and those of other studies strongly support the treatment of arterial hypertension among high-risk persons, including those with symptomatic cerebrovascular disease (Class I Recommendation). There is some evidence to support the use of antihypertensive medications to treat patients without a history of hypertension[3] (Class IIa Recommendation, Level of Evidence B). The desired levels of blood pressure for most patients continue to decline. For most patients, the goal should be a blood pressure <120 mm Hg systolic and <80 mm Hg diastolic[3] (Class IIa Recommendation, Level of Evidence B). Current guidelines recommend that most patients with stroke receive diuretics and either an ACE inhibitor or an ARB[3] (Class I Recommendation, Level of Evidence A).

■ Diabetes Mellitus, Insulin Resistance, and Metabolic Syndrome

Diabetes mellitus promotes both large-artery atherosclerosis and small-artery disease of the brain.[47-50] Stroke is a common vascular complication in both younger insulin-dependent diabetic patients and older persons with type 2 diabetes. Diabetic patients also may have more severe strokes and hyperglycemia also may exacerbate the severity of the neurologic injury.[51] Current recommendations advise careful control of diabetes mellitus and elevated blood glucose concentrations. Choices include increased exercise and diet complemented by oral agents or insulin[3] (Class I Recommendation, Level of Evidence A). The goal is to have the glycosylated hemoglobin (HbA_{1C}) level <7%, with preprandial serum glucose concentrations of <120 mg/dL and bedtime glucose concentrations of approximately 100 to 140 mg/dL[3] (Class IIa Recommendation, Level of Evidence B). One of the goals is to lessen the risk of microvascular disease of the brain. Careful control of blood pressure and other risk factors also is critical even if the patient has not had any ischemic symptoms.

Evidence of insulin resistance, which may be present in nondiabetic patients, also appears to increase the likelihood of atherosclerosis. Insulin resistance increases lipids and affects endothelial function, coagulation, and inflammatory responses.[52-55] Pioglitazone may increase insulin sensitivity and might be useful in preventing vascular disease.[56] However, the utility of this strategy has not been established and clinical trials are under way.

Many Americans are overweight, and obesity is increasingly recognized as an indirect risk factor for vascular disease. Several factors, including truncal obesity, abnormal lipid levels, elevated fasting glucose concentration, and hypertension, are grouped together in an illness called the metabolic syndrome.[57-59] The components of the metabolic syndrome are:

- Waist circumference >40 inches in men or >35 inches in women
- Triglyceride level ≥150 mg/dL
- HDL cholesterol ≤40 mg/dL in men or ≤50 mg/dL in women
- Fasting glucose ≥110 mg/dL
- Blood pressure ≥130/85 mm Hg.

Measures to change lifestyle, including weight loss and increased exercise, are an important primary stroke-prevention strategy[3] (Class IIb Recommendation, Level of Evidence C).

■ Hypercholesterolemia

Hyperlipidemia (hypercholesterolemia) encourages early development of atherosclerosis. The relationship between elevated blood levels of lipids and stroke is hard to establish because cerebrovascular disease occurs in older persons and, in addition, stroke may be due to a large number of nonatherosclerotic vascular diseases.[60,61] However, hyperlipidemia likely is an important factor for stroke secondary to atherosclerosis, especially among middle-aged adults. Patients with ischemic stroke should be evaluated for the presence of hyperlipidemia.

Several clinical trials show that the use of inhibitors of 3-hydroxy-3-methylglutaryl coenzyme A reductase (HMG-CoA/statins) helps lower the risk of ischemic stroke among patients with hyperlipidemia.[62-65] Because the clinical trials have focused on treatment of patients with symptomatic coronary artery disease or asymptomatic, high-risk populations, the rates of stroke are relatively low. Thus demonstration of a statistical difference in stroke prophylaxis is difficult when looking at the results of a single trial (**Table 3.8**). Still, the trials show similar trends and when the data are combined into meta-analyses, the aggregate results prove that the effects in relative risk reduction in stroke are similar to those achieved with antiplatelet aggregating agents.[66] However, because the overall risk of stroke is relatively low in primary prevention studies, the absolute reduction in stroke is not as great as with medications that prevent thromboembolism. The reduction in ischemic events appears relatively soon after starting the statins and the effects seem out of proportion to the degree of reduction in blood levels of cholesterol. These findings suggest that the statins might provide additional therapeutic effects by stabilization of a complex atherosclerotic plaque or possibly by affecting coagulation or platelet function.

Vigorous control of blood lipids by diet and medication also leads to the regression of atherosclerotic lesions in the carotid artery.[64] Aggressive management of hyperlipidemia is a key component for prevention of ischemic stroke[3] (Class I Recommendation, Level of Evidence A) (**Table 3.9**). In most cases, treatment

TABLE 3.8 — Trials of HMG-CoA Reductase Inhibitors in Lowering the Risk of Ischemic Stroke						
Study	Medication	Active Treatment		Control Group	
ACAPS	Lovastatin	0/460	0.0%	2/459	0.4%
CARE	Pravastatin	54/2081	2.4%	78/2078	3.8%
4 S	Simvastatin	75/2221	3.4%	102/2223	4.6%
KAPS	Pravastatin	2/224	0.9%	4/223	1.8%
LIPID	Pravastatin	172/4512	3.8%	198/4502	4.4%
WOSCOPS	Pravastatin	40/3302	1.4%	51/3292	1.5%
Totals		348/12800	2.7%	435/12777	3.4%

Abbreviations: ACAPS, Asymptomatic Carotid Artery Progression Study; CARE, Cholesterol and Recurrent Events; 4 S, Scandinavian Simvastatin Stroke Study; HMG-CoA, 3-hydroxy-3-methylglutaryl coenzyme A reductase; KAPS, Kuopio Atherosclerosis Prevention Study; LIPID, Long-term Intervention With Pravastatin in Ischemic Disease; WOSCOPS, West of Scotland Coronary Prevention Study.

TABLE 3.9 — Recommendations for Treatment of Hypercholesterolemia in Patients With Ischemic Stroke	
Baseline LDL Cholesterol Level	**Desired LDL Cholesterol Level**
≥130 mg/dL	≤100 mg/dL or <70 mg/dL in highest-risk patients
≥160 mg/dL	≤130 mg/dL

should include administration of one of the statins.[3] The goal is to achieve a low-density lipoprotein (LDL) cholesterol level of <100 mg/dL in most patients and a level of <70 mg/dL in very high-risk persons[3] (Class I Recommendation, Level of Evidence A). Patients with a low high-density lipoprotein (HDL) cholesterol may be treated with niacin or gemfibrozil[3] (Class IIb Recommendation, Level of Evidence B). While very low levels of serum cholesterol may be associated with an increased risk of intracranial hemorrhage, there is no evidence that aggressive lowering of cholesterol levels with medications is associated with intracerebral bleeding. Although most patients tolerate the statins, they should be warned about possible side effects, including hepatic dysfunction and myopathy.

■ **Smoking**

Cessation of smoking probably is the single most cost-effective action for lowering the risk of either hemorrhagic or ischemic stroke. Smokers are at increased risk for atherosclerosis, coronary artery disease, and ischemic stroke.[67] Even passive exposure to smoking has been implicated as a risk factor for stroke.[68,69] Although the relationship between smoking and cerebrovascular disease is not as obvious as the correlation with heart disease, tobacco abuse is a strong risk factor for stroke in younger persons.[70]

Smoking also probably increases the risk of stroke in young women taking oral contraceptives.[71] In addition, smoking adds to the risk of intracranial bleeding, including rupture of saccular aneurysms.[72,73] All patients should be encouraged to stop smoking[3] (Class I Recommendation, Level of Evidence C). Among the options for helping a patient to stop smoking are counseling, nicotine products, and medications, such as bupropion[3] (Class IIa Recommendation, Level of Evidence B).

■ **Other Potential Risk Factors**

Other potential risk factors for stroke include:
- Migraine
- Hyperhomocysteinemia
- Use of oral contraceptives
- Obesity
- Lack of exercise
- Excessive alcohol consumption
- Drug abuse
- Sleep disorders, including sleep apnea.

Excessive consumption of alcohol may be associated with an increased risk of intracranial bleeding.[74] Patients who are consuming large amounts of alcohol should be encouraged to reduce or eliminate their alcohol use[3] (Class I Recommendation, Level of Evidence A). Limited alcohol consumption (<2 drinks/day in men and 1 drink/day for nonpregnant women) is acceptable[3] (Class IIb Recommendation, Level of Evidence B). Patients who do not drink alcoholic beverages should be advised to not consume alcohol as a measure to lower the risk of stroke. Elevated blood levels of homocysteine may augment the development of atherosclerosis and associated thrombosis.[75-78] Supplementing the diet with folic acid, vitamin B_{12}, and pyridoxine will lower blood levels of homocysteine. However, the utility of vitamin supplementation for preventing recurrent stroke has not been established. Three clinical trials did not demonstrate a benefit from this treatment approach[79]; another trial is under way.[80] While screening patients for hyperhomocysteinemia may have merit, the level of homocysteine that should prompt vitamin supplementation has not been established (Class I Recommendation, Level of Evidence A). Inflammation also may play a role in the course of atherosclerosis.[81,82] Elevations of high-sensitivity C-reactive protein appear to be associated with an increased risk of stroke.[83,84] This marker of inflammation is associated with other risk factors for stroke. The best therapeutic response to elevated levels of this inflammatory marker has not been determined.

Symptomatic Atherosclerosis in Other Circulations

Evidence of atherosclerotic disease in other vascular territories identifies a person as being at high risk for ischemic stroke.[85,86] Patients who have a history of one of the following conditions should be considered to have a high chance of ischemic cerebrovascular disease:

- MI
- Angina pectoris
- Abdominal aortic aneurysm
- Claudication in the lower extremities.

Conversely, patients with ischemic stroke secondary to atherosclerotic disease also are at high risk for major cardiovascular events. MI is the leading long-term cause of death among persons who survive stroke. Attention to codeveloping coronary artery disease should be part of any long-term treatment plan for patients with stroke. Much of the management of these high-risk patients includes surgical or medical intervention, including antithrombotic agents that are discussed in Chapter 11, *Prevention of Ischemic Stroke or Recurrent Ischemic Stroke.*

Patients at Highest Risk

Persons with the following conditions are at the highest risk for ischemic stroke:

- AF
- Asymptomatic stenosis of the internal carotid artery
- Amaurosis fugax
- TIA
- Previous ischemic stroke.

■ Atrial Fibrillation

AF is the leading cardiac abnormality associated with ischemic stroke.[87] The prevalence of AF is growing and the importance of the cardiac arrhythmia likely will increase in the future. It is the most important predictor of stroke in persons older than 75, particularly among women.[88-90] AF complicates a number of cardiac diseases and the presence of the arrhythmia is associated with an increased chance of cardioembolism. The most common cardiac diseases associated with AF are:

- Coronary artery disease
- Hypertensive heart disease
- Dilated cardiomyopathies
- Rheumatic valvular disease (particularly mitral stenosis)
- Prosthetic cardiac valves (particularly mechanical mitral valve prostheses).

Persons younger than 60 who have AF and no other cardiac disorder (lone AF) appear to be at relatively low risk for stroke.[91] Thus the importance of AF is as an abetting factor leading to the formation of intra-atrial thrombi in a patient with another heart disease.

Both people with chronic, sustained AF and those with an intermittent arrhythmia are at risk, and embolization may complicate new-onset AF. The risk of embolization is relatively low during the first 2 to 3 days after the start of AF. Thereafter, the risk starts to increase. Many patients do not have symptoms corresponding to the onset of the arrhythmia and the time the AF began becomes inferential. Thus determining the onset of AF is problematic. Either electrical or pharmacologic cardioversion may be associated with embolization and, therefore, anticoagulation is prescribed for several weeks before and after correction of the arrhythmia.

Several factors identify those persons with AF who are at greatest risk for embolization:

- Prior TIA or stroke
- Age >75 years, especially women
- History of hypertension or systolic blood pressure >160 mm Hg
- Diabetes mellitus
- Coronary artery disease
- Congestive heart failure
- Left ventricular dysfunction
- Echocardiographic evidence of atrial or ventricular enlargement.

Of these conditions, the most important forecaster for embolism in a patient with AF is a history of ischemic neurologic symptoms or prior embolization.

■ Asymptomatic Cervical (Carotid) Stenosis or Bruit

Severe asymptomatic stenosis of the extracranial portion of the internal carotid artery may be detected after a physician auscultates a cervical bruit. In addition, the narrowing may be detected during the evaluation of:

- Atherosclerotic disease, including coronary artery disease

- Ischemia in the vertebrobasilar circulation
- Ischemia in the contralateral carotid circulation.

The prevalence of severe but asymptomatic stenosis increases with advancing age, and it may be found in both men and women.[92] The presence of previously identified risk factors for atherosclerosis portends an increased likelihood of finding a severe narrowing. Besides being a marker for a high risk for stroke, an asymptomatic carotid artery stenosis also forecasts an increased risk for MI or vascular death.[93,94] The chance of an ipsilateral stroke among patients with narrowing >60% appears to be approximately 2% per year. Ischemic strokes are as likely to occur in the contralateral hemisphere or brain stem as in the hemisphere perfused by stenotic artery.

The chance of stroke probably correlates with the severity of the arterial narrowing; patients with high-grade stenosis are assumed to be at the greatest risk. Those with severely ulcerated stenotic lesions and those with demonstrated progression of the narrowing also may be at high risk. In general, the presence of a carotid stenosis does not predict a high risk of stroke among patients who are undergoing peripheral vascular or general surgical operations.[95,96] Thus prophylactic endovascular or surgical treatment of a carotid narrowing is not recommended prior to another operation.

The risk of stroke among patients with a carotid stenosis may be increased with coronary artery bypass surgery or other major cardiac operations.[97] However, strokes in patients having these procedures usually are not directly related to the carotid lesion. Such patients usually have extensive aortic diseases and embolization of atherosclerotic debris from fracture plaques is a likely explanation for many of these strokes.[98] Doing carotid endarterectomy or carotid angioplasty and stenting to treat an asymptomatic lesion at the time of a major cardiovascular operation is not recommended because of the high rate of serious complications, including stroke or death.[99]

■ Transient Ischemic Attack or Amaurosis Fugax

Patients with ischemic symptoms of either the brain or eye are at the greatest risk for subsequent ischemic stroke. In general, the risk is highest among patients with a previous stroke, higher among patients with a TIA, and high among patients with amaurosis fugax.[100,101] Overall, the risk of a serious stroke within 1 year of a TIA is approximately 10%. The likelihood of a stroke is greatest during the first few days after the event, especially during the first 48 hours.[102] Patients rapidly recovering from a stroke also have a high chance of subsequent neurologic worsening from a recurrent event.[103,104] Thus a recent TIA or minor stroke should be considered as a very high-risk situation. One of these events should prompt rapid evaluation and urgent treatment.

Amaurosis fugax (transient monocular blindness) is an episode of painless and transient monocular visual loss that is secondary to ischemia (**Table 3.10**). Amaurosis fugax most commonly is associated with atherosclerotic disease of the ipsilateral internal carotid artery. The attacks are discrete and brief, usually lasting a few seconds to minutes. Occasionally, postural changes or exposure to bright light may provoke an attack. While the classic description involves the complaint of an ascending or descending curtain that covers part or all of the visual field in one eye, this symptom is relatively uncommon. Patients usually describe the symptoms as a fog, scum, haze, or blurring. Occasionally, the patient will describe a constriction of the visual field, with grayness from the periphery to the center. Complete blindness may occur. Other reported visual phenomena may include sparkles or shimmers that are bright.

A TIA is defined as a transient episode of neurologic dysfunction secondary to ischemia in one of the vascular territories of the brain. These events are discrete. They have a sudden onset and relatively rapid resolution. While the definition of a TIA includes symptoms that may persist for 24 hours, most events are a few minutes in duration. An event that lasts a few seconds usually is not a TIA. Symptoms that wax and wane or those that are relatively nondescript likely are not due to a TIA. The symptoms should reflect dysfunction of one area of the brain. Global symptoms, including confusion, wooziness, light-headedness, or loss of consciousness, usually are not due to a TIA. The symptoms of a TIA, such as weakness, numbness, or incoordination, represent a loss of normal neurologic activity. Positive neurological symptoms, such as scintillating visual phenomena, seizure activity, or involuntary movements, rarely are due to transient brain ischemia. A migration or march of symptoms from one body part to another is uncommon with a TIA. The pattern of symptoms of a TIA in the vertebrobasilar circulation differs from those symptoms that occur with an event in the carotid territory (**Table 3.11**). Approximately 20% to 25% of patients have a headache with the event and this complaint is more likely with events in the posterior circulation. The differential diagnosis of a TIA or amaurosis fugax is outlined in **Table 3.12**. The approach to the evaluation of patients with a TIA is outlined in **Table 3.13**.

- **Warning Leak**
    In general, patients do not have any warning symptoms prior to an intracranial hemorrhage. The exception is among some patients with aneurysmal subarachnoid hemorrhage. These patients may have an unusually severe headache, often associated with nausea, vomiting, and constitutional symptoms a few days before the more severe intracranial bleed-

TABLE 3.10 — Rules of Thumb for the Diagnosis of Transient Ischemic Attack

- The event should have sudden onset and rapid resolution:
  - An event that has an ill-defined onset, waxes and wanes, or slowly worsens probably is not a transient ischemic attack (TIA)
  - An event that has persistent neurologic deficits, however mild, is not a TIA
- The event should last 2 to 20 minutes:
  - An episode of neurologic dysfunction that lasts a few seconds probably is not a TIA
  - An episode of neurologic dysfunction that lasts >1 hour probably is a minor stroke
- The event initially should involve all affected areas relatively simultaneously:
  - An episode that involves the march of symptoms from one body part to another probably is not a TIA
  - On the other hand, a patient may not recognize all the involved areas being affected simultaneously
- The event should involve the focal loss of neurologic function, with symptoms reflecting dysfunction of the cerebral hemisphere, cerebellum, or brain stem
  - An event that produces "positive" phenomena, such as involuntary movements, jerking, or scintillating visual symptoms, usually is not a TIA
  - An event that causes "global" brain symptoms only, such as loss of consciousness, syncope, giddiness, light-headedness, confusion, usually is not a TIA
- Headaches occur with approximately 20% to 25% of TIA
- Ask observers about any overt signs such as limb or facial weakness or speech impairments
- Vertigo in isolation usually is not due to a TIA; ischemic vertigo usually is accompanied by other neurologic symptoms
- Recurrent TIA of any origin often are stereotyped
- Recurrent episodes of unilateral weakness that alternatively affect the right or left side are more likely due to ischemia in the vertebrobasilar circulation than to

Continued

both carotid circulations being symptomatic simultaneously
- Amaurosis fugax rarely occurs at the same time as the cerebral symptoms of a TIA
- Patients and observers often have difficulty differentiating symptoms of dysarthria and aphasia
- Observers often confuse the normal side of the face ("drawn up") with the paralyzed ("drooping") side
- Patients often confuse the symptoms of numbness and weakness; as a result, it should not be assumed that a TIA is purely motor or sensory in nature
- Patients often have difficulty differentiating a visual disturbance in the lateral portion of the visual field (hemianopia) from a monocular visual event (amaurosis fugax), consequently other neurologic symptoms should be sought

ing event[105,106] (**Table 3.14**). The ominous nature of these warning symptoms, which represent a minor hemorrhage from the aneurysm, often is not recognized (**Table 3.15**). Patients with vascular malformations may present with non–stroke-related symptoms, including recurrent (usually localized) headaches or seizures.

REFERENCES

1. Gorelick PB, Sacco RL, Smith DB, et al. Prevention of a first stroke: a review of guidelines and a multidisciplinary consensus statement from the National Stroke Association. *JAMA*. 1999;281:1112-1120.
2. Gorelick PB. Stroke prevention therapy beyond antithrombotics: unifying mechanisms in ischemic stroke pathogenesis and implications for therapy: an invited review. *Stroke*. 2002;33:862-875.
3. Sacco RL, Adams R, Albers G, et al; American Heart Association; American Stroke Association Council on Stroke; Council on Cardiovascular Radiology and Intervention; American Academy of Neurology. Guidelines for prevention of stroke in patients with ischemic stroke or transient ischemic attack: a statement for healthcare professionals from the American Heart Association/American Stroke Association Council on Stroke: co-sponsored by the Council on Cardiovascular Radiology and Intervention: the American Academy of Neurology affirms the value of this guideline. *Stroke*. 2006;37:577-617.

TABLE 3.11 — Symptoms of TIA

Carotid Circulation
- Ipsilateral transient monocular blindness (amaurosis fugax)
- Contralateral weakness, numbness, clumsiness, or heaviness:
  - Hand, hand, and face; hand, arm, and face
  - Rarely one half of the body
- Dysarthria
- Aphasia
- Contralateral homonymous visual loss

Vertebrobasilar Circulation
- Binocular visual loss (one or both fields)
- Diplopia
- Vertigo
- Unilateral or bilateral weakness, numbness, clumsiness, or heaviness:
  - May alternate between right and left sides
  - May be crossed, face ipsilateral, limbs contralateral
- Ataxia
- Dysarthria
- Dysphagia
- Hearing loss
- Drop attack

Abbreviation: TIA, transient ischemic attack.

TABLE 3.12 — Alternative Diagnosis: Transient Ischemic Attacks

- Migraine with focal neurologic symptoms
- Focal seizures with Todd's paralysis
- Syncope or presyncope
- Metabolic disorders (hypoglycemia)
- Mass lesion with waxing and waning symptoms
  - Subdural hematoma
  - Tumor

TABLE 3.13 — Key Questions When Evaluating and Treating a Patient With Suspected TIA or Ischemic Stroke

- Do the symptoms represent a TIA or a stroke?
- Do the symptoms reflect ischemia in the carotid or vertebrobasilar circulation?
- What is the likely cause of the ischemic symptoms?
- Does the patient have symptoms ipsilateral to a severe stenosis of the internal carotid artery; is the patient a "good" candidate for carotid endarterectomy or endovascular treatment?
- What stroke prophylaxis medications were being taken at the time of the last ischemic event?
- Does the patient have a contraindication for a specific medication?

Abbreviation: TIA, transient ischemic attack.

4. Adams HP Jr, Bendixen BH, Kappelle LJ, et al. Classification of subtype of acute ischemic stroke. Definitions for use in a multicenter clinical trial. TOAST. Trial of Org 10172 in Acute Stroke Treatment. *Stroke*. 1993;24:35-41.

5. Gordon DL, Bendixen BH, Adams HP Jr, Clarke W, Kappelle LJ, Woolson RF. Interphysician agreement in the diagnosis of subtypes of acute ischemic stroke: implications for clinical trials. The TOAST Investigators. *Neurology*. 1993;43:1021-1027.

6. Paradowski B, Maciejak A. TOAST classification of subtypes of ischaemic stroke: diagnostic and therapeutic procedures in stroke. A four-year observation. *Cerebrovasc Dis*. 2005;20:319-324.

7. Simons LA, McCallum J, Friedlander Y, Simons J. Risk factors for ischemic stroke: Dubbo Study of the elderly. *Stroke*. 1998;29:1341-1346.

8. Adams HP Jr, Butler MJ, Biller J, Toffol GJ. Nonhemorrhagic cerebral infarction in young adults. *Arch Neurol*. 1986;43:793-796.

9. Kittner SJ. Stroke in the young: coming of age. *Neurology*. 2002;59:6-7.

10. Fullerton HJ, Chetkovich DM, Wu YW, Smith WS, Johnston SC. Deaths from stroke in US children, 1979 to 1998. *Neurology*. 2002;59:34-39.

11. Broderick J, Talbot GT, Prenger E, Leach A, Brott T. Stroke in children within a major metropolitan area: the surprising importance of intracerebral hemorrhage. *J Child Neurol*. 1993;8:250-255.

12. Pavlakis SG, Kingsley PB, Bialer MG. Stroke in children: genetic and metabolic issues. *J Child Neurol*. 2000;15:308-315.

13. Giroud M, Lemesle M, Madinier G, Manceau E, Osseby GV, Dumas R. Stroke in children under 16 years of age. Clinical and etiological difference with adults. *Acta Neurol Scand*. 1997;96:401-406.

14. Hershey LA. Gender differences in cerebrovascular disease. *Neurology*. 1993;3:1-4.

TABLE 3.14 — Rules of Thumb in the Diagnosis of Warning Leak of Subarachnoid Hemorrhage

- Severe headache without other neurologic complaints may be the chief complaint in a patient with a minor SAH:
  - Index of suspicion should be increased when the patient describes the headache as unusually severe
  - An unusually severe headache of abrupt onset (thunderclap) or one that is described as the worst pain of life suggests SAH
  - A headache complicated with loss of consciousness at the onset of the headache suggests SAH
  - An abrupt headache that occurs during exercise suggests SAH
- Patients will look moderately ill but the neurologic examination often is normal, including signs of meningeal irritation
- Most patients have photophobia, phonophobia, nausea, or vomiting
- Most patients do not have motor or sensory or cranial nerve impairments
- Nuchal rigidity may be mild or absent
- Most patients have normal vital signs
- Most patients do not have more than one episode, but a clustering may occur during a few weeks before a major SAH

Abbreviation: SAH, subarachnoid hemorrhage.

15. Natowicz M, Kelley RI. Mendelian etiologies of stroke. *Ann Neurol*. 1987;22:175-192.
16. Kongable GL, Lanzino G, Germanson TP, et al. Gender-related differences in aneurysmal subarachnoid hemorrhage. *J Neurosurg*. 1996;84:43-48.
17. Ischaemic stroke and combined oral contraceptives: results of an international, multicentre, case-control study. WHO Collaborative Study of Cardiovascular Disease and Steroid Hormone Contraception. *Lancet*. 1996;348:498-505.
18. Haemorrhagic stroke, overall stroke risk, and combined oral contraceptives: results of an international, multicentre, case-control study. WHO Collaborative Study of Cardiovascular Disease and Steroid Hormone Contraception. *Lancet*. 1996;348:505-510.
19. Kissela B, Schneider A, Kleindorfer D, et al. Stroke in a biracial population: the excess burden of stroke among blacks. *Stroke*. 2004;35:426-431.

TABLE 3.15 — Differential Diagnosis:
Minor Subarachnoid Hemorrhage

- Migraine headache
- Tension or pressure headache
- Sinusitis
- Cervical spine injury, herniated disk, or arthritis
- Cervical strain or whiplash
- Ischemic stroke
- Flu or viral illness
- Viral meningitis
- Hypertensive encephalopathy
- Drug or alcohol abuse or intoxication

20. Qureshi AI, Safdar K, Patel M, Janssen RS, Frankel MR. Stroke in young black patients. Risk factors, subtypes, and prognosis. *Stroke*. 1995;26:1995-1998.

21. Worrall BB, Johnston KC, Kongable G, Hung E, Richardson D, Gorelick PB. Stroke risk factor profiles in African American women: an interim report from the African-American Antiplatelet Stroke Prevention Study. *Stroke*. 2002;33:913-919.

22. Gillum RF. Epidemiology of stroke in Hispanic Americans. *Stroke*. 1995;26:1707-1712.

23. Bruno A, Qualls C. Risk factors for intracerebral and subarachnoid hemorrhage among Hispanics and non-Hispanic whites in a New Mexico community. *Neuroepidemiology*. 2000;19:227-232.

24. Feldmann E, Daneault N, Kwan E, et al. Chinese-white differences in the distribution of occlusive cerebrovascular disease. *Neurology*. 1990;40:1541-1545.

25. Tentschert S, Greisenegger S, Wimmer R, Lang W, Lalouschek W. Association of parental history of stroke with clinical parameters in patients with ischemic stroke or transient ischemic attack. *Stroke*. 2003;34:2114-2119.

26. Raaymakers TW, Rinkel GJ, Ramos LM. Initial and follow-up screening for aneurysms in families with familial subarachnoid hemorrhage. *Neurology*. 1998;51:1125-1130.

27. Rastenyte D, Tuomilehto J, Sarti C. Genetics of stroke—a review. *J Neurol Sci*. 1998;153:132-145.

28. Nachman RL, Silverstein R. Hypercoagulable states. *Ann Intern Med*. 1993;119:819-827.

29. Price DT, Ridker PM. Factor V Leiden mutation and the risks for thromboembolic disease: a clinical perspective. *Ann Intern Med*. 1997;127:895-903.

30. Petrovic D, Milanez T, Kobal J, Bregar D, Potisk KP, Peterlin B. Prothrombotic gene polymorphisms and atherothrombotic cerebral infarction. *Acta Neurol Scand*. 2003;108:109-113.

31. Voetsch B, Loscalzo J. Genetic determinants of arterial thrombosis. *Arterioscler Thromb Vasc Biol*. 2004;24:216-229.

32. Alexander RW. Theodore Cooper Memorial Lecture. Hypertension and the pathogenesis of atherosclerosis. Oxidative stress and the mediation of arterial inflammatory response: a new perspective. *Hypertension.* 1995;25:155-161.

33. Droste DW, Ritter MA, Dittrich R, et al. Arterial hypertension and ischaemic stroke. *Acta Neurol Scand.* 2003;107:241-251.

34. Nawrot T, Den Hond E, Thijs L, Staessen JA. Isolated systolic hypertension and the risk of vascular disease. *Curr Hypertens Rep.* 2003;5:372-379.

35. Staessen JA, Wang J. Blood-pressure lowering for the secondary prevention of stroke. *Lancet.* 2001;358:1026-1027.

36. Davis BR, Vogt T, Frost PH, et al. Risk factors for stroke and type of stroke in persons with isolated systolic hypertension. Systolic Hypertension in the Elderly Program Cooperative Research Group. *Stroke.* 1998;29:1333-1340.

37. Staessen JA, Thijs L, Gasowski J, Cells H, Fagard RH. Treatment of isolated systolic hypertension in the elderly: further evidence from the systolic hypertension in Europe (Syst-Eur) trial. *Am J Cardiol.* 1998;82:20R-22R.

38. Kaplan NM, Gifford RW Jr. Choice of initial therapy for hypertension. *JAMA.* 1996;275:1577-1580.

39. Iadecola C, Gorelick PB. Hypertension, angiotensin, and stroke: beyond blood pressure. *Stroke.* 2004;35:348-350.

40. Yusuf S, Sleight P, Pogue J, Bosch J, Davies R, Dagenais G. Effects of an angiotensin-converting-enzyme inhibitor, ramipril, on cardiovascular events in high-risk patients. The Heart Outcomes Prevention Evaluation Study Investigators. *N Engl J Med.* 2000;342:145-153.

41. Bosch J, Yusuf S, Pogue J, et al; HOPE Investigators. Heart outcomes prevention evaluation. Use of ramipril in preventing stroke: double blind randomised trial. *BMJ.* 2002;324:699-702.

42. MacMahon S, Rodgers A, Neal B, Woodward M, Chalmers J, on behalf of the PROGRESS Collaborative Group. The lowering of blood pressure after stroke. *Lancet.* 2002;358:1994-1995.

43. Chapman N, Huxley R, Anderson C, et al; Writing Committee for the PROGRESS Collaborative Group. Effects of perindopril-based blood pressure — lowering regimen on the risk of recurrent stroke according to stroke subtype and medical history: the PROGRESS Trial. *Stroke.* 2004;35:116-121.

44. Yusuf S, Sleight P, Pogue J, Bosch J, Davies R, Dagenais G. Effects of an angiotensin-converting-enzyme inhibitor, ramipril, on cardiovascular events in high-risk patients. The Heart Outcomes Prevention Evaluation Study Investigators. *N Engl J Med.* 2000;342:145-153.

45. PROGRESS Collaborative Group. Randomised trial of a perindopril-based blood-pressure-lowering regimen among 6,105 individuals with previous stroke or transient ischaemic attack. *Lancet.* 2001;358:1033-1041.

46. Devereux RB, Dahlof B, Kjeldsen SE, et al; LIFE Study Group. Effects of losartan or atenolol in hypertensive patients without clinically evident vascular disease: a substudy of the LIFE randomized trial. *Ann Intern Med.* 2003;139:169-177.

47. Caplan LR. Diabetes and brain ischemia. *Diabetes.* 1996;45(suppl 3): S95-S97.

48. Davis TM, Millns H, Stratton IM, Holman RR, Turner RC. Risk factors for stroke in type 2 diabetes mellitus: United Kingdom Prospective Diabetes Study (UKPDS) 29. *Arch Intern Med.* 1999;159:1097-1103.

49. Lukovits TG, Mazzone TM, Gorelick TM. Diabetes mellitus and cerebrovascular disease. *Neuroepidemiology*. 1999;18:1-14.

50. Fox CS, Coady S, Sorlie PD, et al. Trends in cardiovascular complications of diabetes. *JAMA*. 2004;292:2495-2499.

51. Di Bonito P, Di Fraia L, Di Gennaro L, et al. Impact of known and unknown diabetes on in-hospital mortality from ischemic stroke. *Nutr Metab Cardiovasc Dis*. 2003;13:148-153.

52. Kernan WN, Inzucchi SE, Viscoli CM, Brass LM, Bravata DM, Horwitz RI. Insulin resistance and risk for stroke. *Neurology*. 2002;59:809-815.

53. Kernan WN, Inzucchi SE, Viscoli CM, et al. Impaired insulin sensitivity among nondiabetic patients with a recent TIA or ischemic stroke. *Neurology*. 2003;60:1447-1451.

54. Sakkinen PA, Wahl P, Cushman M, Lewis MR, Tracy RP. Clustering of procoagulation, inflammation, and fibrinolysis variables with metabolic factors in insulin resistance syndrome. *Am J Epidemiol*. 2000;152:897-907.

55. Facchini FS, Hua N, Abbasi F, Reaven GM. Insulin resistance as a predictor of age-related diseases. *J Clin Endocrinol Metab*. 2001;86:3574-3578.

56. Kernan WN, Inzucchi SE, Viscoli CM, et al. Pioglitazone improves insulin sensitivity among nondiabetic patients with a recent transient ischemic attack or ischemic stroke. *Stroke*. 2003;34:1431-1436.

57. Meigs JB. Epidemiology of the metabolic syndrome, 2002. *Am J Manag Care*. 2002;8(suppl 11):S283-S292.

58. Grundy SM. Obesity, metabolic syndrome, and coronary atherosclerosis. *Circulation*. 2002;105:2696-2698.

59. Reusch JE. Current concepts in insulin resistance, type 2 diabetes mellitus, and the metabolic syndrome. *Am J Cardiol*. 2002;90:19G-26G.

60. Hachinski V. Cholesterol as a risk factor for stroke. *Arch Neurol*. 1999;56:1524.

61. O'Leary DH, Polak JF, Kronmal RA, Manolio TA, Burke GL, Wolfson SK Jr. Carotid-artery intima and media thickness as a risk factor for myocardial infarction and stroke in older adults. Cardiovascular Health Study Collaborative Research Group. *N Engl J Med*. 1999;340:14-22.

62. Plehn JF, Davis BR, Sacks FM, et al. Reduction of stroke incidence after myocardial infarction with pravastatin: the Cholesterol and Recurrent Events (CARE) study. The Care Investigators. *Circulation*. 1999;99:216-223.

63. Blauw GJ, Lagaay AM, Smelt AH, Westendorp RG. Stroke, statins, and cholesterol. A meta-analysis of randomized, placebo-controlled, double-blind trials with HMG-CoA reductase inhibitors. *Stroke*. 1997;28:946-950.

64. Crouse JR. Effects of statins on carotid disease and stroke. *Curr Opin Lipidol*. 1999;10:535-541.

65. Hebert PR, Gaziano JM, Chan KS, Hennekens CH. Cholesterol lowering with statin drugs, risk of stroke, and total mortality. An overview of randomized trials. *JAMA*. 1997;278:313-321.

66. Crouse JR 3rd, Byington RP, Furberg CD. HMG-CoA reductase inhibitor therapy and stroke risk reduction: an analysis of clinical trials data. *Atherosclerosis*. 1998;138:11-24.

67. Inoue T, Oku K, Kimoto K, et al. Relationship of cigarette smoking to the severity of coronary and thoracic aortic atherosclerosis. *Cardiology*. 1995;86:374-379.

68. Otsuka R, Watanabe H, Hirata K, et al. Acute effects of passive smoking on the coronary circulation in healthy young adults. *JAMA*. 2001;286:436-441.

69. You RX, Thrift AG, McNeil JJ, Davis SM, Donnan GA. Ischemic stroke risk and passive exposure to spouses' cigarette smoking. Melbourne Stroke Risk Factor Study (MERFS) Group. *Am J Public Health.* 1999;89:572-575.

70. You RX, McNeil JJ, O'Malley HM, Davis SM, Thrift AG, Donnan GA. Risk factors for stroke due to cerebral infarction in young adults. *Stroke.* 1997;28:1913-1918.

71. Levine SR, Fagan SC, Pessin MS, et al. Accelerated intracranial occlusive disease, oral contraceptives, and cigarette use. *Neurology.* 1991;41:1893-1901.

72. Weir BK, Kongable GL, Kassell NF, Schultz JR, Truskowski LL, Sigrest A. Cigarette smoking as a cause of aneurysmal subarachnoid hemorrhage and risk for vasospasm: a report of the Cooperative Aneurysm Study. *J Neurosurg.* 1998;89:405-411.

73. Thrift AG, McNeil JJ, Donnan GA. The risk of intracerebral haemorrhage with smoking. The Melbourne Risk Factor Study Group. *Cerebrovasc Dis.* 1999;9:34-39.

74. Thrift AG, Donnan GA, McNeil JJ. Heavy drinking, but not moderate or intermediate drinking, increases the risk of intracerebral hemorrhage. *Epidemiology.* 1999;10:307-312.

75. Sacco RL, Anand K, Lee HS, et al. Homocysteine and the risk of ischemic stroke in a triethnic cohort: the Northern Manhattan Study. *Stroke.* 2004;35:2263-2269.

76. Taylor LM Jr, Moneta GL, Sexton GJ, Schuff RA, Porter JM. Prospective blinded study of the relationship between plasma homocysteine and progression of symptomatic peripheral arterial disease. *J Vasc Surg.* 1999;29:8-21.

77. Ridker PM, Manson JE, Buring JE, Shih J, Matias M, Hennekens CH. Homocysteine and risk of cardiovascular disease among postmenopausal women. *JAMA.* 1999;281:1817-1821.

78. Hankey GJ, Eikelboom JW. Homocysteine and stroke. *Lancet.* 2005;365:194-196.

79. Toole JF, Malinow MR, Chambless LE, et al. Lowering homocysteine in patients with ischemic stroke to prevent recurrent stroke, myocardial infarction, and death: the Vitamin Intervention for Stroke Prevention (VISP) randomized controlled trial. *JAMA.* 2004;291:565-575.

80. Hankey GJ, Eikelboom JW. Folic acid-based multivitamin therapy to prevent stroke: the jury is still out. *Stroke.* 2004;35:1995-1998.

81. Ridker PM. Inflammatory biomarkers, statins, and the risk of stroke: cracking a clinical conundrum. *Circulation.* 2002;105:2583-2585.

82. Ridker PM. On evolutionary biology, inflammation, infection, and the causes of atherosclerosis. *Circulation.* 2002;105:2-4.

83. Ridker PM, Hennekens CH, Buring JE, Rifai N. C-reactive protein and other markers of inflammation in the prediction of cardiovascular disease in women. *N Engl J Med.* 2000;342:836-843.

84. Ridker PM, Buring JE, Cook NR, Rifai N. C-reactive protein, the metabolic syndrome, and risk of incident cardiovascular events: an 8-year follow-up of 14,719 initially healthy American women. *Circulation.* 2003;107:391-397.

85. Smith FB, Rumley A, Lee AJ, Leng GC, Fowkes FG, Lowe GD. Haemostatic factors and prediction of ischaemic heart disease and stroke in claudicants. *Br J Haematol.* 1998;100:758-763.

86. Maggioni AP, Franzosi MG, Santoro E, White H, Van de Werf F, Tognoni G.. The risk of stroke in patients with acute myocardial infarction after thrombolytic and antithrombotic treatment. Gruppo Italiano per lo Studio della Sopravvivenza nell'Infarto Miocardico II (GISSI-2), and The International Study Group. *N Engl J Med.* 1992;327:1-6.

87. Wolf PA, Mitchell JB, Baker CS, Kannel WB, D'Agostino RB. Impact of atrial fibrillation on mortality, stroke, and medical costs. *Arch Intern Med.* 1998;158:229-234.

88. Kannel WB, Wolf PA, Benjamin EJ, Levy D. Prevalence, incidence, prognosis, and predisposing conditions for atrial fibrillation: population-based estimates. *Am J Cardiol.* 1998;82:2N-9N.

89. Aronow WS, Ahn C, Kronzon I, Gutstein H. Risk factors for new thromboembolic stroke in patients > or = 62 years of age with chronic atrial fibrillation. *Am J Cardiol.* 1998;82:119-121.

90. Wang TJ, Massaro JM, Levy D, et al. A risk score for predicting stroke or death in individuals with new-onset atrial fibrillation in the community: the Framingham Heart Study. *JAMA.* 2003;290:1049-1056.

91. Scardi S, Mazzone C, Pandullo C, Goldstein D, Poletti A, Humar F. Lone atrial fibrillation: prognostic differences between paroxysmal and chronic forms after 10 years of follow-up. *Am Heart J.* 1999;137:686-691.

92. Josse MO, Touboul PJ, Mas JL, Laplane D, Bousser MG. Prevalence of asymptomatic internal carotid artery stenosis. *Neuroepidemiology.* 1987;6:150-152.

93. Olin JW, Fonseca C, Childs MB, Piedmonte MR, Hertzer NR, Young JR. The natural history of asymptomatic moderate internal carotid artery stenosis by duplex ultrasound. *Vasc Med.* 1998;3:101-108.

94. Risk of stroke in the distribution of an asymptomatic carotid artery. The European Carotid Surgery Trialists Collaborative Group. *Lancet.* 1995;345:209-212.

95. Gerraty RP, Gates PC, Doyle JC. Carotid stenosis and perioperative stroke risk in symptomatic and asymptomatic patients undergoing vascular or coronary surgery. *Stroke.* 1993;24:1115-1118.

96. Ropper AH, Wechsler LR, Wilson LS. Carotid bruit and the risk of stroke in elective surgery. *N Engl J Med.* 1982;307:1388-1390.

97. Safa TK, Friedman S, Mehta M, et al. Management of coexisting coronary artery and asymptomatic carotid artery disease: report of a series of patients treated with coronary bypass alone. *Eur J Vasc Endovasc Surg.* 1999;17:249-252.

98. Roach GW, Kanchuger M, Mangano CM, et al. Adverse cerebral outcomes after coronary bypass surgery. Multicenter Study of Perioperative Ischemia Research Group and the Ischemia Research and Education Foundation Investigators. *N Engl J Med.* 1996;335:1857-1863.

99. Brown KR. Treatment of concomitant carotid and coronary artery disease. Decision-making regarding surgical options. *J Cardiovasc Surg.* 2003;44:395-399.

100. Hankey GJ, Slattery JM, Warlow CP. Transient ischaemic attacks: which patients are at high (and low) risk of serious vascular events? *J Neurol Neurosurg Psychiatry.* 1992;55:640-652.

101. Hornig CR, Lammers C, Buttner T, Hoffmann O, Dorndorf W. Long-term prognosis of infratentorial transient ischemic attacks and minor strokes. *Stroke.* 1992;23:199-204.

102. Johnston SC, Gress DR, Browner WS, Sidney S. Short-term prognosis after emergency department diagnosis of TIA. *JAMA.* 2000;284:2901-2906.

103. Johnston SC, Leira EC, Hansen MD, Adams HP Jr. Early recovery after cerebral ischemia risk of subsequent neurological deterioration. *Ann Neurol*. 2003;54:439-444.

104. Johnston SC, Easton JD. Are patients with acutely recovered cerebral ischemia more unstable? *Stroke*. 2003;34:2446-2450.

105. Jakobsson KE, Saveland H, Hillman J, et al. Warning leak and management outcome in aneurysmal subarachnoid hemorrhage. *J Neurosurg*. 1996;85:995-999.

106. Linn FH, Rinkel GJ, Algra A, van Gijn J. The notion of "warning leaks" in subarachnoid haemorrhage: are such patients in fact admitted with a rebleed? *J Neurol Neurosurg Psychiatry*. 2000;68:332-336.

4

Diagnosis and Evaluation of Patients With Suspected Stroke

The current concept of stroke as a "brain attack" emphasizes rapid diagnosis and evaluation that should be focused, prompt, and accurate.[1] The findings of the emergency evaluation influence both prognosis and treatment. The goals of the initial evaluation are to:

- Determine that the patient's neurologic symptoms are due to stroke
- Localize the area of the brain injury
- Establish the type of stroke:
  - Ischemic
  - Hemorrhagic
- Ascertain the most likely cause of the vascular lesion
- Detect any acute neurologic or medical complications.

Differential Diagnosis of Stroke

The differential diagnosis of stroke is not extensive; the most important alternative diagnosis for ischemic stroke is hemorrhagic stroke and vice versa[2-4] (**Table 4.1**). Trauma should be considered in the occasional patient who is unconscious and for whom no history of the current illness is available, especially if the patient has evidence of intracranial bleeding. Generally, the course of brain tumors, subdural hematomas, and infectious brain diseases is longer than that of stroke. Hypoglycemia may produce focal signs and it should be a diagnostic consideration, especially in any insulin-dependent diabetic

TABLE 4.1 — Differential Diagnosis of Stroke

- Ischemic stroke
- Hemorrhagic stroke
- Craniocerebral trauma
- Subdural hematoma
- Brain abscess
- Encephalitis
- Brain tumor
- Seizure with postictal paralysis
- Metabolic disorder, particularly hypoglycemia
- Migraine

patient.[5] Complicated migraine or seizure with postictal paralysis is a diagnosis of exclusion.

Clinical Features of Stroke

The sudden onset of symptoms and signs of brain dysfunction is the hallmark of all acute cerebrovascular events (**Table 4.2**). While some patients have premonitory symptoms, many are literally struck down without any warning. A scenario, which may occur in approximately 10% of cases, is the presence of neurologic signs upon awakening. In this situation, the time of onset of stroke is not known. While the deficits usually are of maximal severity almost immediately, progression or stepwise deterioration also may occur. A gradual evolution of neurologic impairment over several days or weeks is unusual. Some patients may have early neurologic improvement with subsequent worsening and others will have progressive deterioration, most commonly during the first 24 hours after onset. The outcome among patients with neurologic worsening is poorer than among persons whose impairment is stable.

Progression of the neurologic deficits is especially common among patients with ischemic disease of the posterior circulation. While neurologic worsening is

TABLE 4.2 — Historical Features of Ischemic or Hemorrhagic Stroke

Time Course and Evolution
- Sudden or rapid onset
- Usually reaches maximal intensity in <24 hours
- Gradual or stepwise progression may occur

Focal Neurologic Symptoms
- Cognitive impairments (aphasia, neglect)
- Weakness or incoordination of limbs
- Facial weakness
- Numbness of limbs or face
- Cranial nerve palsies
- Dysarthria

Global Symptoms
- Headache
- Nausea and vomiting
- Altered alertness
  - Syncope
  - Seizure
  - Delirium
  - Stupor or coma
- Elevated blood pressure or abnormal vital signs
- Nuchal rigidity

often considered among patients with ischemia, deterioration secondary to a growth of the hematoma is also seen among patients with hemorrhagic stroke. The causes of neurologic worsening are listed in **Table 4.3**.

The neurologic symptoms of stroke in the carotid or vertebrobasilar circulations reflect the individual vascular territories of the arteries or their branches (**Table 4.4**). Patients have focal neurologic impairments that reflect the area of the brain that is injured. Clinical findings suggest disease in the cerebral hemisphere or the brain stem and/or cerebellum, superficial or deep portions of the cerebral hemisphere, or dominant or nondominant hemisphere (**Table 4.5**, **Table 4.6**, **Table 4.7**, and **Table 4.8**). Signs reflecting dysfunction of

TABLE 4.3 — Causes of Neurologic Worsening: Patients With Stroke

Vascular Causes
- Propagation of intravascular thrombus
- Failure of collateral circulation
- Early recurrent embolism
- Growth of hematoma
- Hemorrhagic transformation of infarction

Neurologic Complications
- Brain edema and increased intracranial pressure
- Hydrocephalus
- Seizures

Medical Complications
- Infections
- Pulmonary embolism
- Cardiac failure
- Electrolyte and metabolic disturbances

several areas of the brain simultaneously are unusual. Nausea, vomiting, headache, seizures, and impairment of consciousness are found in many patients. The features that distinguish ischemic from hemorrhagic stroke are outlined in **Table 4.9**.[4,6-8]

Although many patients with ischemic stroke have headache, an extremely severe headache usually points toward an intracranial hemorrhage[9] (**Table 4.9** and **Table 4.10**). The sudden or explosive onset of an unusually severe headache, often described as the worst headache in the patient's life, points towards a sub-arachnoid hemorrhage (SAH) even in the absence of focal neurologic deficits[6,10,11] (**Table 4.11**). Nausea and vomiting are common with intracranial hemorrhages and may occur with ischemic events in the brain stem or cerebellum, but these signs are unusual with infarctions of the cerebral hemisphere. While patients with major infarctions may be stunned or slow to respond, early depression of consciousness is uncommon with ischemic lesions of the cerebral hemisphere. Rapid

TABLE 4.4 — Territories of the Carotid and Vertebrobasilar Circulations

	Major Branches	Areas Supplied

Carotid Circulation	• Ophthalmic artery
	• Anterior cerebral artery:
	  – Recurrent artery
	  – Cortical branches
	• Anterior choroidal artery
	• Middle cerebral artery:
	  – Lenticulostriate arteries
	  – Cortical branches
	• Posterior cerebral artery (20% of patients)
		• Eye
		• Cerebral hemisphere:
		  – Cortex
		  – Lobar white matter
		  – Deep structures

Vertebrobasilar Circulation	• Posterior inferior cerebellar artery • Anterior inferior cerebellar artery • Internal auditory artery • Superior cerebellar artery • Penetrating branches • Posterior cerebral artery (80% of patients)	• Inner ear • Brain stem • Cerebellum • Cerebral hemisphere • Thalamus

4

TABLE 4.5 — Signs of Ischemic Stroke in the Brain Stem or Cerebellum

Level of Consciousness
- Ranges from alert to coma
- Confusion or agitation uncommon
- No cognitive impairments

Motor Impairments
- Contralateral paresis of the arm and leg:
  - Contralateral hemiparesis
- Quadriparesis
- Crossed paresis: ·
  - Ipsilateral paresis of face, tongue, palate, or pharynx
  - Contralateral weakness of the limbs
- Unilateral or bilateral hyperreflexia
- Unilateral or bilateral Babinski signs
- Dysarthria
- Hoarseness
- Dysphagia with nasal regurgitation
- Ipsilateral ataxia, primarily affecting the arm:
  - Dysmetria
  - Dyssynergia
  - Incoordination
- Gait or truncal instability

Sensory Impairment
- Unilateral sensory loss in the face, arm, and leg
- Bilateral sensory loss in the face
- Crossed sensory loss:
  - Ipsilateral face
  - Contralateral arm and leg
- Dissociated sensory loss:
  - Loss of vibratory sense with preserved pain sense
  - Loss of pain sense with preserved vibratory sense
- Facial pain or dysesthesia
- Absent or depressed corneal or gag reflexes

Continued

Abnormalities of Ocular Motility • Isolated nerve palsy • Conjugate gaze palsy • Internuclear ophthalmoplegia • Skew deviation • Horizontal, vertical, or rotatory nystagmus
Horner syndrome
Vertigo
Unilateral hearing loss
Nausea and vomiting
Headache or neck pain

onset of coma usually suggests an intracranial hemorrhage or a major infarction of the brain stem.[12,13]

Patients with SAH may have syncope, a seizure, or transient loss of consciousness at the time of the aneurysmal rupture, but their consciousness may be restored at the time of evaluation (**Table 4.11**). Agitation or a delirium may be seen in patients with SAH.[14] The presence of signs of meningeal irritation (nuchal rigidity, Brudzinski sign, or Kernig sign) points to an intracranial hemorrhage or an infectious or inflammatory cause of ischemic stroke. The severity and types of neurologic impairments predict the location and extent of the brain injury and forecast prognosis. The impairments also are the foundation for the several scales that are used to assess patients with stroke (**Table 4.12**, **Table 4.13**, and **Table 4.14**).

General Examination of a Patient With Suspected Stroke

The general medical examination focuses on assessment of the cardiovascular system, which might provide evidence for the cause of ischemic stroke and might detect cardiac complications from the cerebrovascular event. Among the findings that are important are:

TABLE 4.6 — Signs of Ischemic Stroke: Cerebral Hemisphere

Left (dominant) Hemisphere
- Right hemiparesis – variable involvement:
  – Face, arm, leg
- Right sensory loss – variable involvement:
  – Face, arm, leg
  – All modalities
  – Decreased graphesthesia
  – Decreased stereognosis
- Right homonymous hemianopia
- Dysarthria
- Aphasia
- Alexia
- Agraphia
- Acalculia
- Apraxia of the left limbs

Right (nondominant) Hemisphere
- Left hemiparesis (same as with left-hemisphere stroke)
- Left-sided sensory loss (same as with left-hemisphere stroke)
- Left homonymous hemianopia
- Dysarthria
- Neglect of the left side of the environment
- Anosognosia
- Asomatognosia
- Loss of prosody of speech
- Blunted affect

- Cardiac murmurs
- Cardiac arrhythmias
- Asymmetry of blood pressure between the two arms
- Asymmetry of peripheral pulses
- Cervical or cranial bruits
- Evidence of embolization elsewhere (splinter hemorrhages, etc).

TABLE 4.7 — Lacunar Syndromes

Pure Motor Hemiparesis
- Contralateral hemiparesis:
  – Usually affects face, arm, and leg equally
  – May have some variation in weakness
- Dysarthria
- No cognitive impairments
- No sensory or visual loss

Pure Sensory Stroke
- Contralateral sensory loss:
  – Usually affects face, arm, and leg equally
  – Affects all sensory modalities
  – May be painful
- No motor loss or dysarthria
- No cognitive or visual impairments

Dysarthria – Clumsy Hand Syndrome
- Dysarthria
- Dysphagia
- Contralateral face and tongue weakness
- Paresis and clumsiness of the contralateral hand

Homolateral Ataxia and Crural Paresis
- Paresis of the contralateral leg
- Prominent ataxia of the contralateral arm and leg

Isolated Sensory/Motor Stroke
- Paresis of the contralateral face, arm, and leg
- Sensory loss of the contralateral face, arm, and leg
- No visual or cognitive impairments

Fisher CM. *Cerebrovasc Dis.* 1991;1:311-320.

Examination of the ocular fundus also is a key part of the examination. The presence of ocular hemorrhages in a comatose patient who has not had overt trauma also points to an intracranial hemorrhage.[15,16] The ocular hemorrhages are found in approximately 20% of cases with severe aneurysmal SAH. Findings of diabetic or hypertensive retinopathy provide clues for the cause of either hemorrhagic or ischemic stroke. A fibrin-platelet embolus or cholesterol embolus also may

	TABLE 4.8 — Localizing Signs: Infarctions of Cerebral Hemisphere		
Impairments	Cortical Infarction*	Deep Infarction†	Major Infarction‡
Consciousness	Alert to stunned	Alert	Drowsy or stupor
Cognitive signs	Prominent	Normal or mild	Prominent
Articulation	Rare dysarthria	Dysarthria	Dysarthria
Visual defect	Contralateral	Rarely found	Contralateral
Gaze paresis	Often present	Rarely found	Prominent
Motor paresis	Contralateral	Contralateral	Contralateral
Pattern	Unequal	Equal	Equal
	Face, arm, leg	Face, arm, leg	Face, arm, leg
Sensory loss	Contralateral	Contralateral	Contralateral
Pattern	Unequal	Equal	Equal
	Face, arm, leg	Face, arm, leg	Face, arm, leg

Motor/sensory loss	Usually both	Isolated motor or sensory	Usually both

* Involvement of the cerebral cortex and lobar white matter.
† Involvement of basal ganglia, thalamus, deep white matter.
‡ Involvement of both cortical and deep structures.

TABLE 4.9 — Features Distinguishing Ischemic From Hemorrhagic Stroke

Features Suggesting Hemorrhagic Stroke
- Early and prolonged unconsciousness
- Prominent headache, nausea, and vomiting
- Retinal hemorrhages
- Nuchal rigidity
- Focal signs do not fit the anatomic pattern of single artery

Features Suggesting Ischemic Stroke
- Stepwise deterioration or progressive worsening
- Waxing and waning of symptoms
- Focal signs fit the anatomic pattern of a single artery
- Focal signs suggest either a cortical or deep location

be found in patients with extracranial atherosclerosis. Increased intracranial pressure may lead to papilledema, although this finding usually is not detected during the first hours after stroke. Signs of trauma (ie, Battle Sign or raccoon eyes) also may provide clues about the patient's impairment. The potential for trauma causing coma should affect the initial clinical evaluation. For example, testing for signs of meningeal irritation may not be done until there is evidence (usually by x-ray or computed tomography [CT]) that there is no cervical spine injury. In addition, the scenario of stroke leading to a head injury through a fall also is a consideration. Conversely, arterial injury leading to infarction is a potential complication of craniocerebral trauma.

Immediate Evaluation of a Patient With Suspected Stroke

Early differentiation of ischemic stroke from hemorrhagic stroke is especially important because it influences acute treatment and subsequent care. A limited number of rapidly performed diagnostic tests are required, while extensive testing to determine the most likely cause of stroke may be performed after admission to the hospital.[17-20] These tests should be performed on an urgent basis because time is critical (**Table 4.15**).

Brain imaging (CT) is the single most important diagnostic test because it is the most reliable way to differentiate ischemic from hemorrhagic stroke (see Chapter 5, *Imaging of the Brain and Blood Vessels in Stroke*). The clinical findings of the two forms of cerebrovascular disease are sufficiently similar to make the diagnosis of brain hemorrhage or infarction problematic when using only the history or physical examination. Patients should not be treated with anticoagulants or thrombolytic agents until CT has helped exclude brain hemorrhage. CT has several advantages that make it attractive for emergency evaluation[17,18,21-25]:

- Widely available
- Relatively inexpensive
- Noninvasive
- Performed rapidly
- Extraordinarily high ability to detect bleeding.

CT does have limitations. It may not detect the early changes of ischemic stroke during the first few hours. In addition, clinicians may miss some of early CT findings.[26,27] CT also may miss small ischemic lesions, particularly in the brain stem.

Because of the strong relationship between heart disease and stroke and because of the nature of early cardiopulmonary complications and their effect on emergency management and outcomes, an electrocardiogram is an important diagnostic test.[28] A chest x-ray may be performed if the patient has evidence of pulmonary dysfunction, but most patients do not need the test.[17] The blood tests listed in **Table 4.15** are used to screen for serious comorbid diseases and acute

TABLE 4.10 — Symptoms and Signs of Hemorrhagic Stroke

Headache

Nausea and Vomiting

Arterial Hypertension and Abnormal Vital Signs

Nuchal Rigidity (may be mild or absent)

Retinal Hemorrhages (approximately 20% of patients)

Altered Consciousness – drowsy, stupor, coma, delirium

Focal Neurologic Impairments – point to area of bleeding

Putamen
- Contralateral hemiparesis
- Contralateral sensory loss
- Contralateral conjugate gaze paresis
- Contralateral homonymous hemianopia
- Aphasia (dominant) or neglect (nondominant)

Thalamus
- Contralateral sensory loss
- Contralateral hemiparesis
- Contralateral or ipsilateral conjugate gaze paresis
- Downward deviation of the eyes
- Small pupils that are sluggishly reactive
- Aphasia (dominant)

Cerebral Hemisphere Lobar White Matter
- Contralateral hemiparesis or sensory loss
- Contralateral gaze paresis
- Contralateral homonymous hemianopia
- Abulia
- Aphasia (dominant) or neglect (nondominant)

Brain Stem (usually pons)
- Quadriparesis or contralateral hemiparesis
- Ipsilateral or bilateral facial paresis
- Locked-in syndrome
- Coma
- Bilateral horizontal gaze paresis
- Ocular bobbing
- Pinpoint pupils
- Hyperthermia and hyperventilation

Continued

Cerebellum
- Truncal and gait ataxia
- Ipsilateral limb ataxia
- Ipsilateral facial weakness and sensory loss
- Ipsilateral conjugate gaze paresis
- Ipsilateral abducens nerve paresis
- Skew deviation
- Small reactive pupils
- Later – development of coma and bilateral weakness, sensory loss

4

complications of stroke. The coagulation tests are used to screen for the presence of an underlying hematologic (coagulation) disorder that could lead to either hemorrhagic or ischemic stroke. The tests also may influence decisions about the use of thrombolytic agents or other interventions to treat stroke.

Examination of the cerebrospinal fluid (CSF) is an important ancillary diagnostic test to search for bleeding in the evaluation of patients with suspected SAH.[6,29,30] This test is not necessary if a CT scan demonstrates bleeding. Because the clinical features of SAH are sufficiently unique, most patients with suspected ischemic stroke do not need to have evaluation of the CSF to exclude a ruptured aneurysm. Lumbar puncture is an invasive procedure that has some potential morbidity and it should not be performed if the clinical or brain imaging findings suggest a large lesion causing mass effect because of the potential for herniation. A CSF examination to screen for a cause of ischemic stroke, such as an inflammatory or infectious disease, may be done after the patient's condition has been stabilized.

Subsequent Diagnostic Testing

Although several other diagnostic tests are available, their utility in emergency care has not been established. They may be obtained after emergency

TABLE 4.11 — Symptoms and Signs of Subarachnoid Hemorrhage

- Headache:
  - Sudden or cataclysmic onset
  - Unusually severe
  - Described as worst headache in life
- Pain in neck, face, eye, or ear
- Loss of consciousness (especially at onset of symptoms):
  - Transient loss of consciousness
  - Syncope
  - Seizure
  - Prolonged unresponsiveness
  - Confusion
  - Agitation
- Nausea and vomiting
- Photophobia and phonophobia
- Focal neurologic signs (usually are absent or mild):
  - Oculomotor nerve palsy (pupil involved)
  - Hemiparesis
  - Paraparesis
  - Incontinence
- Elevated blood pressure and abnormal vital signs
- Nuchal rigidity
- Retinal hemorrhages (approximately 20% of patients)

treatment and admission to the hospital. **Figure 4.1**, **Figure 4.2**, **Figure 4.3**, and **Figure 4.4** provide algorithms for the additional evaluation of patients with either hemorrhagic or ischemic stroke.

Magnetic resonance imaging (MRI) is gaining in popularity for the initial evaluation of patients with stroke. It is more sensitive than CT for detecting smaller ischemic lesions, particularly those in the posterior fossa. Advances in MRI technology allow evaluation of perfusion, diffusion, and metabolic studies of the brain. The use of diffusion-weighted imaging allows for rapid detection of an ischemic lesion. The changes may be detected within minutes to hours of the onset of stroke.[31,32]

TABLE 4.12 — National Institutes of Health Stroke Scale

Level of consciousness	0-3 points
Orientation questions	0-2 points
Responses to commands	0-2 points
Eye movements	0-2 points
Visual fields	0-3 points
Facial motor activity	0-3 points
Right upper extremity motor activity	0-4 points
Left upper extremity motor activity	0-4 points
Right lower extremity motor activity	0-4 points
Left lower extremity motor activity	0-4 points
Sensory function	0-2 points
Limb coordination (ataxia)	0-2 points
Articulation	0-2 points
Language	0-3 points
Neglect	0-2 points
Brott T, et al. *Stroke*. 1989;20:864-870.	

MRI is being used to evaluate patients with intracerebral hemorrhage or SAH.[33,34] MRI also may be used to assess the presence of an underlying arterial or venous occlusion (see Chapter 5, *Imaging of the Brain and Blood Vessels in Stroke*). The role of MRI in emergency evaluation likely will increase. In particular, mismatches between perfusion and other imaging sequences may become a key early diagnostic finding in determining eligibility for emergency treatment. Already, one clinical trial has used this mismatch technology to help select patients treated with desmoteplase.[35] Still, MRI is not needed for emergency treatment of most patients with stroke. It should be reserved for atypical or problematic cases in which the

TABLE 4.13 — Hunt and Hess Scale: Subarachnoid Hemorrhage	
Grade 1	• Asymptomatic or mild headache
Grade 2	• Moderate to severe headache • Nuchal rigidity • Oculomotor nerve palsy
Grade 3	• Confusion or drowsiness • Mild focal neurologic signs
Grade 4	• Stupor • Hemiparesis
Grade 5	• Coma, moribund • Extensor posturing
Hunt WE, Hess RM. *J Neurosurg.* 1968;28:14-20.	

location or the nature of the brain lesion is critical in making decisions about management. In addition, there are limitations with MRI including:

- It is not widely available on an emergency basis
- It is more expensive and may take time to perform
- Patients who are agitated or confused may not tolerate the procedure
- Patients who have claustrophobia may not tolerate the procedure
- Patients with pacemakers or foreign bodies cannot have the procedure.

The cerebral vasculature also may be examined with several diagnostic tests[20] (see Chapter 5, *Imaging of the Brain and Blood Vessels in Stroke*). While these tests usually are not performed during the initial evaluation, most patients with either hemorrhagic or ischemic stroke will have at least one of the vascular imaging tests done after admission to the hospital. Some of these studies are done on an emergency basis.

TABLE 4.14 — Glasgow Coma Scale	
Best Response in Eye Opening	
Spontaneous	4 points
To speech	3 points
To pain	2 points
No response	1 points
Best Motor Response	
Obeys commands	6 points
Localizes	5 points
Withdraws in response to pain	4 points
Flexor response to pain	3 points
Extensor response to pain	2 points
No movement	1 points
Best Verbal Response	
Normal conversation	5 points
Confused	4 points
Inappropriate words	3 points
Incomprehensible sounds	2 points
No speech	1 points
Langfitt TW. *J Neurosurg.* 1979;48:673-678.	

These tests would be aimed at detecting aneurysms, vascular malformations, or arterial occlusions that might necessitate early surgical intervention. While digital subtraction arteriography (DSA) has been the preferred method to assess the vasculature, there have been advances in computed tomographic angiography (CTA), magnetic resonance angiography (MRA), and Doppler ultrasonography.[36-44]

Imaging of the heart often is advised because of the high prevalence of cardiac disease that may be the source of emboli in people with ischemic stroke.[45]

TABLE 4.15 — Emergency Diagnostic Studies: Evaluation of Patient With Suspected Stroke

- Computed tomography (CT) of the brain without contrast
- Electrocardiogram (ECG)
- Complete blood count including platelet count
- Prothrombin time (international normalized ratio [INR])
- Activated partial thromboplastin time (aPTT)
- Blood glucose
- Serum chemistries, including electrolytes
- Cervical spine x-ray (if unconscious and trauma is suspected)
- Chest x-ray (if active pulmonary disease is suspected)
- Arterial blood gases (if hypoxia is suspected)
- Cerebrospinal fluid examination (if subarachnoid hemorrhage is suspected and CT is negative for bleeding)

Transthoracic (TTE) and transesophageal (TEE) echocardiography are the two most widely ordered cardiac imaging tests.[46,47] If another obvious source for stroke, such as an arterial dissection or atherosclerotic stenosis, is found or if the results of the cardiac imaging tests are not likely to alter management, these studies might not be necessary. On the other hand, cardiac imaging may be informative in young people with ischemic symptoms or in those who have other evidence suggesting a cardiac source for embolization.

In general, TTE has a low yield in detecting cardiac abnormalities; it is most likely to reveal abnormalities of the left ventricle. The test would be ordered if a mural thrombus following a myocardial infarction (MI), a left ventricular aneurysm, or an akinetic left ventricular segment were suspected. TEE is particularly useful in detecting abnormalities in the left atrium (**Figure 4.5**). TEE also is used to discover advanced or complex atherosclerotic plaques of the proximal aorta. Supplementing the TEE with intravenous contrast may permit detection of communication between the right and left atria, which may support the diagnosis of paradoxical embolization.[48,49] TEE is a moderately invasive study that may be complicated by cardiac arrhythmias or esophageal injury. Other cardiac imaging options include cine-CT or gated MRI. These tests are not done widely.

Additional tests are ordered on a case-by-case basis and are performed to screen for specific risk factors or causes of stroke. Some of these tests are expensive, and generally, they are of low yield. Among the tests is a fasting lipid profile to screen for hyperlipidemia as a risk factor for accelerated atherosclerosis. Special tests to screen for acquired or inherited prothrombotic disorders that promote arterial or venous thrombosis or coagulopathy that leads to serious hemorrhage may be ordered if the cause of stroke is not obvious[50] (**Table 4.16**). The tests also could be done if a patient has a personal or family history of the following conditions that suggest a prothrombotic disease:

- Recurrent arterial or venous thromboembolism:
  - Stroke or MI at a young age
  - Deep vein thrombosis
  - Pulmonary embolism
  - Spontaneous abortion
- Livedo reticularis
- Clinical features suggestive of systemic lupus erythematosus.

Abnormalities of the initial coagulation tests (activated partial thromboplastin time [aPTT], international normalized ratio [INR], platelet count) may prompt a more detailed assessment of the coagulation system. Levels of these factors may be perturbed following stroke or the use of antithrombotic agents. For instance, antithrombin III may be lowered following the use of heparin. Warfarin use is associated with reduction in levels of proteins C and S. These factors should be measured during convalescence when the patient is no longer taking the medications.

FIGURE 4.1 — Evaluation for Suspected Stroke

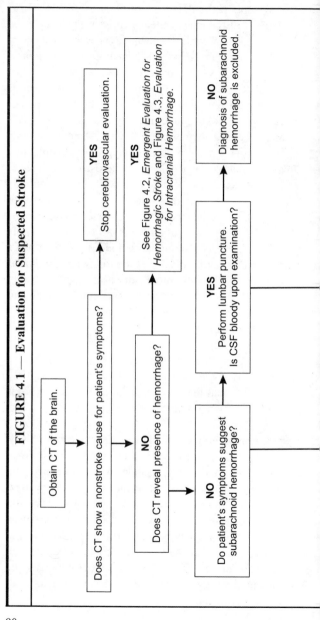

Obtain CT of the brain.

Does CT show a nonstroke cause for patient's symptoms?

YES
Stop cerebrovascular evaluation.

NO
Does CT reveal presence of hemorrhage?

YES
See Figure 4.2, *Emergent Evaluation for Hemorrhagic Stroke* and Figure 4.3, *Evaluation for Intracranial Hemorrhage.*

NO
Do patient's symptoms suggest subarachnoid hemorrhage?

YES
Perform lumbar puncture.
Is CSF bloody upon examination?

NO
Diagnosis of subarachnoid hemorrhage is excluded.

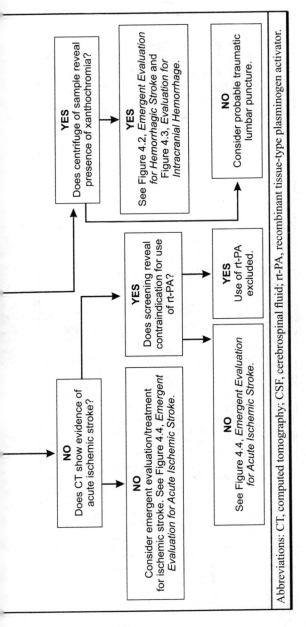

Does CT show evidence of acute ischemic stroke?

NO — Does CT show evidence of acute ischemic stroke?

NO
Consider emergent evaluation/treatment for ischemic stroke. See Figure 4.4, *Emergent Evaluation for Acute Ischemic Stroke.*

YES
Does screening reveal contraindication for use of rt-PA?

NO
See Figure 4.4, *Emergent Evaluation for Acute Ischemic Stroke.*

YES
Use of rt-PA excluded.

YES
Does centrifuge of sample reveal presence of xanthochromia?

YES
See Figure 4.2, *Emergent Evaluation for Hemorrhagic Stroke* and Figure 4.3, *Evaluation for Intracranial Hemorrhage.*

NO
Consider probable traumatic lumbar puncture.

Abbreviations: CT, computed tomography; CSF, cerebrospinal fluid; rt-PA, recombinant tissue-type plasminogen activator.

4

91

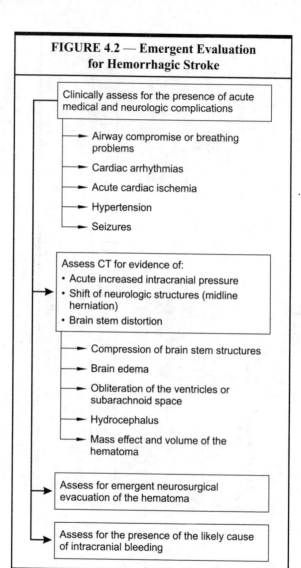

FIGURE 4.2 — Emergent Evaluation for Hemorrhagic Stroke

Clinically assess for the presence of acute medical and neurologic complications

- Airway compromise or breathing problems
- Cardiac arrhythmias
- Acute cardiac ischemia
- Hypertension
- Seizures

Assess CT for evidence of:
• Acute increased intracranial pressure
• Shift of neurologic structures (midline herniation)
• Brain stem distortion

- Compression of brain stem structures
- Brain edema
- Obliteration of the ventricles or subarachnoid space
- Hydrocephalus
- Mass effect and volume of the hematoma

Assess for emergent neurosurgical evacuation of the hematoma

Assess for the presence of the likely cause of intracranial bleeding

Abbreviation: CT, computed tomography.

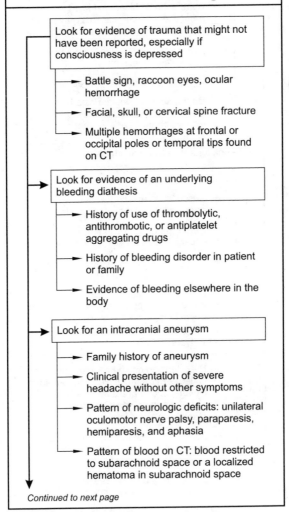

FIGURE 4.3 — Evaluation for Intracranial Hemorrhage

Look for evidence of trauma that might not have been reported, especially if consciousness is depressed

- Battle sign, raccoon eyes, ocular hemorrhage
- Facial, skull, or cervical spine fracture
- Multiple hemorrhages at frontal or occipital poles or temporal tips found on CT

Look for evidence of an underlying bleeding diathesis

- History of use of thrombolytic, antithrombotic, or antiplatelet aggregating drugs
- History of bleeding disorder in patient or family
- Evidence of bleeding elsewhere in the body

Look for an intracranial aneurysm

- Family history of aneurysm
- Clinical presentation of severe headache without other symptoms
- Pattern of neurologic deficits: unilateral oculomotor nerve palsy, paraparesis, hemiparesis, and aphasia
- Pattern of blood on CT: blood restricted to subarachnoid space or a localized hematoma in subarachnoid space

Continued to next page

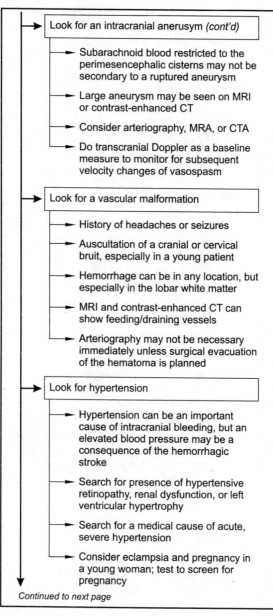

Look for an intracranial anerusym *(cont'd)*

- Subarachnoid blood restricted to the perimesencephalic cisterns may not be secondary to a ruptured aneurysm
- Large aneurysm may be seen on MRI or contrast-enhanced CT
- Consider arteriography, MRA, or CTA
- Do transcranial Doppler as a baseline measure to monitor for subsequent velocity changes of vasospasm

Look for a vascular malformation

- History of headaches or seizures
- Auscultation of a cranial or cervical bruit, especially in a young patient
- Hemorrhage can be in any location, but especially in the lobar white matter
- MRI and contrast-enhanced CT can show feeding/draining vessels
- Arteriography may not be necessary immediately unless surgical evacuation of the hematoma is planned

Look for hypertension

- Hypertension can be an important cause of intracranial bleeding, but an elevated blood pressure may be a consequence of the hemorrhagic stroke
- Search for presence of hypertensive retinopathy, renal dysfunction, or left ventricular hypertrophy
- Search for a medical cause of acute, severe hypertension
- Consider eclampsia and pregnancy in a young woman; test to screen for pregnancy

Continued to next page

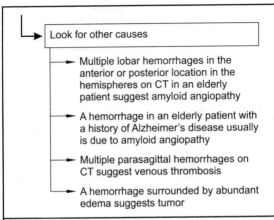

Look for other causes

→ Multiple lobar hemorrhages in the anterior or posterior location in the hemispheres on CT in an elderly patient suggest amyloid angiopathy

→ A hemorrhage in an elderly patient with a history of Alzheimer's disease usually is due to amyloid angiopathy

4

→ Multiple parasagittal hemorrhages on CT suggest venous thrombosis

→ A hemorrhage surrounded by abundant edema suggests tumor

Abbreviations: CT, computed tomography; CTA, computed tomographic angiography; MRA, magnetic resonance angiography; MRI, magnetic resonance imaging.

Screening for a multisystem vasculitis is performed when the cause of stroke is not otherwise obvious. Examination of the CSF also may be helpful if an inflammatory or infectious process of the central nervous system is suspected as the cause of brain ischemia. Cultures of blood may be indicated if infective endocarditis is a potential explanation for an ischemic stroke. Serologic studies also are used to screen for infectious causes of stroke.

REFERENCES

1. Hill MD, Hachinski V. Stroke treatment: time is brain. *Lancet.* 1998;352(suppl 3):SIII10-SIII14.
2. Norris JW, Hachinski VC. Misdiagnosis of stroke. *Lancet.* 1982;1:328-331.
3. The Members of the Lille Stroke Program. Misdiagnoses in 1,250 consecutive patients admitted to an acute stroke unit. *Cerebrovasc Dis.* 1997;7:284-288.
4. Harrison MJ. Clinical distinction of cerebral haemorrhage and cerebral infarction. *Postgrad Med J.* 1980;56:629-632.
5. Wallis WE, Donaldson I, Scott RS, Wilson J. Hypoglycemia masquerading as cerebrovascular disease (hypoglycemic hemiplegia). *Ann Neurol.* 1985;18:510-512.

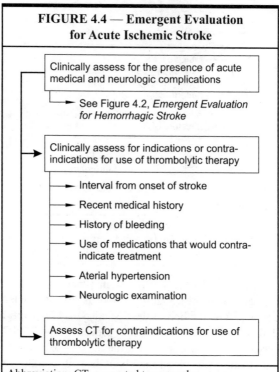

FIGURE 4.4 — Emergent Evaluation for Acute Ischemic Stroke

Clinically assess for the presence of acute medical and neurologic complications

→ See Figure 4.2, *Emergent Evaluation for Hemorrhagic Stroke*

Clinically assess for indications or contra-indications for use of thrombolytic therapy

→ Interval from onset of stroke

→ Recent medical history

→ History of bleeding

→ Use of medications that would contra-indicate treatment

→ Aterial hypertension

→ Neurologic examination

Assess CT for contraindications for use of thrombolytic therapy

Abbreviation: CT, computed tomography.

6. van Gijn J, Rinkel GJ. Subarachnoid haemorrhage: diagnosis, causes and management. *Brain*. 2001;124:249-278.

7. Weir CJ, Murray GD, Adams FG, Muir KW, Grosset DG, Lees KR. Poor accuracy of stroke scoring systems for differential clinical diagnosis of intracranial haemorrhage and infarction. *Lancet*. 1994;344:999-1002.

8. Besson G, Robert C, Hommel M, Perret J. Is it clinically possible to distinguish nonhemorrhagic infarct from hemorrhagic stroke? *Stroke*. 1995;26:1205-1209.

9. Ferro JM, Melo TP, Oliveira V, et al. A multivariate study of headache associated with ischemic stroke. *Headache*. 1995;35:315-319.

10. Adams HP Jr, Jergenson DD, Kassell NF, Sahs AL. Pitfalls in the recognition of subarachnoid hemorrhage. *JAMA*. 1980;244:794-796.

11. Edlow JA, Caplan LR. Avoiding pitfalls in the diagnosis of subarachnoid hemorrhage. *N Engl J Med*. 2000;342:29-36.

12. St Louis EK, Wijdicks EF, Li H, Atkinson JD. Predictors of poor outcome in patients with a spontaneous cerebellar hematoma. *Can J Neurol Sci*. 2000;27:32-36.

13. Wijdicks EF, St Louis E. Clinical profiles predictive of outcome in pontine hemorrhage. *Neurology*. 1997;49:1342-1346.

TABLE 4.16 — Special Diagnostic Tests of Coagulation to Screen for Prothrombotic Cause of Ischemic Stroke

- Antiphospholipid antibodies:
  - Lupus anticoagulant
- Sickle cell screen and hemoglobin electrophoresis
- Serum fibrinogen
- D dimer
- Fibrin degradation products
- Proteins C and S
- Antithrombin III
- Factor V Leiden
- Prothrombin gene mutation

4

14. Ferro JM, Caeiro L, Verdelho A. Delirium in acute stroke. *Curr Opin Neurol.* 2002;15:51-55.

15. Frizzell RT, Kuhn F, Morris R, Quinn C, Fisher WS 3rd. Screening for ocular hemorrhages in patients with ruptured cerebral aneurysms: a prospective study of 99 patients. *Neurosurgery.* 1997;41:529-533.

16. Keane JR. Retinal hemorrhage: its significance in 100 patients with acute encephalopathy of unknown cause. *Arch Neurol.* 1979;36:691-694.

17. Adams HP Jr, Adams RJ, Brott T, et al. Guidelines for the early management of patients with ischemic stroke. A scientific statement from the Stroke Council of the American Stroke Association. *Stroke.* 2003;34:1056-1083.

18. Adams H, Adams R, del Zoppo G, Goldstein LB; Stroke Council of the American Heart Association; American Stroke Association. Guidelines for the early management of patients with ischemic stroke: 2005 guidelines update: a scientific statement from the Stroke Council of the American Heart Association/American Stroke Association. *Stroke.* 2005;36:916-923.

19. Broderick JP, Adams HP, Jr, Barsan W, et al. Guidelines for the management of spontaneous intracerebral hemorrhage: a statement for healthcare professionals from a special writing group of the Stroke Council, American Heart Association. *Stroke.* 1999;30:905-915.

20. Culebras A, Kase CS, Masdeu JC, et al. Practice guidelines for the use of imaging in transient ischemic attacks and acute stroke. A report of the Stroke Council, American Heart Association. *Stroke.* 1997;28:1480-1497.

21. Grond M, von Kummer R, Sobesky J, Schmulling S, Heiss WD. Early computed-tomography abnormalities in acute stroke. *Lancet.* 1997;350:1595-1596.

22. von Kummer R, Nolte PN, Schnittger H, Thron A, Ringelstein EB. Detectability of cerebral hemisphere ischaemic infarcts by CT within 6 h of stroke. *Neuroradiology.* 1996;38:31-33.

23. von Kummer R, Allen KL, Holle R, et al. Acute stroke: usefulness of early CT findings before thrombolytic therapy. *Radiology.* 1997;205:327-333.

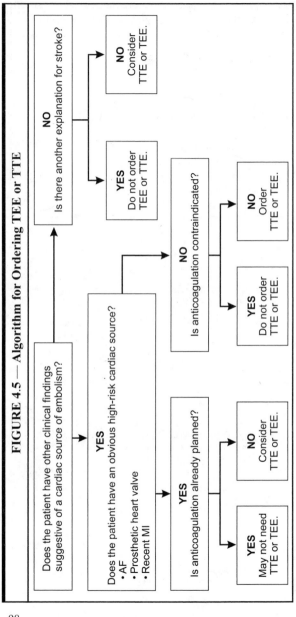

FIGURE 4.5 — Algorithm for Ordering TEE or TTE

Does the patient have other clinical findings suggestive of a cardiac source of embolism?

YES

Does the patient have an obvious high-risk cardiac source?
- AF
- Prosthetic heart valve
- Recent MI

YES

Is anticoagulation already planned?

YES
May not need TTE or TEE.

NO
Consider TTE or TEE.

NO

Is anticoagulation contraindicated?

YES
Do not order TTE or TEE.

NO
Order TTE or TEE.

NO

Is there another explanation for stroke?

YES
Do not order TEE or TTE.

NO
Consider TTE or TEE.

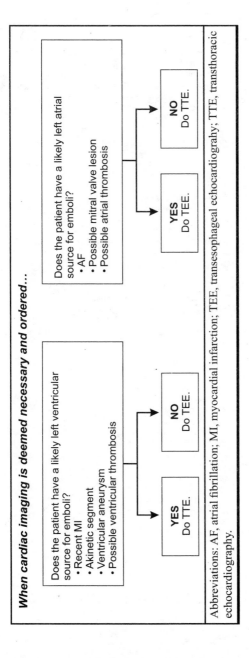

When cardiac imaging is deemed necessary and ordered...

Does the patient have a likely left ventricular source for emboli?
• Recent MI
• Akinetic segment
• Ventricular aneurysm
• Possible ventricular thrombosis

YES
Do TTE.

NO
Do TEE.

Does the patient have a likely left atrial source for emboli?
• AF
• Possible mitral valve lesion
• Possible atrial thrombosis

YES
Do TEE.

NO
Do TTE.

Abbreviations: AF, atrial fibrillation; MI, myocardial infarction; TEE, transesophageal echocardiograhy; TTE, transthoracic echocardiography.

24. von Kummer R, Patel S. Neuroimaging in acute stroke. *J Stroke Cerebrovasc Dis*. 1999;8:127-138.

25. Brainin M, Olsen TS, Chamorro A, et al; EUSI Executive Committee; EUSI Writing Committee. Organization of stroke care: education, referral, emergency management and imaging, stroke units and rehabilitation. European Stroke Initiative. *Cerebrovasc Dis*. 2004;17(suppl 2):1-14.

26. Grotta JC, Chiu D, Lu M, et al. Agreement and variability in the interpretation of early CT changes in stroke patients qualifying for intravenous rtPA therapy. *Stroke*. 1999;30:1528-1533.

27. Wardlaw JM, Dorman PJ, Lewis SC, Sandercock PA. Can stroke physicians and neuroradiologists identify signs of early cerebral infarction on CT? *J Neurol Neurosurg Psychiatry*. 1999;67:651-653.

28. Vandenberg B, Biller J. Cardiac evaulation of the patient with stroke. *Cerebrovasc Dis*. 1991;1(suppl 1):73-82.

29. Vermeulen M, van Gijn J. The diagnosis of subarachnoid hemorrhage. *J Neurol Neurosurg Psychiatry*. 1990;53:365-372.

30. Morgenstern LB, Luna-Gonzales H, Huber JC Jr, et al. Worst headache and subarachnoid hemorrhage: prospective, modern computed tomography and spinal fluid analysis. *Ann Emerg Med*. 1998;32:297-304.

31. Kidwell CS, Chalela JA, Saver JL, et al. Comparison of MRI and CT for detection of acute intracerebral hemorrhage. *JAMA*. 2004;292:1823-1830.

32. Lovblad KO. Diffusion-weighted MRI: back to the future. *Stroke*. 2002;33:2204-2205.

33. Schellinger PD, Fiebach JB, Hoffmann K, et al. Stroke MRI in intracerebral hemorrhage: is there a perihemorrhagic penumbra? *Stroke*. 2003;34:1674-1679.

34. Wiesmann M, Mayer TE, Yousry I, Medele R, Hamann GF, Bruckmann H. Detection of hyperacute subarachnoid hemorrhage of the brain by using magnetic resonance imaging. *J Neurosurg*. 2002;96:684-689.

35. Hacke W, Albers G, Al-Rawi Y, et al; DIAS Study Group. The Desmoteplase in Acute Ischemic Stroke Trial (DIAS): a phase II MRI-based 9-hour window acute stroke thrombolysis trial with intravenous desmoteplase. *Stroke*. 2005;36:66-73.

36. Wildermuth S, Knauth M, Brandt T, Winter R, Sartor K, Hacke W. Role of CT angiography in patient selection for thrombolytic therapy in acute hemispheric stroke. *Stroke*. 1998;29:935-938.

37. Velthuis BK, Van Leeuwen MS, Witkamp TD, Ramos LM, Berkelbach van Der Sprenkel JW, Rinkel GJ. Computerized tomography angiography in patients with subarachnoid hemorrhage: from aneurysm detection to treatment without conventional angiography. *J Neurosurg*. 1999;91:761-767.

38. Dehdashti AR, Rufenacht DA, Delavelle J, Reverdin A, de Tribolet N. Therapeutic decision and management of aneurysmal subarachnoid haemorrhage based on computed tomographic angiography. *Br J Neurosurg*. 2003;17:46-53.

39. Hirai T, Korogi Y, Suginohara K, et al. Clinical usefulness of unsubtracted 3D digital angiography compared with rotational digital angiography in the pretreatment evaluation of intracranial aneurysms. *AJNR Am J Neuroradiol*. 2003;24:1067-1074.

40. Nonent M, Serfaty JM, Nighoghossian N, et al; CARMEDAS Study Group. Concordance rate differences of 3 noninvasive imaging techniques to measure carotid stenosis in clinical routine practice: results of the CARMEDAS multicenter study. *Stroke*. 2004;35:682-686.

41. Derex L, Nighoghossian N, Hermier M, et al. Magnetic resonance imaging: significance of early ischemic changes on computed tomography. *Cerebrovasc Dis*. 2004;18:232-235.

42. Mallouhi A, Felber S, Chemelli A, et al. Detection and characterization of intracranial aneurysms with MR angiography: comparison of volume-rendering and maximum-intensity-projection algorithms. *AJR Am J Roentgenol*. 2003;180:55-64.

43. Alexandrov AV. Imaging cerebrovascular diseases with ultrasound. *Cerebrovasc Dis*. 2003;16:1-3.

44. Alexandrov AV. Ultrasound identification and lysis of clots. *Stroke*. 2004;35(11 suppl 1):2722-2725.

45. Beattie JR, Cohen DJ, Manning WJ, Douglas PS. Role of routine transthoracic echocardiography in evaluation and management of stroke. *J Intern Med*. 1998;243:281-291.

46. Cohen A, Chauvel C. Transesophageal echocardiography in the management of transient ischemic attack and ischemic stroke. *Cerebrovasc Dis*. 1996;6(suppl 1):15-25.

47. Albers GW, Comess KA, DeRook FA, et al. Transesophageal echocardiographic findings in stroke subtypes. *Stroke*. 1994;25:23-28.

48. Schneider B, Zienkiewicz T, Jansen V, Hofmann T, Noltenius H, Meinertz T. Diagnosis of patent foramen ovale by transesophageal echocardiography and correlation with autopsy findings. *Am J Cardiol*. 1996;77:1202-1209.

49. Serena J, Segura T, Perez-Ayuso MJ, Bassaganyas J, Molins A, Davalos A. The need to quantify right-to-left shunt in acute ischemic stroke: a case-control study. *Stroke*. 1998;29:1322-1328.

50. Bushnell C, Siddiqi Z, Morgenlander JC, Goldstein LB. Use of specialized coagulation testing in the evaluation of patients with acute ischemic stroke. *Neurology*. 2001;56:624-627.

5

Imaging of the Brain and Blood Vessels in Stroke

Imaging of the brain is a crucial step in the assessment of persons with suspected stroke[1,2] (**Table 5.1** and **Table 5.2**). Brain imaging helps in the determination of the type and cause of stroke.[3-5] Imaging also provides information about the condition of the brain because it helps differentiate tissue that is damaged irreversibly from areas that have the potential for recovery. The results of brain imaging may guide emergency and subsequent treatment and may help predict outcomes. In deciding when and how to order an imaging study, it should be clear in advance to what extent the results of the study will affect the patient's care. Imaging tests should be scheduled in parallel with emergency medical management. If the imaging facility is informed in advance, the scanner could be kept free for a stroke emergency. Emergency life-support may be continued while the patient is undergoing the study. While a detailed neurologic examination is not needed before the brain imaging test is done, localizing the stroke to the cerebral hemisphere or the posterior fossa assists in tailoring the imaging techniques.

Computed Tomography (CT) of the Brain

In current practice, CT is the emergency brain imaging test of choice.[1,2] The results of CT affect management. Patients should not receive emergency thrombolytic or antithrombotic therapy until CT has excluded the possibility of a hemorrhage (**Table 5.3** and **Table 5.4**). Emergency CT also provides data that

TABLE 5.1 — Imaging Techniques for Assessment of a Patient With Suspected Stroke

- Computed tomography (CT) of the brain
- Computed tomographic angiography (CTA)
  - CT perfusion imaging (PI)
- Magnetic resonance imaging (MRI):
  - T1, T2, FLAIR, T2*
  - Diffusion weighted imaging (DWI)
  - Magnetic resonance perfusion imaging
- Magnetic resonance angiography (MRA)
- Transcranial Doppler ultrasound (TDU)
- Duplex imaging of the extracranial carotid artery
- Digital subtraction angiography (DSA)
- Single photon emission CT (SPECT)
- Positron emission tomography (PET)

are crucial for urgent treatment of primary intracerebral hemorrhage.[6,7]

CT should be performed primarily without contrast enhancement. CT angiography (CTA) and CT perfusion imaging require a bolus contrast injection. Modern scanners are so quick that motion artifacts usually are not a problem. If necessary, a specific section may be repeated easily. Artifacts may blur the lower portion of the posterior fossa and an infarction of the brain stem may be missed. Image windows should be adjusted so that the gray and white matter may be distinguished. The cortical layer, basal ganglia, and thalamus have higher x-ray attenuation than does the white matter. Net water uptake immediately after severe hypoperfusion and subsequent hypoattenuation may blur the margins of these structures in acute stroke. Swelling of brain tissue with obliteration of the cortical sulci can be found in areas with low perfusion pressure and compensatory arterial dilatation.[8]

Arterial occlusion may be visible on nonenhancing CT as a hyperattenuating segment of an artery (hyperdense artery sign, dot sign), whereas only fibrin-rich

TABLE 5.2 — What Can Be Imaged in Patients With Acute Stroke?	
Imaging Test	**Imaging Results**
CT	Brain tissue, CSF space, skull, brain tissue perfusion
MRI	Brain tissue, CSF space, brain tissue proton diffusion and perfusion, brain function, vascular imaging
CTA	Blood vessels in neck or brain (arteries and veins)
MRA	Same as CTA
Arteriography	Same as CTA
Ultrasonography	Arteries and veins in the neck
TDU	Arteries and veins of the brain
SPECT	Brain tissue perfusion
PET	Brain tissue perfusion and metabolism
MRS	Brain tissue metabolism
Abbreviations: CSF, cerebrospinal fluid; CT, computed tomography; CTA, computed tomographic angiography; MRA, magnetic resonance angiography; MRI, magnetic resonance imaging; MRS, magnetic resonance spectroscopy; PET, positron emission tomography; SPECT, single photon emission computed tomography; TDU, transcranial Doppler ultrasound.	

thrombi attenuate x-rays higher than brain tissue in contrast to white, platelet-rich thrombi.[9]

If craniocerebral trauma is possible, additional bone window sequences may be performed to search for skull fractures, subdural air or blood, or effusion in the nasal sinuses or the middle ear.

Parenchymal hemorrhage is readily seen as a hyperattenuated, space-occupying mass (**Figure 5.1**). CT has a yield of nearly 100% in finding acute hemorrhages in the cerebral hemisphere, cerebellum, or brain stem — even small lesions may be detected. The find-

TABLE 5.3 — Key Questions for Brain Imaging in Patients With Stroke

- Any intracranial pathology?
- Pathology appropriate to the clinical symptoms?
- Old brain lesions and vascular pathology characterizing underlying disease?
- Parenchymal hypoattenuation with arterial pattern?
- Hyperattenuation of arterial segments?
- Parenchymal hypoattenuation with arterial pattern?
- Parenchymal hypoattenuation with venous pattern?
- Hyperattenuation with venous sinus?
- Hyperattentuation consistent with blood?
- Pattern of hemorrhage (parenchymal, intraventricular, subarachnoid, subdural, or epidural)?
- Size of lesion and main location?
- Abnormal or enlarged vessels?
- Blockage of cerebrospinal fluid with secondary hydrocephalus?
- Brain edema with mass effect or effacement of the cisterns?
- Evidence of midbrain distortion or compression?

ings of subarachnoid hemorrhage (SAH) may be subtle and might be missed by CT or by physicians evaluating the test[10-12] (**Figure 5.2**). If blood is intermixed with the cerebrospinal fluid (CSF), the density will be similar to the adjacent brain. In most cases, the blood is restricted to the basal cisterns, interhemispheric fissure, and sylvian fissure. The blood may be localized or diffuse. The sensitivity of CT in detecting subarachnoid blood declines from approximately 90% of the day of bleeding to approximately 50% at 1 week.[12] CT also may miss blood in the subarachnoid space in alert patients who have only headache. A shift of midline structures without an obvious space-occupying process is suspicious for a subdural hematoma isodense to the brain parenchyma. Another clue for an isodense subdural hematoma will be the obliteration of the sulci on the side of the brain (**Figure 5.3**).

TABLE 5.4 — Recommendations for Performance of CT in Patients With Suspected Stroke

- Alert the radiologist and technician rapidly so that the patient may be evaluated as quickly as possible
- Continue life-support measures
- Perform an unenhanced study first
- Obtain thin (<5-mm) transaxial sections from the posterior fossa and the base of the cerebral hemispheres
- Continue with 8-mm sections for the rest of the cerebral hemispheres
- Observe the images when they appear on the monitor
- Repeat sections if the image cannot be interpreted because of artifacts
- Change window and level if gray/white matter differentiation is not clear
- If necessary, continue with a contrast-enhanced CT study

Abbreviation: CT, computed tomography.

Depending upon the location and extent of the brain ischemia, CT appears normal in one third of patients with acute ischemic stroke.[3] CT detects ischemic lesions with a sensitivity of 65% and a specificity of 90% within 6 hours of onset of stroke.[13,14] The extent of the infarction as detected by CT also provides prognostic information.[15] Important information is provided if the CT is normal and no subtle signs of evolving brain infarction or brain edema are present. Intracranial bleeding, brain tumor, and a focal suppurative process generally are excluded. If the CT is negative and the clinical findings are not consistent with encephalitis, migraine, hypoglycemia, or a somatization disorder, ischemic stroke is the most likely diagnosis. Severe brain ischemia may cause edema, which may be detected by CT within 1 to 2 hours following stroke.[14] If the patient is examined within the first 6 hours of stroke, a normal CT study means that

FIGURE 5.1 — Cerebral Hematoma

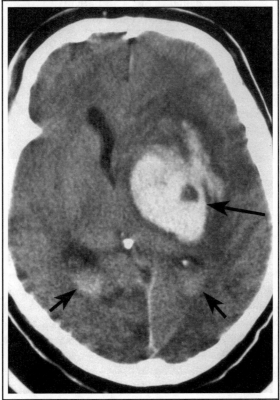

A computed tomography (CT) scan of a 48-year-old man who had parenchymal hemorrhage in the left basal ganglia following the intra-arterial administration of urokinase. Note the fluid level (long arrow) in the coagulum. Blood is also seen within the posterior horns of the ventricles (short arrows), which signifies intraventricular extension of the hemorrhage.

the ischemic process may not have caused irreversible tissue damage and an increase in brain perfusion may rescue tissue and function.

Increases in brain water content decrease x-ray attenuation. The earliest signs of ischemic brain edema on CT consist of slight hypoattenuation of the gray matter that causes a loss of the anatomic margins between the cortex and adjacent white matter. Such subtle hypoattenuation also occurs in the basal ganglia within 3 hours of onset of a stroke secondary to occlusion of the proximal segment of the middle cerebral artery (**Figure 5.4**). Large hypoattenuated areas detected within 6 hours of onset of stroke portend that treatment with thrombolytic agents likely will not be effective because life-threatening brain edema already is developing[14] (**Figure 5.5**). Most ischemic strokes involving the occlusion of the pial arteries that cause wedge-shaped lesions respect a described vascular territory. A hypodensity that is round or that does fit an arterial pattern probably is not ischemic in origin. Border-zone ischemic lesions usually are found in a scattered pattern at the junction of the perfusion beds of the major cerebral arteries; these lesions extend from the cortical surface into deeper lobar white matter issue (**Figure 5.6**). Lacunar strokes usually are smaller than 0.5 cm in diameter and are oval in shape.

In interpreting a CT scan, the terms "hypoattenuation" and "hyperattenuation" are preferred to the terms "hypodensity" and "hyperdensity." Hypoattenuation and hyperattenuation mean a decrease or increase in x-ray attenuation compared with the normal attenuation of the brain. To assess such changes in x-ray attenuation, brain tissue or vascular structures should be compared with other portions of the same structure or with the contralateral counterparts (**Table 5.5**).

Hemorrhagic transformation of an infarction may be subtle because it consists of a mixture of hypoattenuating brain edema and blood. To which extent such

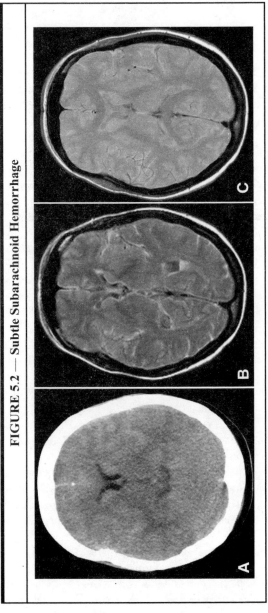

FIGURE 5.2 — Subtle Subarachnoid Hemorrhage

A. A computed tomography (CT) scan of a young woman with headache for 2 days showing hyperattenuating cerebrospinal fluid (CSF) within the frontal interhemispheric fissure and in the fourth ventricle (not shown).

B. On magnetic resonance imaging (MRI) in the same patient, using a fluid attenuated inversion recovery sequence (FLAIR), the CSF has an abnormal hyperintense signal in almost all brain fissures. Note the level between dark CSF and CSF intermixed with blood in both posterior horns of the lateral ventricles.

C. A similar phenomenon is observed on proton density weighted (PDw) MRI (same patient): The signal of CSF appears normal in the anterior horns of both lateral ventricles. It is higher in the brain fissures and posterior horns.

D. The T2w MRI (same patient) is relatively insensitive for blood within the CSF. Note the low signal in the posterior horns of the lateral ventricles with fluid level representing blood.

5

FIGURE 5.3 — Subdural Hematoma

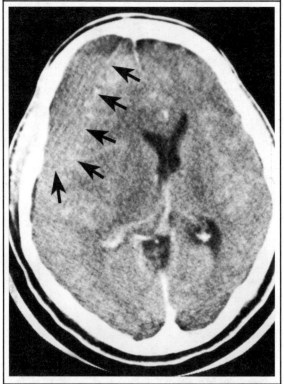

A computed tomography (CT) scan of a 54-year-old man admitted because of headache and mild hemiparesis. Severe mass effect with shift of midline structures from right to left is caused by a large right frontal subdural hematoma (arrows). Note that the density of the hematoma increases slightly from anterior to posterior because of the increasing concentration of red blood cells.

FIGURE 5.4 — Early Stages of Ischemic Infarction

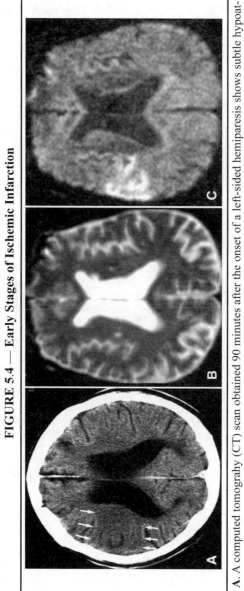

A. A computed tomography (CT) scan obtained 90 minutes after the onset of a left-sided hemiparesis shows subtle hypoattenuation of the right frontal cortex (arrows). **B.** The T2w sequence in the same patient appears normal 30 minutes later. **C.** The diffusion weighted imaging (DWI) shows hyperintensity (decreased proton diffusion) in the area indicated by CT that is more easily detected than hypoattenuation on CT.

FIGURE 5.5 — Large Middle Cerebral Artery Territory Infarction

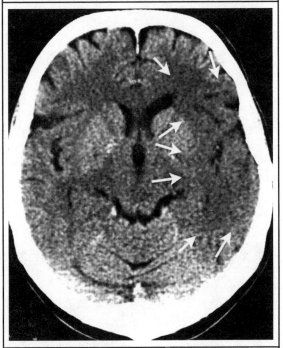

An unenhanced computed tomography (CT) scan of a 68-year-old woman obtained 180 minutes after the onset of aphasia and right hemiparesis. An area of parenchymal hypoattenuation (arrows) involves almost the entire territory of the left middle cerebral artery (MCA).

FIGURE 5.6 — Watershed Infarctions

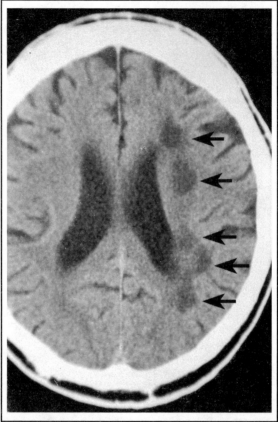

A computed tomography (CT) scan of a 73-year-old man with a known occlusion of the left internal carotid artery who had progressive increase in a right hemiparesis. The imaging study shows a chain of ischemic (border-zone/watershed) lesions (arrows) in the central white matter of the left hemisphere in the terminal area of supply of the left middle cerebral artery (MCA).

TABLE 5.5 — How to Interpret a CT Scan in a Patient With a Suspected Stroke

- Look for blood within the brain, ventricle, subarachnoid space, or subdural or epidural spaces
- If blood is visible, assess the location and check for abnormal vessels, venous sinuses, mass effect, or blockage of cerebrospinal fluid pathways
- If blood is visible, do a contrast-enhanced scan to look for aneurysm, tumor, or vascular malformation
- If blood is in the subarachnoid space, do CTA or arteriography to screen for an aneurysm
- If blood is absent, ischemia is the probable cause of the patient's symptoms
- Look for patterns of old, well-demarcated ischemic lesions
- Look for vascular pathology such as calcification, dilation, or elongation of vessels
- Look for segmental hyperattenuation of arteries (dense artery or dot sign)
- Look for subtle territorial hypoattenuation of the cortical gray matter or basal ganglia
- Look for compression of the effacement of sulci on the cerebral cortex
- Look for mass effect and assess the extent of the hypoattenuated volume
- If the hypoattenuated territory appears unusual or is bilateral, assess for venous thrombosis

Abbreviations: CT, computed tomography; CTA, computed tomographic angiography.

hemorrhages may cause clinical symptoms in addition to ischemic neurologic dysfunction is unclear. It appears that only hemorrhagic transformation associated with space-occupying effect or intraventricular or subarachnoid extension may independently cause clinical deterioration.[16,17] Magnetic resonance imaging (MRI), particularly gradient echo studies, is more sensitive than CT in detecting hemorrhagic transformation.

When parenchymal hemorrhage (clot with space-occupying effect) usually is easy to detect, small hemorrhages or blood in the subarachnoid space may be missed if the scan is not examined carefully. Localization of the blood provides clues to the cause of hemorrhage.[3] A hematoma in the basal ganglia, thalamus, internal capsule, brain stem, or cerebellum typically is hypertensive in origin. Blood adjacent to the brain's surface is suspicious for a vascular malformation or, in an elderly person, for cerebral amyloid angiopathy. In the latter situation, the hemorrhages often are located in the frontal and occipital poles or are multiple. Hemorrhages secondary to trauma are most commonly located at the tips of the temporal, frontal, or occipital lobes. Hemorrhages secondary to anticoagulants or thrombolytic agents often are inhomogeneous with fluid levels. Old ischemic lesions that reflect risk factors such as hypertension sometimes accompany parenchymal hematomas. Acutely, hemorrhages usually show hyperattenuation without surrounding edema. The presence of abundant edema may represent an underlying primary or metastatic brain tumor. A hemorrhage embedded within a hypoattenuated area covering an arterial territory also may be secondary to transformation of an ischemic lesion. The finding, particularly when it is bilaterally located in parasagittal areas, is suspicious for sagittal sinus thrombosis. Multiple hemorrhagic lesions may be seen with bleeding diatheses or metastatic disease.

Sequential CT studies may show enlargement of the hematoma, which is correlated with neurologic worsening and poorer outcomes.[18,19] The size of the hematoma also affects prognosis; a large (>2.5-cm) hematoma in the cerebellum or deep in the cerebral hemisphere may pose a life-threatening lesion. Intraparenchymal hemorrhages also may disrupt the ependyma and lead to intraventricular bleeding; the presence of intraventricular hemorrhage predicts a less-

5

favorable prognosis. Intraventricular hemorrhage also is found among patients with SAH. Isolated intraventricular bleeding may be secondary to an arteriovenous malformation. Blood restricted to the subarachnoid space is the hallmark of SAH.[10] The most common causes are:

- Ruptured saccular (berry) aneurysm
- Ruptured nonsaccular aneurysm
- Ruptured cerebral vein
- Trauma.

If the subarachnoid blood is at its most dense in the basal cisterns, an aneurysm is the most probable cause. The location of the blood in the subarachnoid space gives a hint as to the site of the ruptured aneurysm. The amount of subarachnoid blood is also predictive of the development of vasospasm and brain ischemia.[20]

Magnetic Resonance Imaging

MRI has a great potential to provide information in the setting of acute stroke.[21-27] Besides imaging of the brain, MRI also provides information about the CSF spaces and intracranial vessels. MRI is able to detect the following:

- Proton diffusion through brain tissue
- Pathology (edema, necrosis, hemorrhage) of brain tissue
- Brain perfusion
- Flow velocity
- Spectra of brain metabolites
- Functionally activated brain areas.

The limitations of MRI are described in Chapter 4, *Diagnosis and Evaluation of Patients With Suspected Stroke*. Patients who are acutely ill and need supportive care, who are unable to cooperate, or who need continuous observation may not be able to tolerate

MRI.[28,29] In addition, MRI was thought to be inferior to CT in detection of brain hemorrhage, particularly SAH. This concern reduced the use of MRI in patients with acute stroke. However, with modern sequences and technology, MRI has been shown to be highly sensitive and specific for detection of intracranial bleeding.[30-34] These data suggest that MRI could be substituted for CT in the emergency evaluation of patients with suspected stroke. A multimodal MRI program could be used to assess the brain and vasculature in patients with acute stroke.[35,36] Some physicians and researchers are using the findings of MRI to select patients to treat with thrombolytic agents.[23,37,38]

MRI measures the resonance of protons that are manipulated by magnetic-field strengths representing brain tissue contrasts. Diffusion-weighted imaging (DWI), perfusion imaging (PI), and magnetic resonance spectroscopy (MRS) require advanced technology with high (>1 Tesla) field-strength and strong and quick magnetic gradients. Shrinking of the extracellular fluid space after ischemia (20–30 mL/100 g × min) is associated with disturbed diffusion in the affected area. Such disturbance of diffusion may normalize spontaneously or after treatment with thrombolytic agents.[39,40] Scanners using a high-field strength can detect changes in DWI almost immediately after an arterial occlusion. DWI may detect abnormalities in patients with a transient ischemic attack (TIA); the finding suggests an area of brain injury.[41] The sequences may be performed within a few seconds to minutes. Thus DWI may be used to detect the early changes of ischemic brain edema and to differentiate these areas from normal tissue or old ischemic tissue (**Figure 5.7**). Like hypoattenuation on CT, diminished proton diffusion on MRI, if detected >2 hours after the onset of stroke, means, in most cases, that the brain tissue is irreversibly damaged. Thus DWI sequences are well suited for early detection of ischemic brain lesions and the exclusion

FIGURE 5.7 — Old and Acute Ischemic Lesions

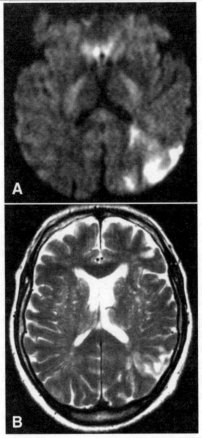

A. Diffusion weighted imaging (DWI) in a patient with severe stenosis of the right extracranial internal carotid artery (ICA) and slight right-sided hemiparesis shows hyperintensity within the border area and between the territories of left middle cerebral artery (MCA) and posterior cerebral artery (PCA). **B**. The T2w image in the same patient shows, in addition to the acute left border-zone infarct, multiple small ischemic lesions in both basal ganglia, indicating small-vessel disease.

of other possible brain illnesses in seriously ill patients. Differences in the size of the lesions seen on DWI and perfusion sequences (mismatch) may correspond to the ischemic penumbra, tissue that is ischemic but might be salvageable with early intervention.[42]

Conventional spin-echo sequences show relatively low sensitivity in finding ischemic lesions early in persons with suspected acute stroke (**Figure 5.4**). As with CT, brain perfusion may be imaged after injection of a contrast agent, and local contrast kinetics may be calculated.[30,43] Parameter images, representing the period from contrast entry to the concentration peak, seem to be robust (**Figure 9.2**). Quantification faces similar problems since other methods based on tracer kinetics and these techniques are regarded as experimental. Functional MRI and MRS also are considered to be experimental in the setting of acute stroke. While MRI is an important imaging adjunct for evaluation of some patients with hemorrhagic stroke, it usually is reserved for atypical or problematic cases in which the location or the nature of the brain lesion is critical for decisions in emergency management. Gradient-echo sequences on MRI may help detect small areas of prior bleeding (microhemorrhages) that may influence acute management, including the administration of thrombolytic agents, but the relationship between the presence of microhemorrhages and the subsequent risk of major bleeding is not known.[44,45]

Guidelines for performing and interpreting MRI in a patient with acute stroke are outlined in **Table 5.6** and **Table 5.7**. First, proton DWI would be performed as a quick screening technique. If a high-quality DWI study cannot be obtained, a FLAIR or a proton–density weighted sequence is an alternative; these studies show brain tissue edema with high sensitivity. A gradient-echo or T2-weighted sequence may be used to exclude hemorrhage. The usual T2- and T1-weighted sequences may provide good tissue contrast and high resolution

TABLE 5.6 — Recommendations for Use of Magnetic Resonance Imaging in Patients With Suspected Stroke

- Choose a high-field (>1 Tesla) scanner if possible
- Organize professional personnel for close observation of the patient and to maintain life-support during the test
- Use fast spin-echo and gradient-echo techniques if the patient cannot cooperate
- Obtain proton diffusion weighted imaging
- Obtain proton density-, T1-, and T2-weighted images without contrast
- Obtain additional sagittal plane scans to image the brain stem
- Use FLAIR sequence to detect tissue edema and blood products in the CSF
- Use gradient-echo sequence to detect areas of hemorrhage within the brain
- Continue with MRA to examine for the underlying vascular lesion
- If necessary, perform a contrast-enhanced, T1-weighted study

Abbreviations: CSF, cerebrospinal fluid; FLAIR, fluid attenuated inversion recovery; MRA, magnetic resonance angiography.

of cerebral structures. Ischemic lesions present as areas with abnormal high signal on proton-density and T2-weighted images and associated low signal on T1-weighted images. The T1-weighted image may be normal if the ischemia has affected the myelin of neural axons without associated tissue necrosis. As with CT, a normal tissue signal on MRI may be consistent with brain ischemia above the level that leads to structural changes.

Arteries and veins normally appear black (flow void) on spin-echo sequences on MRI. The course of the arteries branching from the circle of Willis, the internal carotid arteries curving through the base of

**TABLE 5.7 — Guide to Interpretation of
Magnetic Resonance Imaging Studies
in Patients With Suspected Stroke**

- Understand the MRI technique responsible for the tissue contrast
- Identify the brain tissue lesions with abnormal signal
- Decide whether the lesion is caused by ischemia or other pathology
- Differentiate old vs new ischemic lesions
- Consider whether a lesion may be secondary to another lesion (Wallerian degeneration)
- Screen for the appearance of the normal black signal (flow void) in the cranial arteries and veins
- Look for abnormal vessels
- Screen the CSF signal within the ventricles, cisterns, and sulci on all available scans
- Look for subtle cortical swelling, especially on PD-weighted images
- Assess the stage of any blood products seen
- Assess for mass effects or any secondary brain stem lesions

Abbreviations: CSF, cerebrospinal fluid; MRI, magnetic resonance imaging; PD, proton density.

the skull and the cavernous sinus, and the vertebral arteries at the level of the foramen magnum may be assessed. A careful assessment of the lower MRI sections is important to identify the flow voids in both internal carotid arteries. The internal carotid artery at the base of the skull is the most common site for an arterial dissection. A semilunar-shaped hyperintense segment with a peripheral dark flow void is diagnostic of an arterial dissection (**Figure 5.8**). A segmental increase in a vessel's signal indicates either slow or absent flow, which may be secondary to a thromboembolic occlusion (**Figure 5.9**). Because the fresh intraluminal thrombus has a low signal on MRI, it may not be distinguishable from slow-flowing blood on spin-echo sequences. Therefore, vascular imaging often

FIGURE 5.8 — Carotid Dissections

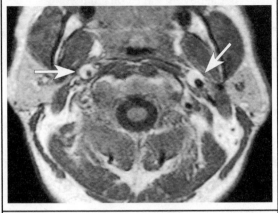

A magnetic resonance imaging (MRI) study in a 48-year-old man shows dissections of both internal carotid arteries *(arrows)*.

is required in patients with presumed acute arterial or venous obstruction.

Acute intraparenchymal hemorrhage appears isodense on T1-weighted images and hyperintense on T2-weighted images[46] (**Figure 5.10**). A hematoma needs to be differentiated from a brain tumor. The MRI signals of a parenchymal hemorrhage change over time due to different magnetization properties of the predominant blood degradation products (**Table 5.8**). The MRI is well suited to assess the age of a hematoma (**Figure 5.11**). Blood within brain tumors of the CSF does not always follow the stages outlined in **Table 5.8** because of other factors affecting the time course of blood deoxygenation and degradation in these situations.

FIGURE 5.9 — Occlusion of Middle Cerebral Artery Trunk

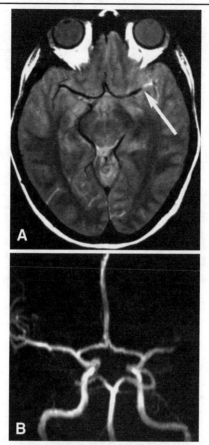

A. Proton density weighted (PDw) magnetic resonance imaging (MRI) in a 37-year-old woman 4 hours after onset of right-sided hemiparesis and aphasia. The image shows the lack of signal void due to flow in the left middle cerebral artery (MCA) trunk (arrow). **B**. The arterial obstruction is as well depicted by time-of-flight magnetic resonance angiography (MRA).

FIGURE 5.10 — Acute Hemorrhage Into the Precentral Gyrus

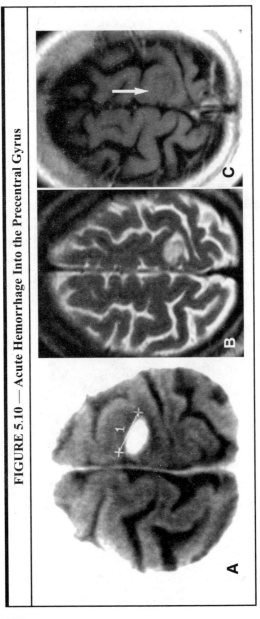

A. A computed tomography (CT) scan of a 54-year-old physician, who realized a weakness in his right leg 8 hours before, shows a small bleeding into the parasagittal portion of his left precentral gyrus. Digital subtraction angiography (DSA) later excluded an arteriovenous malformation. **B**. The T2w magnetic resonance imaging (MRI) was obtained soon after the CT scan to check for abnormal vessels and venous obstructions. It shows the hematoma with hyperintense signal. **C**. The T2w MRI after injection of contrast shows isointensity of the hematoma *(arrow)*.

5

TABLE 5.8 — Magnetic Resonance Imaging Signals of Blood Degradation Products		
Time After Hemorrhage	Blood Product	T1 Signal	T2 Signal
4–6 hours	Oxyhemoglobin	Isointense	Hyperintense
1–3 days	Deoxyhemoglobin	Isointense	Hyper-/hypointense
4–7 days	Methemoglobin (intracellular)	Hyperintense	Hypointense
1–4 weeks	Methemoglobin (extracellular)	Hyperintense	Hyperintense
>4 weeks	Hemosiderin	Hypointense	Hypointense

FIGURE 5.11 — Bilateral Subacute Cerebral Hematomas

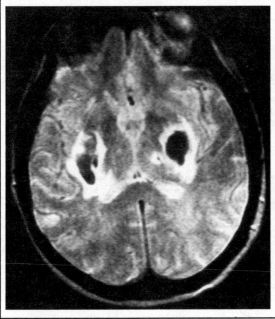

A T2-weighted magnetic resonance imaging (MRI) study in a 73-year-old man with bilateral thalamic hemorrhage that had occurred 3 days earlier. The low signal in the center of the hemorrhage represents deoxyhemoglobin. The surrounding high signal represents brain tissue edema. The image proves that the hemorrhage occurred in both thalamic nuclei.

Vascular Imaging

Whereas brain imaging provides information about the downstream sequelae and location of ischemia and bleeding and the chance for tissue for functional recovery, vascular imaging provides information about the upstream cause of ischemic or hemorrhagic stroke. In addition, the results of vascular imaging will guide choices for secondary prophylaxis. The initial unenhanced CT or MRI already may provide important information about the cranial arteries and veins, such as an intraluminal thrombus or mural hematoma (**Table 5.9**).

Carotid Duplex and Transcranial Doppler Ultrasonography Studies

Duplex scanning and transcranial Doppler (TCD) ultrasonography are noninvasive tests that in experienced hands, may reliably screen both extracranial and intracranial arteries.[47] Carotid duplex scanning is

---

TABLE 5.9 — Sequence of Vascular Imaging Tests: Patients With Acute Stroke

- Imaging of the brain should be performed first (CT or MRI)
- Consider vascular imaging if:
  - Results would alter acute management
  - Patient has unexplained symptoms suggesting brain stem dysfunction
  - Patient may need an acute intra-arterial intervention
  - Patient has SAH or unexplained intraparenchymal hemorrhage
- Consider the following sequence:
  - If available, do CTA after CT
  - If MRI is performed, do MRA
  - If available, consider carotid duplex or TCD
  - DSA may be done if other tests are unavailable
  - DSA may be done if other tests are inconclusive
  - DSA may be done in conjunction with an intra-arterial intervention

Abbreviations: CT, computed tomography; CTA, computed tomographic angiography; DSA, digital subtraction angiography; MRA, magnetic resonance angiography; MRI, magnetic resonance imaging; SAH, subarachnoid hemorrhage; TCD, transcranial Doppler ultrasonography.

---

relatively inexpensive and widely available. It is used to assess the origin of the internal carotid artery in the neck. It generally is a preliminary diagnostic step in the assessment of a patient with an ischemic stroke or TIA who might be a candidate for either carotid endarterectomy (CEA) or carotid angioplasty and stenting.[47,48] The absence of a severe narrowing generally eliminates consideration of a CEA. However, duplex scanning may be vulnerable to errors in technique. The degree of narrowing may be either over- or underestimated. A carotid duplex study may not differentiate a very high-grade stenosis from an occlusion (**Figure 5.12**). If uncertainties persist about the severity of narrowing, the results of the carotid duplex study may be complemented by MRA or digital subtraction arteriography. In many locations, the decision for CEA now is based on the results of carotid duplex alone or in combination with MRA.

TCD examines the major intracranial arteries at the base of the brain.[47] Its most widely accepted indication is for the sequential assessment of patients with recent SAH to screen for vasospasm before signs of cerebral ischemia appear.[49] Changes in flow velocity may appear up to 24 hours before the neurologic signs. TCD is being used to screen for arterial occlusions and to monitor response to thrombolytic therapy, including recanalization.[50-52] Still, the role of TCD as part of the emergency assessment of patients with ischemic stroke has not been established. TCD also has been used to monitor for embolization during carotid operations and as a measure of risk of embolization in patients with cardiac lesions. TCD has limitations; for example, the skull of approximately 15% of patients may not permit adequate ultrasound imaging. The use of echo-contrast substances may improve the detection of flow in clinically relevant arteries from 70% to 90%.[53]

FIGURE 5.12 — Duplex Ultrasound of Right Internal Carotid Artery Stenosis

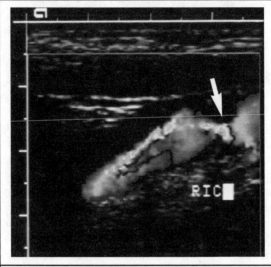

Tight stenosis of right internal carotid artery (arrow) just distal to the carotid bifurcation.

Courtesy of Dr. Georg Gahn, Dept of Neurology, University of Technology, Dresden, Germany.

Magnetic Resonance Angiography and Venography

Magnetic resonance angiography (MRA) and venography (MRV) using time-of-flight (TOF) or phase contrast (PC) sequences may be used to screen large intracranial and extracranial arteries and veins. After injection of a contrast bolus, the brain-supplying vessels are imaged from the arch of the aorta to the circle of Willis within 10 seconds. These contrast-enhanced images are independent of flow velocity and turbulence in comparison to TOF and PC techniques and thus reflect vascular morphology and pathology more reliably that the other methods. MRA may be performed in conjunction with conventional MRI brain imaging. MRA is rapidly becoming the method of choice for a quick overview of the major arteries in the neck and brain.[54-56] It is used to search for arterial occlusions, aneurysms, and vascular malformations (**Figure 5.13**). MRA may overestimate the degree of arterial narrowing in patients with stenosis and it may miss smaller aneurysms. MRV greatly expedites the evaluation of patients with suspected venous thrombosis.[57,58]

Computed Tomographic Angiography

CTA requires spiral CT techniques and a bolus injection of a contrast agent.[59] Thus persons with allergic reactions to iodine or renal dysfunction usually cannot be studied with CTA. Using the spiral technique, patients may be imaged immediately after a conventional CT scan. The interval from the time of the injection of the bolus of contrast to the scanning determines whether cranial arteries or veins are imaged. CTA appears to be reliable in visualizing:

- Obstruction of major intracranial arteries
- Intracranial saccular aneurysms
- Arteriovenous malformations
- Obstruction of cortical veins or venous sinuses.

CTA is an excellent way to determine whether the occlusion of a major artery is the cause of stroke, differentiating between basilar and middle cerebral artery occlusion, and assessing whether spontaneous recanalization has occurred (**Figure 5.14**). If SAH is demonstrated by CT, CTA may be used to screen for an intracranial aneurysm.[60,61] CTA can reconstruct a 3-dimensional image of the aneurysm, its neck, and its relationship to adjacent intracranial arteries. If CTA does not demonstrate an aneurysm, digital subtraction angiography (DSA) should be performed. CTA also can

FIGURE 5.13 — Magnetic Resonance Angiography in
Venous Sinus Thrombosis Before and After Treatment With Heparin

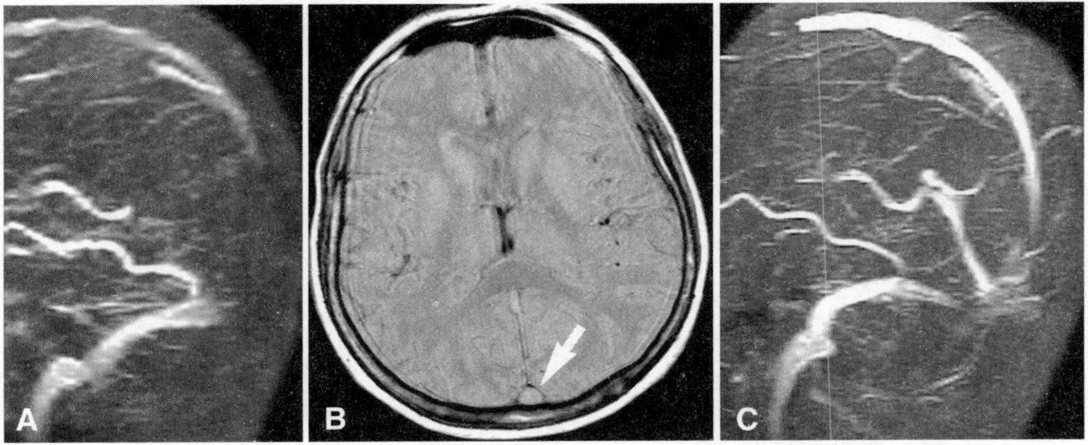

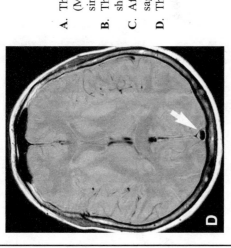

A. Three-dimensional phase contrast (PC) magnetic resonance angiography (MRA) shows obstruction of the posterior third of the superior sagittal sinus and the sinus rectus.

B. The proton-density weighted (PDw) image of the same MRA directly shows the thrombus within the superior sagittal sinus.

C. After 10 days of full anticoagulation with intravenous heparin, the superior sagittal sinus and the sinus rectus are recanalized.

D. The PDw image proves that the thrombus has disappeared.

FIGURE 5.14 — Computed Tomographic Angiography of a Carotid Artery Occlusion

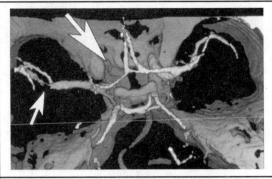

The 3-dimensional reconstruction of computed tomographic angiography (CTA) (viewed from above) shows occlusion of the left internal carotid artery (large arrow) and a stenosis of the distal middle cerebral artery (MCA) trunk (small arrow) in a 42-year-old man with aphasia and paresis of the right upper extremity. A subsequent arteriogram confirmed dissection of the left internal carotid artery with distal occlusion but an open distal MCA.

be used to screen for the presence of occlusive disease of the internal carotid artery.[62]

Digital Subtraction Angiography

DSA is the conventional method for evaluating the extracranial and intracranial vasculature. It is available in many medical institutions and has replaced conventional arteriography.[63-65] DSA now is used for regular diagnostic studies or as part of neurointerventional procedures. DSA may be used in one or two planes and with rotational angiography, which requires a workstation for 3-D reconstructions (**Figure 5.15**). The first obtained image from the test is electronically subtracted from all subsequent images; a procedure that results in views of the vascular tree alone because the

FIGURE 5.15 — 3-D Reconstruction of Rotational Digital Subtraction Angiography in a Patient With Basilar Aneurysm

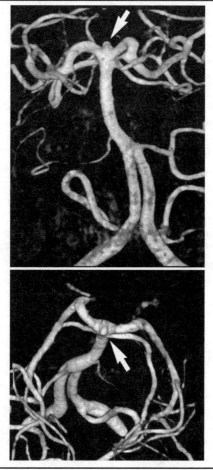

Two views of a rotational digital subtraction angiography (DSA) after 3-D reconstruction. Note the small aneurysm at the tip of the basilar artery *(arrows)*.

skull and soft tissues are subtracted. DSA requires the following steps:

- Arterial puncture and insertion of an intra-arterial catheter by a physician with specialized training
- An intra-arterial injection of a contrast agent
- Good cooperation from the patient to avoid motion-induced artifacts
- General anesthesia in uncooperative patients.

An advantage of DSA is that only small amounts of contrast at low iodine concentrations are required to examine all cranial vessels. In contrast to CTA and MRA, it provides hemodynamic information by following the contrast bolus through the arterial tree. Because conventional arteriography and DSA are invasive procedures, they may be accompanied by serious complications, including stroke. The likelihood of major morbidity or mortality is approximately 0.5% to 1%.[66] The risk of DSA is not increased in the setting of acute stroke.

Despite being invasive and expensive, DSA should be considered the most reliable method for examining the intracranial and extracranial vasculature. It remains the standard with which other vascular imaging procedures are compared. DSA remains the preferred test for evaluation of the source of intracranial bleeding. An underlying vascular malformation, aneurysm, or vasculitis may be demonstrated best by DSA.[3] Usually the procedure is performed when the patient's condition is stabilized. Because early clipping or endovascular treatment often is recommended for patients with ruptured aneurysms, DSA is performed as a surgical procedure for persons with SAH. If a transarterial occlusion of the aneurysm is possible, the intervention may be performed immediately after the diagnostic DSA, thus avoiding a second procedure. If an aneurysm is not visualized by DSA, a second procedure usually is done approximately 10 days after the first study because an aneurysm may be obscured in the first days after SAH (**Figure 8.1**). Patients with a perimesencephalic pattern of SAH on CT have a more benign illness that is not due to a ruptured aneurysm; a single DSA usually is adequate in this situation.

While several other vascular imaging tests help in screening for a vascular malformation in a patient with an intraparenchymal hemorrhage, DSA usually is required to judge the operability of the vascular lesion. These tests often are recommended when a CT scan demonstrates an intraparenchymal hematoma. Generally, DSA is not performed when a hematoma is found deep in the brain in a patient with chronic hypertension. On the other hand, DSA is recommended when a lobar hemorrhage is found.[67]

DSA also is a key component of intra-arterial interventions used to treat cerebrovascular disease including:

- Administration of thrombolytic agents
- Mechanical thrombolysis
- Angioplasty and placement of stents
- Balloon occlusion of a parent artery
- Placement of coils in an aneurysm
- Injection of occlusive materials into the nidus of a vascular malformation
- Injection of particles into brain tumors.

Because it does involve some risks, DSA should be recommended only when the results are likely to answer clinically relevant questions or to influence decisions about management that cannot be addressed satisfactorily by less-invasive vascular imaging methods. **Table 5.9** outlines the criteria that suggest when vascular imaging may be helpful. Because these tests are relatively time-consuming and expensive, they should be performed after the brain imaging study (CT or MRI) and only if clinically useful conclusions may be drawn from the results of the studies. Imaging the arteries may be very important in a person with an ischemic stroke syndrome and a normal brain imaging test. The site of the arterial occlusion and the capacity of collaterals to maintain perfusion may be assessed; this information may help predict the extent and severity of brain ischemia. The location of the arterial occlusion indicates which vascular territory is jeopardized. In addition, the location of the arterial occlusion and the presence of collateral channels may influence prognosis and decisions about acute treatment (**Table 5.10**). This information may influence decisions about interventions to restore perfusion to the brain.

Perfusion Imaging

Following the same principles, PI is feasible with CT and MRI after injection of contrast bolus. MRI is superior to CT in that it is less invasive and covers the whole brain. Current CT technology can display up to four brain sections. PI directly shows areas of the brain that have disturbed perfusion. Exact quantification of cerebral blood flow (CBF), cerebral blood volume (CBV), and mean transient time (MTT) is problematic because the arterial input function of the voxel under study cannot be determined. Nevertheless, a localized area with prolonged MTT and decreased CBF may indicate an increased risk for ischemic necrosis. Increases in CBV signal compensatory arterial dilatation, whereas decreases in CBV point to exhaustion of the cerebral perfusion reserve and high risk of irreversible injury. The impact of PI on predicting outcomes after stroke and on the decision for acute treatment has not been established.

TABLE 5.10 — System for Stratification of Patients With Acute Stroke: Initial Site of Occlusion and Collateral Flow

Grade	Site of Occlusion/Collaterals
0	No occlusion
1	M-3 segment of middle cerebral artery A-2; segment of anterior cerebral artery or distal single basilar or vertebral artery branch
2	M-2 segment of middle cerebral artery A-1 or A-2 segments of anterior cerebral artery 2 or branches of basilar or vertebral artery
3	Proximal (M-1) segment of middle cerebral artery
A	Lenticulostriate arteries spared or leptomeningeal collateral vessels visualized
B	No sparing of lenticulostriate arteries and no leptomeningeal vessels visualized
4	Internal carotid artery with collaterals; basilar artery (partial filling or collaterals)
A	Collaterals fill the middle cerebral artery or antegrade filling of the basilar artery
B	Collaterals fill the anterior cerebral artery but not the middle cerebral artery; retrograde filling of the basilar artery
5	Internal carotid artery with no collaterals; basilar artery with no collaterals
Adapted from: Qureshi AI. *Lancet*. 2004;363:804-813.	

5

REFERENCES

1. Adams HP Jr, Adams RJ, Brott T, et al. Guidelines for the early management of patients with ischemic stroke. A scientific statement from the Stroke Council of the American Stroke Association. *Stroke.* 2003;34:1056-1083.

2. Adams H, Adams R, del Zoppo G, Goldstein LB; Stroke Council of the American Heart Association; American Stroke Association. Guidelines for the early management of patients with ischemic stroke: 2005 guidelines update: a scientific statement from the Stroke Council of the American Heart Association/American Stroke Association. *Stroke.* 2005;36:916-923.

3. Culebras A, Kase CS, Masdeu JC, et al. Practice guidelines for the use of imaging in transient ischemic attacks and acute stroke. A report of the Stroke Council, American Heart Association. *Stroke.* 1997;28:1480-1497.

4. Marler J R, Jones PW, Emr M. Proceedings of a national symposium on rapid identification and treatment of acute stroke. 1997.

5. Kidwell CS, Villablanca JP, Saver JL. Advances in neuroimaging of acute stroke. *Curr Atheroscler Rep.* 2000;2:126-135.

6. Mayer SA, Brun NC, Broderick J, et al; Europe/AustralAsia NovoSeven ICH Trial Investigators. Safety and feasibility of recombinant factor VIIa for acute intracerebral hemorrhage. *Stroke.* 2005;36:74-79.

7. Mayer SA, Brun NC, Begtrup K, et al; Recombinant Activated Factor VII Intracerebral Hemorrhage Trial Investigators. Recombinant activated factor VII for acute intracerebral hemorrhage. *N Engl J Med.* 2005;352:777-785.

8. Na DG, Kim EY, Ryoo JW, et al. CT sign of brain swelling without concomitant parenchymal hypoattenuation: comparison with diffusion- and perfusion-weighted MR imaging. *Radiology.* 2005;235:992-948.

9. Kirchhof K, Welzel T, Mecke C, Zoubaa S, Sartor K. Differentiation of white, mixed, and red thrombi: value of CT in estimation of the prognosis of thrombolysis phantom study. *Radiology.* 2003;228:126-130.

10. Vermeulen M, van Gijn J. The diagnosis of subarachnoid hemorrhage. *J Neurol Neurosurg Psychiatry.* 1990;53:365-372.

11. Schievink WI. Intracranial aneurysms. *N Engl J Med.* 1997;336:25-40.

12. Adams HP Jr, Kassell NF, Torner JC, Sahs AL. CT and clinical correlations in recent aneurysmal subarachnoid hemorrhage: a preliminary report of the Cooperative Aneurysm Study. *Neurology.* 1983;33:981-988.

13. von Kummer R, Allen KL, Holle R, et al. Acute stroke: usefulness of early CT findings before thrombolytic therapy. *Radiology.* 1997;205: 327-333.

14. von Kummer R, Bozzao L, Zeumer H, Manelfe C. *Early CT Diagnosis of Hemispheric Brain Infarction.* Heidelberg: Springer Verlag; 1995.

15. Barber PA, Demchuk AM, Zhang J, et al. Computed tomographic parameters predicting fatal outcome in large middle cerebral artery infarction. *Cerebrovasc Dis.* 2003;16:230-235.

16. Fiorelli M, Bastianello S, von Kummer R, et al. Hemorrhagic transformation within 36 hours of a cerebral infarct: relationships with early clinical deterioration and 3-month outcome in the European Cooperative Acute Stroke Study I (ECASS I) cohort. *Stroke.* 1999;30:2280-2284.

17. Berger C, Fiorelli M, Steiner T, et al. Hemorrhagic transformation of ischemic brain tissue: asymptomatic or symptomatic? *Stroke.* 2001;32:1330-1335.

18. Broderick JP, Brott TG, Tomsick T, Barsan W, Spilker J. Ultra-early evaluation of intracerebral hemorrhage. *J Neurosurg*. 1990;72:195-199.

19. Brott T, Broderick J, Kothari R, et al. Early hemorrhage growth in patients with intracerebral hemorrhage. *Stroke*. 1997;28:1-5.

20. Adams HP Jr, Kassell NF, Torner JC. Usefulness of computed tomography in predicting outcome after aneurysmal subarachnoid hemorrhage: a preliminary report of the Cooperative Aneurysm Study. *Neurology*. 1985;35:1263-1267.

21. Baird AE, Warach S. Magnetic resonance imaging of acute stroke. *J Cereb Blood Flow Metab*. 1998;18:583-609.

22. Warach S. Stroke neuroimaging. *Stroke*. 2003;34:345-347.

23. Warach S. Thrombolysis in stroke beyond three hours: targeting patients with diffusion and perfusion MRI. *Ann Neurol*. 2002;51:11-13.

24. Mullins ME, Schaefer PW, Sorensen AG, et al. CT and conventional diffusion-weighted MR imaging in acute stroke: study in 691 patients at presentation to the emergency department. *Radiology*. 2002;224:353-360.

25. Fiebach JB, Schellinger PD. Comparison of CT with diffusion-weighted MRI in patients with hyperacute stroke. *Neuroradiology*. 2002;44:448.

26. Fiebach JB, Schellinger PD, Gass A, et al; Kompetenznetzwerk Schlaganfall B5. Stroke magnetic resonance imaging is accurate in hyperacute intracerebral hemorrhage: a multicenter study on the validity of stroke imaging. *Stroke*. 2004;35:502-506.

27. Molina CA, Saver JL. Extending reperfusion therapy for acute ischemic stroke: emerging pharmacological, mechanical, and imaging strategies. *Stroke*. 2005;36:2311-2320.

28. Barber PA, Hill MD, Eliasziw M, et al; ASPECTS Study Group. Imaging of the brain in acute ischaemic stroke: comparison of computed tomography and magnetic resonance diffusion-weighted imaging. *J Neurol Neurosurg Psychiatry*. 2005;76:1528-1533.

29. Hand PJ, Wardlaw JM, Rowat AM, Haisma JA, Lindley RI, Dennis MS. Magnetic resonance brain imaging in patients with acute stroke: feasibility and patient related difficulties. *J Neurol Neurosurg Psychiatry*. 2005;76:1525-1527.

30. Kidwell CS, Chalela JA, Saver JL, et al. Comparison of MRI and CT for detection of acute intracerebral hemorrhage. *JAMA*. 2004;292:1823-1830.

31. Schellinger PD, Fiebach JB, Hoffmann K, et al. Stroke MRI in intracerebral hemorrhage: is there a perihemorrhagic penumbra? *Stroke*. 2003;34:1674-1679.

32. Wiesmann M, Mayer TE, Yousry I, Medele R, Hamann GF, Bruckmann H. Detection of hyperacute subarachnoid hemorrhage of the brain by using magnetic resonance imaging. *J Neurosurg*. 2002;96:684-689.

33. Linfante I, Llinas RH, Caplan LR, Warach S. MRI features of intracerebral hemorrhage within 2 hours from symptom onset. *Stroke*. 1999;30:2263-2267.

34. Mitchell P, Wilkinson ID, Hoggard N, et al. Detection of subarachnoid haemorrhage with magnetic resonance imaging. *J Neurol Neurosurg Psychiatry*. 2001;70:205-211.

35. Kidwell CS, Alger JR, Saver JL. Beyond mismatch: evolving paradigms in imaging the ischemic penumbra with multimodal magnetic resonance imaging. *Stroke*. 2003;34:2729-2735.

36. Kidwell CS, Alger JR, Saver JL. Evolving paradigms in neuroimaging of the ischemic penumbra. *Stroke*. 2004;35(suppl 1):2662-2665.

37. Hacke W, Albers G, Al-Rawi Y, et al; DIAS Study Group. The Desmoteplase in Acute Ischemic Stroke Trial (DIAS): a phase II MRI-based 9-hour window acute stroke thrombolysis trial with intravenous desmoteplase. *Stroke*. 2005;36:66-73.

38. Hjort N, Butcher K, Davis SM, et al; UCLA Thrombolysis Investigators. Magnetic resonance imaging criteria for thrombolysis in acute cerebral infarct. *Stroke*. 2005;36:388-397.

39. Kidwell CS, Alger JR, Di Salle F, et al. Diffusion MRI in patients with transient ischemic attacks. *Stroke*. 1999;30:1174-1180.

40. Kidwell CS, Saver JL, Mattiello J, et al. Thrombolytic reversal of acute human cerebral ischemic injury shown by diffusion/perfusion magnetic resonance imaging. *Ann Neurol*. 2000;47:462-469.

41. Inatomi Y, Kimura K, Yonehara T, Fujioka S, Uchino M. Hyperacute diffusion-weighted imaging abnormalities in transient ischemic attack patients signify irreversible ischemic infarction. *Cerebrovasc Dis*. 2005;19:362-368.

42. Prosser J, Butcher K, Allport L, et al. Clinical-diffusion mismatch predicts the putative penumbra with high specificity. *Stroke*. 2005;36:1700-1704.

43. Koenig M, Klotz E, Luka B, Venderink DJ, Spittler JF, Heuser L. Perfusion CT of the brain: diagnostic approach for early detection of ischemic stroke. *Radiology*. 1998;209:85-93.

44. Kidwell CS, Saver JL, Villablanca JP, et al. Magnetic resonance imaging detection of microbleeds before thrombolysis: an emerging application. *Stroke*. 2002;33:95-98.

45. Kakuda W, Thijs VN, Lansberg MG, et al; DEFUSE Investigators. Clinical importance of microbleeds in patients receiving IV thrombolysis. *Neurology*. 2005;65:1175-1178.

46. Bradley WG Jr. MR appearance of hemorrhage in the brain. *Radiology*. 1993;189:15-26.

47. Alexandrov AV. Imaging cerebrovascular diseases with ultrasound. *Cerebrovasc Dis*. 2003;16:1-3.

48. Moneta GL, Edwards JM, Chitwood RW, et al. Correlation of North American Symptomatic Carotid Endarterectomy Trial (NASCET) angiographic definition of 70% to 99% internal carotid artery stenosis with duplex scanning. *J Vasc Surg*. 1993;17:152-157.

49. Sloan MA, Haley EC Jr, Kassell NF, et al. Sensitivity and specificity of transcranial Doppler ultrasonography in the diagnosis of vasospasm following subarachnoid hemorrhage. *Neurology*. 1989;39:1514-1518.

50. Alexandrov AV, Demchuk AM, Felberg RA, et al. High rate of complete recanalization and dramatic clinical recovery during tPA infusion when continuously monitored with 2-MHz transcranial Doppler monitoring. *Stroke*. 2000;31:610-614.

51. Alexandrov AV, Grotta JC. Arterial reocclusion in stroke patients treated with intravenous tissue plasminogen activator. *Neurology*. 2002;59:862-867.

52. Gahn G, von Kummer R. Ultrasound in acute stroke: a review. *Neuroradiology*. 2001;43:702-711.

53. Gahn G, Gerber J, Hallmeyer S, et al. Contrast-enhanced transcranial color-coded duplex sonography in stroke patients with limited bone windows. *AJNR Am J Neuroradiol*. 2000;21:509-514.

54. Nonent M, Serfaty JM, Nighoghossian N, et al; CARMEDAS Study Group. Concordance rate differences of 3 noninvasive imaging techniques to measure carotid stenosis in clinical routine practice: results of the CARMEDAS multicenter study. *Stroke*. 2004;35:682-686.

55. Derex L, Nighoghossian N, Hermier M, Adeleine P, Froment JC, Trouillas P. Early detection of cerebral arterial occlusion on magnetic resonance angiography: predictive value of the baseline NIHSS score and impact on neurological outcome. *Cerebrovasc Dis*. 2002;13:225-229.

56. Nederkoorn PJ, Elgersma OE, Mali WP, Eikelboom BC, Kappelle LJ, van der Graaf Y. Overestimation of carotid artery stenosis with magnetic resonance angiography compared with digital subtraction angiography. *J Vasc Surg*. 2002;36:806-813.

57. Biousse V, Tong F, Newman NJ. Cerebral venous thrombosis. *Curr Treat Options Cardiovasc Med*. 2003;5:181-192.

58. Lee SK, terBrugge KG. Cerebral venous thrombosis in adults: the role of imaging evaluation and management. *Neuroimaging Clin North Am*. 2003;13:139-152.

59. Knauth M, von Kummer R, Jansen O, Hahnel S, Dorfler A, Sartor K. Potential of CT angiography in acute ischemic stroke. *AJNR Am J Neuroradiol*. 1997;18:1001-1010.

60. Velthuis BK, Van Leeuwen MS, Witkamp TD, Ramos LM, Berkelbach van Der Sprenkel JW, Rinkel GJ. Computerized tomography angiography in patients with subarachnoid hemorrhage: from aneurysm detection to treatment without conventional angiography. *J Neurosurg*. 1999;91:761-767.

61. Dehdashti AR, Rufenacht DA, Delavelle J, Reverdin A, de Tribolet N. Therapeutic decision and management of aneurysmal subarachnoid haemorrhage based on computed tomographic angiography. *Br J Neurosurg*. 2003;17:46-53.

62. Lubezky N, Fajer S, Barmeir E, Karmeli R. Duplex scanning and CT angiography in the diagnosis of carotid artery occlusion: a prospective study. *Eur J Vasc Endovasc Surg*. 1998;16:133-136.

63. Fieschi C, Argentino C, Lenzi GL, Sacchetti ML, Toni D, Bozzao L. Clinical and instrumental evaluation of patients with ischemic stroke within the first six hours. *J Neurol Sci*. 1989;91:311-321.

64. Caplan LR, Wolpert SM. Angiography in patients with occlusive cerebrovascular disease: views of a stroke neurologist and neuroradiologist. *AJNR Am J Neuroradiol*. 1991;12:593-601.

65. Rothwell PM, Gibson RJ, Villagra R, Sellar R, Warlow CP. The effect of angiographic technique and image quality on the reproducibility of measurement of carotid stenosis and assessment of plaque surface morphology. *Clin Radiol*. 1998;53:439-443.

66. Endarterectomy for asymptomatic carotid artery stenosis. Executive Committee for the Asymptomatic Carotid Atherosclerosis Study. *JAMA*. 1995;273:1421-1428.

67. Toffol GJ, Biller J, Adams HP Jr, Smoker WR. The predicted value of arteriography in nontraumatic intracerebral hemorrhage. *Stroke*. 1986;17:881-883.

6

Emergency Medical Management of Stroke

The emergency management of patients with acute stroke parallels the approach used to treat patients with acute myocardial infarction (MI).[1] Acute cardiovascular and cerebrovascular events have many similarities. These life-threatening conditions usually are of arterial origin (most commonly an acute arterial occlusion) and they are accompanied by complications that add to both morbidity and mortality. Treatment of patients with either acute stroke or MI often involves emergency measures to restore perfusion and may include either pharmacologic thrombolysis or mechanical measures. Several potentially life-threatening medical or neurologic complications occur within the first hours after the vascular event.[2] Both acute stroke and acute MI may be treated successfully and outcomes may be improved. Like management of those persons with MI, modern stroke care requires urgent treatment.

Emergency Life-Support

■ Airway and Breathing

The administration of basic life-support is a crucial first step in the emergency treatment of patients with stroke[1,3-10] (**Table 6.1**). Most patients do not need immediate endotracheal intubation, ventilatory assistance, or urgent cardiac care. However, patients with a massive stroke leading to a decreased level of consciousness or those persons with a stroke causing prominent bulbar dysfunction likely will need protection of the airway. Patients having seizures secondary to the acute stroke also will need airway protection.

TABLE 6.1 — Components of General Emergency Treatment of Patients With Acute Stroke

- Monitor vital signs and do frequent neurologic assessments
- Protect the airway and, if necessary, do endotracheal intubation
- Do frequent suctioning if the patient is retaining secretions
- Monitor pulse oximetry
- Give ventilatory assistance and supplemental oxygen if hypoxic
- Monitor cardiac rhythm
- Treat serious cardiac arrhythmias
- Treat fever
- Assess blood glucose concentration
- Treat hyperglycemia or hypoglycemia
- Start intravenous fluids (normal saline) via an access
- Treat seizures with anticonvulsants

Patients with intracranial hemorrhages and those with infarctions in the brain stem or cerebellum often experience vomiting. Securing the airway helps forestall the complication of aspiration pneumonia. While no clinical trial has tested the utility of airway protection in the setting of stroke, it is unlikely that any such study will ever be done. Placement of an oropharyngeal or nasopharyngeal airway usually is not adequate; there is general agreement that an endotracheal tube should be placed if the airway is threatened[4,7] (Class I Recommendation, Level of Evidence C).

Abnormalities of respiratory rate or rhythm may be prominent in patients who have depressed consciousness. The respiratory disturbances may be secondary to dysfunction of the respiratory centers in the brain stem or delayed responses to hypoxia or hypercarbia. While respiratory arrest may occur most commonly in the setting of a massive hemorrhage, hypoventilation may develop in a large number of patients. The resulting hypoxia and hypercarbia may worsen the patient's neurologic status or aggravate the development of increased intracranial pressure (ICP) by promoting vasodilation. Ventilatory assistance may be started if hypoventilation occurs.[11] A small study found that supplemental oxygen did not improve outcomes of most patients with acute stroke.[12] However, patients with stroke should be monitored with a pulse oximetry device. If the blood oxygen concentration falls below 95%, oxygen could be given.[13] Until evidence shows that early supplemental oxygen improves outcomes after stroke, most patients with acute cerebrovascular disease do not need this intervention (Class III Recommendation, Level of Evidence C).

■ Hyperbaric Oxygen

While hyperbaric oxygen is used to treat patients with neurologic symptoms secondary to air embolization or Caisson disease, there is no evidence that this intervention is effective in stroke.[14] Data from a small trial suggest that hyperbaric oxygen therapy may be harmful.[15] At present, hyperbaric oxygen is not recommended for treatment of patients with ischemic stroke (Class III Recommendation, Level of Evidence B).

■ Fever

Fever is relatively uncommon during the first hours after stroke but its presence is associated with poorer neurologic outcomes.[16-18] It may result from complications, such as aspiration pneumonia, or it may be a manifestation of an infectious cause of stroke, such as infective endocarditis. Patients with intracranial hemorrhage also may have hemorrhage secondary to disturbances of the thermoregulatory center of the hypothalamus.[19,20] While central fever does happen, another source of the elevated temperature should be sought and the cause treated.

149

Treating fever may improve prognosis of patients with stroke.[21] Potential interventions include antipyretic medications and cooling devices. Several small studies have tested the utility of antipyretic medications, such as aspirin, ibuprofen, or acetaminophen, in improving outcomes after stroke; results are inconclusive.[22-25] Additional research on this strategy likely will be done. Currently, evaluation to determine the cause of fever and treatment of an elevated body temperature is reasonable (Class I Recommendation, Level of Evidence C). Induced hypothermia as a potential neuroprotection strategy is discussed in Chapter 10, *Acute Treatment of Ischemic Stroke: Neuroprotection.*

■ **Cardiac Complications, Including Arrhythmias**

A clinically silent MI is a potential source of emboli and, as a result, an ischemic stroke may be the initial clinical presentation of the cardiac lesion. While heart disease is a leading cause of stroke, cardiac disorders are important, potential life-endangering complications of both hemorrhagic and ischemic cerebrovascular events.[26-33] In particular, myocardial ischemia, cardiac arrhythmias, cardiac failure, and pulmonary edema are potential complications of intracranial hemorrhages.[34-37] Both electrocardiographic (ECG) and serum enzyme changes consistent with MI may be detected. Acute myocardial injury and arrhythmias are potential causes of sudden death among patients with major strokes (**Table 6.2**). Cardiac monitoring to detect abnormal rhythms should be part of the initial observation of all patients with possible stroke. No trials have tested the use of medications to protect the heart or to prevent arrhythmias among persons with stroke. Still, there is consensus that patients with acute hemorrhagic or ischemic stroke should have cardiac monitoring for at least 24 hours and therapies should be administered when arrhythmias are detected[3] (Class I Recommendation, Level of Evidence C). There are no data to support the

TABLE 6.2 — Cardiac Abnormalities Associated With Acute Stroke

Electrocardiographic Abnormalities
- Pathologic Q waves
- Loss of R waves
- Elevation or depression of ST segment
- QT prolongation
- Negative T waves
- Abnormal U waves

Arrhythmias
- Sinus bradycardia
- Supraventricular premature contractions
- Supraventricular tachycardia
- Atrial fibrillation
- Sinoatrial block
- Atrioventricular dissociation
- Atrioventricular block
- Idioventricular rhythm
- Unifocal or multifocal ventricular premature contractions
- Nonsustained ventricular tachycardia
- Torsades de pointes ventricular tachycardia
- Ventricular flutter or fibrillation

Abbreviations: QT, electrocardiographic interval from the beginning of the QRS complex and the end of the T wave; ST, electrocardiographic wave segment.

prophylactic administration of medications to prevent cardiac injury or rhythm disorders.

Arterial Hypertension

Many patients, especially those with intracranial hemorrhage, have an elevated blood pressure during the first hours following stroke. An elevated blood pressure is associated with a poor outcome.[38-40] Some of the association of increased mortality and morbidity following stroke with arterial hypertension may reflect the seriousness of the brain injury instead of the elevated blood pressure itself. The causes of arterial hypertension following stroke include the following:

- Pre-existing hypertension
- Pain, nausea, and vomiting
- Confusion or anxiety
- Stress of the stroke
- Increased intracranial pressure
- Physiologic responses in an attempt to increase perfusion to the brain.

Because cerebrovascular autoregulation is lost in the setting of acute stroke, blood flow becomes pressure-dependent. The brain may need an elevated blood pressure to limit the scope of the ischemic injury. Sudden lowering of blood pressure might result in worsening of neurologic impairments.[41,42] Rapid treatment of blood pressure may be associated with poor neurologic outcomes.[38,43] On the other hand, lowering the blood pressure may reduce the formation of brain edema, lessen the development of a hemorrhagic transformation of an infarction, diminish growth of an acute hemorrhage, prevent additional vascular damage, and forestall early recurrent stroke. Urgent antihypertensive therapy also may be needed to treat patients who also have hypertensive encephalopathy, aortic dissection, acute renal failure, acute pulmonary edema, or acute myocardial ischemia.[41] In general, the blood pressure is treated more aggressively in persons with hemorrhagic stroke than in those with ischemic stroke. The elevated blood pressure may promote growth of an intraparenchymal hematoma or increase the chances of early recurrent hemorrhage. Normally, arterial hypertension declines spontaneously during the first hours after stroke, even without any specific treatment.[43]

■ Treatment of Acute Arterial Hypertension

There are several issues related to the management of arterial hypertension during the setting of acute stroke[44-46] (**Table 6.3**). Unfortunately, data to address these issues are not definitive. Treatment of anxiety, pain, nausea, vomiting, and increased intracranial pressure may lower the blood pressure. Several small studies have tested calcium channel blocking agents, angiotensin-converting enzyme inhibitors, diuretics, β-blockers, or nitrates, but the results are inconclusive.[47-50] A trial tested the angiotensin receptor blocker candesartan when started within 1 day of onset of stroke.[51] While the trial found a lower mortality (at 1 year) among patients treated with candesartan, it is unclear how the acute treatment had such a delayed evidence of efficacy. A trial testing the utility of anti-hypertensive therapy in the setting of stroke is under way.[52]

**TABLE 6.3 — Issues Related to
Emergency Management of
Arterial Hypertension Associated With Stroke**

- Continue taking medications that were used prior to stroke?
  - Should some be discontinued?
  - Should there be a delay before restarting?
- Administer another (new) antihypertensive agent?
- Level of blood pressure that would require treatment?
- Which medication should be administered?

The treatment of arterial hypertension in the setting of acute stroke has not been established with certainty. A reasonable approach is not to overreact to arterial hypertension and to gradually lower the blood pressure. In general, a systolic blood pressure that would lead to treatment would be >180 mm Hg.[38] A systolic blood pressure >185 mm Hg or a diastolic blood pressure >110 mm Hg is a contraindication for administration of recombinant tissue-type plasminogen activator (rt-PA) for treatment of acute ischemic stroke.[3,4,53,54] Treatment of the arterial hypertension may allow a patient to be treated with thrombolytic therapy (**Table 6.4**) (Class 1 Recommendation, Level of Evidence C). Unless measures to restore reperfusion are planned, there is a consensus to avoid aggressive treatment of arterial hypertension unless the diastolic blood pressure is >120 mm Hg or systolic blood pressure is >220 mm Hg[4] (Class 1 Recommendation, Level of Evidence C). These levels probably are too high. In addition, lower levels of blood pressure should mandate antihypertensive therapy among patients with brain hemorrhage.[55,56] Careful management of arterial hypertension is a crucial part of the management of patients who receive thrombolytic therapy. Violations of the blood pressure criteria for selection of patients to treat with rt-PA may be associated with an increased risk of hemorrhagic complications.[57-59]

Given the relatively short interval from onset of ischemic stroke, treatment of arterial hypertension may be problematic. Still, in many cases, time may be sufficient to determine that the blood pressure has stabilized and is within criteria for treatment with rt-PA. While there is the concern that lowering the blood pressure may decrease perfusion and exacerbate the ischemia, these effects may be counteracted by the benefits of restoring blood flow that accompanies thrombolytic therapy.

The possibility of an elevated blood pressure increasing the likelihood of symptomatic hemorrhagic transformation after rt-PA treatment requires that monitoring and control of the blood pressure be aggressive during and following the administration of the thrombolytic agent[3,4] (**Table 6.4**). Elevated blood pressure increasing the risk of hemorrhagic transformation of a large infarction also may occur even if the patient does not receive thrombolytic or antithrombotic agents.

If no other medical conditions contraindicate a specific therapy, choices for initial emergency therapy include labetalol, nicardipine, sodium nitroprusside, or topical nitroglycerin (Class IIa Recommendation, Level of Evidence C). The medications may be used to treat an acute hypertensive emergency in the setting of either hemorrhagic or ischemic stroke. These agents usually act rapidly to lower blood pressure and their duration of action is relatively brief. As a result, their dosage may be adjusted if the blood pressure decline is excessive or if neurologic worsening is noted. Some of the medications do require close monitoring of blood pressure either with an intra-arterial catheter or a non-invasive system. Placement of an intra-arterial catheter may be difficult immediately after the use of a thrombolytic agent because of the bleeding risk. Because of its prolonged effects on blood pressure, sublingual administration of nifedipine is not recommended[3,60] (Class III Recommendation, Level of Evidence B).

■ **Initiation of Long-Term Treatment of Arterial Hypertension**

Many patients with stroke will need long-term antihypertensive treatment, which will need to be started after the acute vascular event. Data about the timing of the initiation of antihypertensive therapy following stroke are limited. The results of one recent trial suggest that medications may be started within 24 hours after stroke in many patients[51] (Class I Recommendation, Level of Evidence B). The selection of medications will be influenced by the following factors:

- The patient's neurologic status
- Severity of neurologic impairment
- Presence of increased intracranial pressure
- Ability to swallow medications
- Presence of concomitant diseases
- Indications for specific medications
- Contraindications for specific medications

TABLE 6.4 — Approach to Elevated Blood Pressure in Acute Ischemic Stroke

Blood Pressure Level (mm Hg)	Treatment
Not eligible for thrombolytic therapy	
Systolic ≤220 OR Diastolic ≤120	Observe unless other end-organ involvement (eg, aortic dissection, acute myocardial infarction, pulmonary edema, hypertensive encephalopathy) Treat other symptoms of stroke (eg, headache, pain, agitation, nausea, vomiting) Treat other acute complications of stroke, including hypoxia, increased intracranial pressure, seizures, or hypoglycemia
Systolic ≤220 OR Diastolic 121–140	Labetalol 10-20 mg IV for 1-2 min May repeat or double every 10 min (max dose 300 mg) OR Nicardipine 5 mg/h IV infusion as initial dose; titrate to desired effect by increasing 2.5 mg/h every 5 min to max of 15 mg/h Aim for a 10% to 15% reduction of blood pressure
Diastolic >140	Nitroprusside 0.5 µg/kg⁻¹/min⁻¹ IV infusion as initial dose with continuous blood pressure monitoring Aim for a 10% to 15% reduction in blood pressure
Eligible for thrombolytic therapy	
Pretreatment	
Systolic >185 OR Diastolic >110	Labetalol 10-20 mg IV for 1-2 min May repeat 1 time or nitropaste 1-2 inches

156

During and after treatment	
1. Monitor blood pressure	Check blood pressure every 15 min for 2 h, then every 30 min for 6 h, and finally every hour for 16 h
2. Diastolic >140	Sodium nitroprusside 0.5 μg/kg^{-1}/min^{-1} IV infusion as initial dose and titrate to desired blood pressure
3. Systolic >230 OR Diastolic 121–140	Labetalol 10 mg IV for 1-2 min May repeat or double labetalol every 10 min to a maximum dose of 300 mg, or give the initial labetalol bolus, then start labetalol drip at 2–8 mg/min OR Nicardipine 5 mg/h IV infusion as initial dose and titrate to desired effect by increasing 2.5 mg/h every 5 min to maximum of 15 mg/h; if blood pressure is not controlled by labetalol, consider sodium nitroprusside
4. Systolic 180–230 OR Diastolic 105–120	Labetalol 10 mg IV for 1-2 min May repeat or double labetalol every 10-20 min to a maximum dose of 300 mg or give initial labetalol dose, then start labetalol drip at 2-8 mg/min
Adams HP Jr, et al. *Stroke.* 2005;36:916-921.	

6

- Medications previously used for treatment of hypertension.

Arterial Hypotension

While arterial hypotension (systolic <100 mm Hg or diastolic <70 mm Hg) is found rarely among persons with acute stroke, its presence is associated with an increased likelihood of neurologic worsening, poor neurologic outcome, or death.[38,61] If hypotension is present, a possible explanation should be sought. Possible explanations are:
- Volume depletion
- Aortic dissection
- Blood loss
- Decreased cardiac output
- Cardiac arrhythmia.

Treatment of hypotension includes volume replacement with saline or blood products (Class IIa Recommendation, Level of Evidence C). If severe hypotension persists, a vasopressor, such as dopamine, may be used.

Hyperglycemia and Hypoglycemia

Because hypoglycemia may produce impairments in consciousness or focal neurologic signs that mimic stroke and because low blood concentrations of glucose may exacerbate any brain injury, rapid assessment of the blood glucose level is an important emergency assessment. Although there are no data demonstrating the efficacy of correction of hypoglycemia in management of patients with stroke, rapid correction of a low blood glucose level is recommended[3] (Class I Recommendation, Level of Evidence A).

Elevated blood concentrations are relatively common findings following acute stroke; in most

158

cases, the elevations are moderate.[62,63] Both a history of diabetes and the presence of hyperglycemia at the time of stroke are associated with poor outcomes following stroke.[64-67] Some of the association of hyperglycemia and its negative prognostic implications may be related to a stress response to a serious neurologic event.[68] Still, persistent hyperglycemia appears to be an independent predictor of poor outcomes and neurological worsening following stroke.[67,69] Many patients will have a spontaneous decline in blood glucose levels in the hours after stroke.[63] While there is a strong rationale for aggressive treatment of hyperglycemia following stroke, the level of blood glucose that would mandate emergency treatment has not been established.[3] Conversely, there are no data to demonstrate that aggressive management of hyperglycemia will improve outcomes after stroke. Small clinical trials have looked at the utility of infusions of insulin, glucose, and potassium that might be effective in achieving relative normal glucose levels.[63,70,71] Pending more definitive data, it seems reasonable to treat hyperglycemia in the setting of acute stroke. The goal should be to lower levels to <200 mg/dL (Class IIa Recommendation, Level of Evidence B).

Seizures

While seizures complicate approximately 5% of strokes, status epilepticus is uncommon.[72,73] Still, seizures intensify metabolic demands and augment the brain injury from stroke. They also are a neurologic emergency, which may be life endangering. Seizures are most common among patients with subarachnoid hemorrhage (SAH) and those with cortical (embolic) infarctions. Seizures may occur at the time of onset of stroke or may occur during both the acute period and convalescence.

Besides basic life-support measures, emergency parenteral administration of anticonvulsants is recommended for treatment of a patient who is having seizures. Patients who are not actively seizing but who have had a seizure with their ictus should also receive anticonvulsants.[74] Fosphenytoin and phenytoin are the most commonly prescribed anticonvulsants. Depending upon the extent of seizure activity, the medication may be given rapidly or administered over the first 4 to 6 hours. Short-acting benzodiazepines may be given to those patients who are having active seizures or status epilepticus. Because the overall risk of seizures complicating stroke is relatively low, prophylactic administration of anticonvulsants to those patients who have not had seizures is not recommended[3] (Class III Recommendation, Level of Evidence C). Some physicians include prophylactic administration of anticonvulsants in their medical management of patients with recent SAH because of the concern that the stress of a seizure might promote early recurrent aneurysmal rupture. The utility of this strategy has not been established.

Brain Edema and Increased Intracranial Pressure

Brain edema and increased ICP are important complications of acute hemorrhagic or ischemic stroke; they are leading causes of death within the first week after the cerebrovascular events.[75] Elevated ICP may worsen brain ischemia by reducing cerebral perfusion pressure. In addition, pressure gradients between compartments of the cranial vault may lead to herniation and secondary brain stem injury. Elevations of ICP usually are the result of brain edema or the mass effect of a hematoma.

Brain edema and increased ICP are not major problems in those patients with small or discrete infarctions or hematomas. Rather, these complications are noted among patients with multilobar infarctions or large hematomas. In addition, large infarctions or hematomas of the posterior fossa may block cerebrospinal fluid (CSF) pathways leading to acute hydrocephalus or cause secondary brain stem compression. In addition, intraventricular hemorrhage or SAH also may be complicated with acute hydrocephalus. These are the patients who need to be observed for the development of an increased ICP. In general, the time course for increased ICP is more acute among patients with intracranial hemorrhages; patients may be symptomatic within the first hours. Usually, the course of brain edema and increased ICP is slower in patients with ischemic strokes of the cerebral hemisphere; the symptoms usually evolve over the first 2 to 4 days. Those patients with large infarctions or hematomas of the cerebellum or brain stem also may rapidly develop signs of increased ICP.

Papilledema, the usual physical finding of increased ICP, appears over several hours; thus it usually is not found among patients with a recent stroke. Increased ICP should be considered if a patient has a depression of consciousness or if a previously alert patient has become drowsy or stuporous. Changes in consciousness are the most sensitive early signs. In addition, an increase in blood pressure and slowing of the heart rate may be signs of intracranial hypertension. Signs of herniation, such as a unilateral oculomotor (III) nerve palsy, appear late in the course. The presence of an oculomotor nerve palsy in an alert or drowsy patient probably does not represent a unilateral herniation syndrome; a more likely situation is a ruptured aneurysm of the posterior communicating artery or the basilar artery that is directly affecting the nerve.

Brain imaging is particularly helpful in management of patients with suspected increases in ICP. These studies may demonstrate mass effects of the stroke or hydrocephalus. Because the results of the studies may influence decisions in treatment, such as placement of a ventricular catheter to drain CSF or surgical resection of a mass, they should be done quickly.

■ Medical Management

Management of brain edema and increased ICP after stroke includes both prophylactic and urgent interventions[76] (**Table 6.5**). Prophylactic measures include elevation of the head of the patient's bed and positioning of the head in order to expedite venous drainage. Modest fluid restriction often is prescribed. The usual 24-hour restriction is 1.5 to 2 L. Potential hypo-osmolar fluids, such as 5% dextrose in water, should be avoided. Measures to control or treat fever, hypoxia, and hypercarbia are complemented by therapies to treat nausea, vomiting, pain, or agitation. Although controversy persists, to date there are no data showing that corticosteroids are effective in controlling brain edema following stroke.[77-79] Their use is not recommended[3] (Class III Recommendation, Level of Evidence B).

Most patients at highest risk for markedly elevated ICP already will have been intubated to protect their airway. If not, those patients with neurologic deterioration secondary to brain edema or increased ICP should have emergency intubation and hyperventilation. The goal is to lower the blood level of the partial pressure of carbon dioxide (pCO_2) to approximately 30 mm Hg. Carbon dioxide is a potent vasodilator and lowering its concentration may cause vasoconstriction of the vascular compartment and a brief drop in ICP. Excessive lowering of the pCO_2 with resultant vasoconstriction might lead to ischemia. Hyperventilation has an immediate but nonsustained effect; it should not be considered as definitive treatment. Other therapies are needed in this situation.

TABLE 6.5 — Prevention and Treatment of Increased Intracranial Pressure Following Stroke

General Prevention
- Control fever, agitation, nausea, and vomiting
- Treat hypoxia, hypercarbia, or seizures
- Modest fluid restriction (approximately 1.5 L/day to 2 L/day)
- Avoid potential hypoosmolar intravenous fluids, such as 5% dextrose in water
- Avoid hyperrotation of head to prevent venous obstruction
- Elevate head of bed to augment venous drainage

Acute Treatment
- Intubation to protect the airway
- Hyperventilation to lower pCO_2 to approximately 30 mm Hg
- Administer 20% mannitol at a dose of 0.5–1 gm/kg:
  - Given over approximately 20 to 30 minutes
  - May be repeated 0.25 mg/kg every 6 hours
  - Usual maximal daily dose is 2 g/kg
  - Replace lost fluids
  - Hypertonic saline (3%) may be an alternative
- Administer furosemide, 20 to 40 mg given intravenously
- Monitor ICP to assess changes
- Drainage of CSF via a ventricular catheter

Surgical Procedures
- Evacuation of a hematoma
- Resection of an area of infarcted brain
- Craniectomy with removal of large section of skull

Abbreviations: CSF, cerebrospinal fluid; ICP, intracranial pressure.

Intravenous administration of furosemide (20 mg to 40 mg) may lower ICP through its diuretic effect. Furosemide may be used in an emergency situation but it should be considered as an adjunct to other measures to control brain edema and ICP. Osmotic therapy (hypertonic saline, mannitol, or glycerol) may be given to patients with clinically significant brain edema and elevated ICP following stroke[80-87] (Class IIa Recommendation, Level of Evidence B). Clinical experience suggests that these agents may lessen the morbidity and mortality of malignant brain edema. The regimen for the use of mannitol is described in **Table 6.5**. The ICP usually begins to decline within 20 minutes of starting an infusion and the effects usually persist for approximately 4 to 6 hours. Alternative interventions include hypertonic saline or glycerol, although experience with these therapies is less than with mannitol. These agents may be associated with a hyperosmolar state, which is most likely to occur with repeated doses. In order to lessen the likelihood of this side effect, intravenous fluids usually are administered to compensate for losses that are occurring.

■ Surgical Treatment

If secondary hydrocephalus is present, drainage of CSF may be achieved through the insertion of an intra-ventricular catheter.[88,89] Removal of a small amount of fluid may lower ICP dramatically. In particular, ventricular drainage may help control ICP in a patient with a mass-producing cerebellar hematoma or infarction. It may eliminate the need for surgical evacuation of the cerebellar lesion. Continuous CSF drainage may be performed, especially in patients with SAH. Repeated lumbar punctures could be done if the patient does not have a mass, but this intervention has limited applicability after stroke. Other potential therapies to treat malignant brain edema and increased ICP include hypothermia and barbiturate-induced coma.[90-92] Neither of these interventions has established utility. Despite aggressive medical management, many patients with malignant brain edema or increased ICP do not have favorable outcomes.[76,93]

■ Surgical Treatment of a Large Hematoma or Infarction Causing Mass Effects

Operative evacuation of a large hematoma or infarction may be a lifesaving procedure in a patient with increased ICP, and a patient with a mass-producing intraparenchymal hematoma or infarction may be considered for surgery. If the hematoma is secondary to anticoagulants or thrombolytic therapy, surgery should not be performed until the effects of the medications have been reversed. Large (>2.5 cm in diameter) infarctions or hematomas of the cerebellar hemisphere are especially amenable to surgical treatment.[94-98] Secondary compression of the brain stem, the fourth ventricle, and the aqueduct of Sylvius may be eased by removal of the cerebellar mass. Because decompensation may happen abruptly, patients with large cerebellar strokes are monitored closely and surgery is performed quickly if deterioration is detected.

There is uncertainty about the utility of operative evacuation of large hematomas of the cerebral hemisphere. Surgical treatment of hemorrhages in the basal ganglia or thalamus may be associated with considerable morbidity or mortality. Several small clinical trials did not demonstrate any real benefit from surgical evacuation of a hematoma.[99-103] Recently, a large clinical trial failed to show any significant improvement in outcomes with early surgical management of hemispheric hematomas.[104] These data suggest that the role of surgery in management of large, deep hemispheric hematomas producing mass effects or increased ICP is limited (Class III Recommendation, Level of Evidence A). Stereotactic evacuation of a hematoma, possibly including the instillation of a thrombolytic agent to

165

promote fibrinolysis, has been evaluated[105,106] (Class IIb Recommendation, Level of Evidence B). This approach has not been evaluated sufficiently to know if it truly is useful. Large subarachnoid clots also may be evacuated; in most instances, this is conjunction with surgical repair of a ruptured aneurysm.

Surgical decompression may be offered to patients with multilobar infarctions of large hematomas that have not responded to medical interventions.[92,107-110] During the operation, the surgeon may remove a section of necrotic brain, most commonly the temporal lobe, to provide room for adjacent tissues to swell. A section of bone also is removed to give additional room for swelling. Decompressive craniectomy without resection of brain tissue also may be done; in this situation, the brain may herniate through the hole in the skull. These operations may be lifesaving measures and some patients may have reasonable outcomes. Still, the usefulness of these surgical therapies has not been established because survival may be associated with devastating neurologic sequelae. In most cases, the patient cannot give consent. In such circumstances, the family will need to make the decision. They should be informed that that while some patients may achieve good outcomes, there is the potential for serious morbidity even if the operation is successful. Operations are recommended most frequently for younger patients with nondominant hemisphere strokes (Class IIa Recommendation, Level of Evidence B).

Palliative Care

Some patients have such serious brain injury from either a hemorrhagic or ischemic stroke that their prognosis is extremely poor even with aggressive medical and surgical treatment. In such circumstances, the family and physician may opt not to institute measures that will only prolong the dying of the patient. Such difficult decisions need to be made with the wishes of the patient in mind and should reflect the cultural, religious, and personal beliefs of the patient and family.

REFERENCES

1. EEC Committee, EEC Subcommittees, ECC Task Forces; Authors of Final Evidence Evaluation Worksheets 2005 International Consensus on Cardiopulmonary Resuscitation and Emergency Cardiovascular Care With Treatment Recommendations Conference. 2005 American Heart Association guidelines for cardiopulmonary resuscitation and emergency cardiovascular care. Part 9: adult stroke. *Circulation*. 2005;112(suppl): IV-111–IV-120.

2. van der Worp HB, Kappelle LJ. Complications of acute ischaemic stroke. *Cerebrovasc Dis*. 1998;8:124-132.

3. Adams HP Jr, Adams RJ, Brott T, et al. Guidelines for the early management of patients with ischemic stroke. A scientific statement from the Stroke Council of the American Stroke Association. *Stroke*. 2003;34:1056-1083.

4. Adams H, Adams R, del Zoppo G, Goldstein LB; Stroke Council of the American Heart Association; American Stroke Association. Guidelines for the early management of patients with ischemic stroke: 2005 guidelines update a scientific statement from the Stroke Council of the American Heart Association/American Stroke Association. *Stroke*. 2005;36:916-923.

5. Bushnell CD, Phillips-Bute BG, Laskowitz DT, Lynch JR, Chilukuri V, Borel CO. Survival and outcome after endotracheal intubation for acute stroke. *Neurology*. 1999;52:1374-1381.

6. Hacke W, Kaste M, Skyhoj Olsen T, Bogousslavsky J, Orgogozo JM. Acute treatment of ischemic stroke. European Stroke Initiative (EUSI). *Cerebrovasc Dis*. 2000;10(suppl 3):22-33.

7. Hacke W, Krieger D, Hirschberg M. General principles in the treatment of acute ischemic stroke. *Cerebrovasc Dis*. 1991;1(suppl 1):93-99.

8. Grotta J, Pasteur W, Khwaja G, Hamel T, Fisher M, Ramirez A. Elective intubation for neurologic deterioration after stroke. *Neurology*. 1995;45:640-644.

9. Gruber A, Reinprecht A, Gorzer H, et al. Pulmonary function and radiographic abnormalities related to neurological outcome after aneurysmal subarachnoid hemorrhage. *J Neurosurg*. 1998;88:28-37.

10. Milhaud D, Popp J, Thouvenot E, Heroum C, Bonafé A. Mechanical ventilation in ischemic stroke. *J Stroke Cerebrovasc Dis*. 2004;13:183-188.

11. Gujjar AR, Deibert E, Manno EM, Duff S, Diringer MN. Mechanical ventilation for ischemic stroke and intracerebral hemorrhage: indications, timing, and outcome. *Neurology*. 1998;51:447-451.

12. Ronning OM, Guldvog B. Should stroke victims routinely receive supplemental oxygen? A quasi-randomized controlled trial. *Stroke*. 1999;30:2033-2037.

13. Treib J, Grauer MT, Woessner R, Morgenthaler M. Treatment of stroke on an intensive stroke unit: a novel concept. *Intensive Care Med*. 2000;26:1598-1611.

167

14. Nighoghossian N, Trouillas P. Hyperbaric oxygen in the treatment of acute ischemic stroke: an unsettled issue. *J Neurol Sci.* 1997;150:27-31.

15. Rusyniak DE, Kirk MA, May JD, et al; Hyperbaric Oxygen in Acute Ischemic Stroke Trial Pilot Study. Hyperbaric oxygen therapy in acute ischemic stroke: results of the Hyperbaric Oxygen in Acute Ischemic Stroke Trial Pilot Study. *Stroke.* 2003;34:571-574.

16. Hajat C, Hajat S, Sharma P. Effects of poststroke pyrexia on stroke outcome: a meta-analysis of studies in patients. *Stroke.* 2000;31:410-414.

17. Kammersgaard LP, Jorgensen HS, Rungby JA, et al. Admission body temperature predicts long-term mortality after acute stroke: the Copenhagen Stroke Study. *Stroke.* 2002;33:1759-1762.

18. Zaremba J. Hyperthermia in ischemic stroke. *Med Sci Monit.* 2004;10: RA148-RA153.

19. Schwarz S, Hafner K, Aschoff A, Schwab S. Incidence and prognostic significance of fever following intracerebral hemorrhage. *Neurology.* 2000;54:354-361.

20. Oliveira-Filho J, Ezzeddine MA, Segal AZ, et al. Fever in subarachnoid hemorrhage: relationship to vasospasm and outcome. *Neurology.* 2001;56:1299-1304.

21. Jorgensen HS, Reith J, Nakayama H, Kammersgaard LP, Raaschou HO, Olsen TS. What determines good recovery in patients with the most severe strokes? The Copenhagen Stroke Study. *Stroke.* 1999;30:2008-2012.

22. Sulter G, Elting JW, Maurits N, Luyckx GJ, De Keyser J. Acetylsalicylic acid and acetaminophen to combat elevated body temperature in acute ischemic stroke. *Cerebrovasc Dis.* 2004;17:118-122.

23. Kasner SE, Wein T, Piriyawat P, et al. Acetaminophen for altering body temperature in acute stroke: a randomized clinical trial. *Stroke.* 2002;33:130-134.

24. Dippel DW, van Breda EJ, van der Worp HB, et al. Timing of the effect of acetaminophen on body temperature in patients with acute ischemic stroke. *Neurology.* 2003;61:677-679.

25. Dippel DW, van Breda EJ, van der Worp HB, et al; PISA-Investigators. Effect of paracetamol (acetaminophen) and ibuprofen on body temperature in acute ischemic stroke PISA, a phase II double-blind, randomized, placebo-controlled trial [ISRCTN98608690]. *BMC Cardiovasc Disord.* 2003;3:2

26. Chua HC, Sen S, Cosgriff RF, Gerstenblith G, Beauchamp NJ Jr, Oppenheimer SM. Neurogenic ST depression in stroke. *Clin Neurol Neurosurg.* 1999;101:44-48.

27. Myers MG, Norris JW, Hachinski VC, Weingert ME, Sole MJ. Cardiac sequelae of acute stroke. *Stroke.* 1982;13:838-842.

28. Korpelainen JT, Sotaniemi KA, Huikuri HV, Myllya VV. Abnormal heart rate variability as a manifestation of autonomic dysfunction in hemispheric brain infarction. *Stroke.* 1996;27:2059-2063.

29. Korpelainen JT, Sotaniemi KA, Makikallio A, Huikuri HV, Myllyla VV. Dynamic behavior of heart rate in ischemic stroke. *Stroke.* 1999;30:1008-1013.

30. Orlandi G, Fanucchi S, Strata G, et al. Transient autonomic nervous system dysfunction during hyperacute stroke. *Acta Neurol Scand.* 2000;102:317-321.

31. Tokgozoglu SL, Batur MK, Topuoglu MA, Saribas O, Kes S, Oto A. Effects of stroke localization on cardiac autonomic balance and sudden death. *Stroke.* 1999;30:1307-1311.

32. Colivicchi F, Bassi A, Santini M, Caltagirone C. Cardiac autonomic derangement and arrhythmias in right-sided stroke with insular involvement. *Stroke*. 2004;35:2094-2098.

33. Colivicchi F, Bassi A, Santini M, Caltagirone C. Prognostic implications of right-sided insular damage, cardiac autonomic derangement, and arrhythmias after acute ischemic stroke. *Stroke*. 2005;36:1710-1715.

34. Yuki K, Kodama Y, Onda J, Emoto K, Morimoto T, Uozumi T. Coronary vasospasm following subarachnoid hemorrhage as a cause of stunned myocardium. Case report. *J Neurosurg*. 1991;75:308-311.

35. Zaroff JG, Rordorf GA, Newell JB, Ogilvy CS, Levinson JR. Cardiac outcome in patients with subarachnoid hemorrhage and electrocardiographic abnormalities. *Neurosurgery*. 1999;44:34-39.

36. Di Pasquale G, Andreoli A, Lusa AM, et al. Cardiologic complications of subarachnoid hemorrhage. *J Neurosurg Sci*. 1998;42:33-36.

37. Di Pasquale G, Pinelli G, Andreoli A, Manini GL, Grazi P, Tognetti F. Torsade de pointes and ventricular flutter-fibrillation following spontaneous cerebral subarachnoid hemorrhage. *Int J Cardiol*. 1988;18:163-172.

38. Castillo J, Leira R, Garcia MM, Serena J, Blanco M, Davalos A. Blood pressure decrease during the acute phase of ischemic stroke is associated with brain injury and poor stroke outcome. *Stroke*. 2004;35:520-526.

39. Vemmos KN, Tsivgoulis G, Spengos K, et al. Pulse pressure in acute stroke is an independent predictor of long-term mortality. *Cerebrovasc Dis*. 2004;18:30-36.

40. Aslanyan S, Fazekas F, Weir CJ, Horner S, Lees KR; GAIN International Steering Committee and Investigators. Effect of blood pressure during the acute period of ischemic stroke on stroke outcome: a tertiary analysis of the GAIN International Trial. *Stroke*. 2003;34:2420-2425.

41. Johnston KC, Mayer SA. Blood pressure reduction in ischemic stroke: a two-edged sword? *Neurology*. 2003;61:1030-1031.

42. Goldstein LB. Blood pressure management in patients with acute ischemic stroke. *Hypertension*. 2004;43:137-141.

43. Oliveira-Filho J, Silva SC, Trabuco CC, Pedreira BB, Sousa EU, Bacellar A. Detrimental effect of blood pressure reduction in the first 24 hours of acute stroke onset. *Neurology*. 2003;61:1047-1051.

44. Verstappen A, Thijs V. What do we (not) know about the management of blood pressure in acute stroke? *Curr Neurol Neurosci Rep*. 2004;4:505-509.

45. Chalmers J. Blood pressure in acute stroke: in search of evidence. *J Hypertens*. 2005;23:277-278.

46. Hillis AE. Systemic blood pressure and stroke outcome and recurrence. *Curr Atheroscler Rep*. 2004;6:274-280.

47. Bath P. High blood pressure as a risk factor and prognostic predictor in acute ischaemic stroke: when and how to treat it? *Cerebrovasc Dis*. 2004;17(suppl 1):51-57.

48. Chalmers J. Trials on blood pressure-lowering and secondary stroke prevention. *Am J Cardiol*. 2003;91:3G-8G.

49. Rodriguez-Garcia JL, Botia E, de La Sierra A, Villanueva MA, Gonzalez-Spinola J. Significance of elevated blood pressure and its management on the short-term outcome of patients with acute ischemic stroke. *Am J Hypertens*. 2005;18:379-384.

50. Eames PJ, Robinson TG, Panerai RB, Potter JF. Bendrofluazide fails to reduce elevated blood pressure levels in the immediate post-stroke period. *Cerebrovasc Dis*. 2005;19:253-259.

51. Schrader J, Luders S, Kulschewski A, et al; Acute Candesartan Cilexetil Therapy in Stroke Survivors Study Group. The ACCESS Study: evaluation of Acute Candesartan Cilexetil Therapy in Stroke Survivors. *Stroke*. 2003;34:1699-1703.

52. Potter J, Robinson T, Ford G, et al; The CHHIPS Trial Group. CHHIPS (Controlling Hypertension and Hypotension Immediately Post-Stroke) pilot trial: rationale and design. *J Hypertens*. 2005;23:649-655.

53. Tissue plasminogen activator for acute ischemic stroke. The National Institute of Neurological Disorders and Stroke rt-PA Stroke Study Group. *N Engl J Med*. 1995;333:1581-1587.

54. Brott T, Lu M, Kothari R, et al. Hypertension and its treatment in the NINDS rt-PA Stroke Trial. *Stroke*. 1998;29:1504-1509.

55. Mayberg MR, Batjer HH, Dacey R, et al. Guidelines for the management of aneurysmal subarachnoid hemorrhage. A statement for healthcare professionals from a special writing group of the Stroke Council, American Heart Association. *Circulation*. 1994;90:2592-2605.

56. Broderick JP, Adams HP Jr, Barsan W, et al. Guidelines for the management of spontaneous intracerebral hemorrhage: a statement for healthcare professionals from a special writing group of the Stroke Council, American Heart Association. *Stroke*. 1999;30:905-915.

57. Katzan IL, Graber TM, Furlan AJ, et al. Cuyahoga County Operation Stroke speed of emergency department evaluation and compliance with National Institutes of Neurological Disorders and Stroke time targets. *Stroke*. 2003;34:799-800.

58. Lopez-Yunez AM, Bruno A, Williams LS, Yilmaz E, Zurru C, Biller J. Protocol violations in community-based rTPA stroke treatment are associated with symptomatic intracerebral hemorrhage. *Stroke*. 2001;32:12-16.

59. Katzan IL, Hammer MD, Furlan AJ, Hixson ED, Nadzam DM; Cleveland Clinic Health System Stroke Quality Improvement Team. Quality improvement and tissue-type plasminogen activator for acute ischemic stroke: a Cleveland update. *Stroke*. 2003;34:799-800.

60. Grossman E, Messerli FH, Grodzicki T, Kowey P. Should a moratorium be placed on sublingual nifedipine capsules given for hypertensive emergencies and pseudoemergencies? *JAMA*. 1996;276:1328-1331.

61. Leonardi-Bee J, Bath PM, Phillips SJ, Sandercock PA; IST Collaborative Group. Blood pressure and clinical outcomes in the International Stroke Trial. *Stroke*. 2002;33:1315-1320.

62. Williams LS, Rotich J, Qi R, et al. Effects of admission hyperglycemia on mortality and costs in acute ischemic stroke. *Neurology*. 2002;59:67-71.

63. Gray CS, Hildreth AJ, Alberti GK, O'Connell JE; GIST Collaboration. Poststroke hyperglycemia: natural history and immediate management. *Stroke*. 2004;35:122-126.

64. Bruno A, Biller J, Adams HP Jr, et al. Acute blood glucose level and outcome from ischemic stroke. Trial of ORG 10172 in Acute Stroke Treatment (TOAST) Investigators. *Neurology*. 1999;52:280-284.

65. Alvarez-Sabin J, Molina CA, Ribo M, et al. Impact of admission hyperglycemia on stroke outcome after thrombolysis: risk stratification in relation to time to reperfusion. *Stroke*. 2004;35:2493-2498.

66. Leigh R, Zaidat OO, Suri MF, et al. Predictors of hyperacute clinical worsening in ischemic stroke patients receiving thrombolytic therapy. *Stroke*. 2004;35:1903-1907.

67. Lindsberg PJ, Roine RO. Hyperglycemia in acute stroke. *Stroke*. 2004;35:363-364.

68. Capes SE, Hunt D, Malmberg K, Pathak P, Gerstein HC. Stress hyperglycemia and prognosis of stroke in nondiabetic and diabetic patients: a systematic overview. *Stroke*. 2001;32:2426-2432.

69. Baird TA, Parsons MW, Phanh T, et al. Persistent poststroke hyperglycemia is independently associated with infarct expansion and worse clinical outcome. *Stroke*. 2003;34:2208-2214.

70. Scott JF, Robinson GM, French JM, O'Connell JE, Alberti KG, Gray CS. Blood pressure response to glucose potassium insulin therapy in patients with acute stroke with mild to moderate hyperglycaemia. *J Neurol Neurosurg Psychiatry*. 2001;70:401-404.

71. Bruno A, Saha C, Williams LS, Shankar R. IV insulin during acute cerebral infarction in diabetic patients. *Neurology*. 2004;62:1441-1442.

72. Labovitz DL, Hauser WA, Sacco RL. Prevalence and predictors of early seizure and status epilepticus after first stroke. *Neurology*. 2001;57:200-206.

73. Bladin CF, Alexandrov AV, Bellavance A, et al. Seizures after stroke: a prospective multicenter study. *Arch Neurol*. 2000;57:1617-1622.

74. Gilad R, Lampl Y, Eschel Y, Sadeh M. Antiepileptic treatment in patients with early postischemic stroke seizures: a retrospective study. *Cerebrovasc Dis*. 2001;12:39-43.

75. Pullicino PM, Alexandrov AV, Shelton JA, Alexandrova NA, Smurawska LT, Norris JW. Mass effect and death from severe acute stroke. *Neurology*. 1997;49:1090-1095.

76. McDonald C, Carter BS. Medical management of increased intracranial pressure after spontaneous intracerebral hemorrhage. *Neurosurg Clin North Am*. 2002;13:335-338.

77. Norris JW. Steroids may have a role in stroke therapy. *Stroke*. 2004; 35:228-229.

78. Poungvarin N. Steroids have no role in stroke therapy. *Stroke*. 2004; 35:229-230.

79. Poungvarin N, Bhoopat W, Viriyavejakul A, et al. Effects of dexamethasone in primary supratentorial intracerebral hemorrhage. *N Engl J Med*. 1987;316:1229-1233.

80. Suarez JI. Hypertonic saline for cerebral edema and elevated intracranial pressure. *Cleve Clin J Med*. 2004;71(suppl 1):S9-S13.

81. Qureshi AI, Suarez JI. Use of hypertonic saline solutions in treatment of cerebral edema and intracranial hypertension. *Crit Care Med*. 2000;28:3301-3313.

82. Tseng MY, Al-Rawi PG, Pickard JD, Rasulo FA, Kirkpatrick PJ. Effect of hypertonic saline on cerebral blood flow in poor-grade patients with subarchnoid hemorrhage. *Stroke*. 2003;34:1389-1396.

83. Manno EM, Adams RE, Derdeyn CP, Powers WJ, Diringer MN. The effects of mannitol on cerebral edema after large hemispheric cerebral infarct. *Neurology*. 1999;52:583-587.

84. Cruz J, Minoja G, Okuchi K. Major clinical and physiological benefits of early high doses of mannitol for intraparenchymal temporal lobe hemorrhages with abnormal pupillary widening: a randomized trial. *Neurosurgery*. 2002;51:628-637.

85. Bereczki D, Mihalka L, Szatmari S, et al. Mannitol use in acute stroke: case fatality at 30 days and 1 year. *Stroke*. 2003;34:1730-1735.

86. Sakamaki M, Igarashi H, Nishiyama Y, et al. Effect of glycerol on ischemic cerebral edema assessed by magnetic resonance imaging. *J Neurol Sci*. 2003;209:69-74.

171

87. Righetti E, Celani MG, Cantisani TA, Sterzi R, Boysen G, Ricci S. Glycerol for acute stroke: a Cochrane systematic review. *J Neurol.* 2002;249:445-451.

88. Greenberg J, Skubick D, Shenkin H. Acute hydrocephalus in cerebellar infarct and hemorrhage. *Neurology.* 1979;29:409-413.

89. Horwitz NH, Ludolph C. Acute obstructive hydrocephalus caused by cerebellar infarction. Treatment alternatives. *Surg Neurol.* 1983;20:13-19.

90. Schwab S, Schwarz S, Spranger M, Keller E, Bertram M, Hacke W. Moderate hypothermia in the treatment of patients with severe middle cerebral artery infarction. *Stroke.* 1998;29:2461-2466.

91. Schwab S, Spranger M, Schwarz S, Hacke W. Barbiturate coma in severe hemispheric stroke: useful or obsolete? *Neurology.* 1997;48:1608-1613.

92. Georgiadis D, Schwarz S, Aschoff A, Schwab S. Hemicraniectomy and moderate hypothermia in patients with severe ischemic stroke. *Stroke.* 2002;33:1584-1588.

93. Berrouschot J, Sterker M, Bettin S, Koster J, Schneider D. Mortality of space-occupying ('malignant') middle cerebral artery infarction under conservative intensive care. *Intensive Care Med.* 1998;24:620-623.

94. Wijdicks EF, St Louis EK, Atkinson JD, Li H. Clinician's biases toward surgery in cerebellar hematomas: an analysis of decision-making in 94 patients. *Cerebrovasc Dis.* 2000;10:93-96.

95. Chen HJ, Lee TC, Wei CP. Treatment of cerebellar infarction by decompressive suboccipital craniectomy. *Stroke.* 1992;23:957-961.

96. Mathew P, Teasdale G, Bannan A, Oluoch-Olunya D. Neurosurgical management of cerebellar haematoma and infarct. *J Neurol Neurosurg Psychiatry.* 1995;59:287-292.

97. St.Louis EK, Wijdicks EF, Li H. Predicting neurologic deterioration in patients with cerebellar hematomas. *Neurology.* 1998;51:1364-1369.

98. Yanaka K, Matsumaru Y, Nose T. Management of spontaneous cerebellar hematomas: a prospective treatment protocol. *Neurosurgery.* 2002;51:524-525.

99. Rabinstein AA, Atkinson JL, Wijdicks EF. Emergency craniotomy in patients worsening due to expanded cerebral hematoma: to what purpose? *Neurology.* 2002;58:1367-1372.

100. Juvela S, Heiskanen O, Poranen A. The treatment of spontaneous intracerebral hemorrhage. A prospective randomized trial of surgical and conservative treatment. *J Neurosurg.* 1989;70:755-758.

101. Batjer HH, Reisch JS, Allen BC, Plaizier LJ, Su CJ. Failure of surgery to improve outcome in hypertensive putaminal hemorrhage. A prospective randomized trial. *Arch Neurol.* 1990;47:1103-1106.

102. Morgenstern LB, Demchuk AM, Kim DH, Frankowski RF, Grotta JC. Rebleeding leads to poor outcome in ultra-early craniotomy for intracerebral hemorrhage. *Neurology.* 2001;56:1294-1299.

103. Zuccarello M, Brott T, Derex L, et al. Early surgical treatment for supratentorial intracerebral hemorrhage: a randomized feasibility study. *Stroke.* 1999;30:1833-1839.

104. Mendelow AD, Gregson BA, Fernandes HM, et al; STICH investigators. Early surgery versus initial conservative treatment in patients with spontaneous supratentorial intracerebral haematomas in the International Surgical Trial in Intracerebral Haemorrhage (STICH): a randomised trial. *Lancet.* 2005;365:387-397.

105. Marquardt G, Wolff R, Sager A, Janzen RW, Seifert V. Subacute stereotactic aspiration of haematomas within the basal ganglia reduces occurrence of complications in the course of haemorrhagic stroke in non-comatose patients. *Cerebrovasc Dis.* 2003;15:252-257.

106. Montes JM, Wong JH, Fayad PB, Awad IA. Stereotactic computed tomographic-guided aspiration and thrombolysis of intracerebral hematoma: protocol and preliminary experience. *Stroke.* 2000;31:834-840.

107. Doerfler A, Forsting M, Reith W, et al. Decompressive craniectomy in a rat model of "malignant" cerebral hemispheric stroke: experimental support for an aggressive therapeutic approach. *J Neurosurg.* 1996;85:853-859.

108. Carter BS, Ogilvy CS, Candia GJ, Rosas HD, Buonanno F. One-year outcome after decompressive surgery for massive nondominant hemispheric infarction. *Neurosurgery.* 1997;40:1168-1175.

109. Rieke K, Schwab S, Krieger D, et al. Decompressive surgery in space-occupying hemispheric infarction: results of an open, prospective trial. *Crit Care Med.* 1995;23:1576-1587.

110. Schwab S, Hacke W. Surgical decompression of patients with large middle cerebral artery infarcts is effective. *Stroke.* 2003;34:2304-2305.

6

7

General Management After Admission to the Hospital

Admission to the Hospital

Almost all patients with acute ischemic or hemorrhagic stroke should be hospitalized. Patients need to be observed for changes in their neurologic status. They may need continued treatment with medical interventions started in the emergency department. They may require surgery or other urgent therapies. Evaluation for the cause of stroke, rehabilitation, and initiation of therapies to prevent recurrent stroke also are needed. Approximately 10% to 20% of patients will have neurologic worsening during the first hours after stroke and the outcomes among these persons are worse than those found in patients whose condition remains stable. Deterioration may occur in patients with either hemorrhagic or ischemic stroke.

In general, those patients with the most severe neurologic impairments are at the greatest risk for deterioration or major medical or neurologic complications.[1-5] The leading causes for neurologic worsening that follows acute stroke are outlined in **Table 7.1**. Because immediate actions in response to neurologic worsening may lessen the risk of mortality or major morbidity, patients should be in the hospital and preferably in a unit that specializes in stroke care. Admission to the hospital may not be necessary if a patient did not seek medical attention for several days following a stroke. Such patients most likely will have had a mild event, and evaluation and treatment may be performed on an outpatient basis.

TABLE 7.1 — Leading Causes of Neurologic Worsening Following Acute Stroke

• Increased intracranial pressure
  – Growth of hematoma
  – Brain edema
  – Acute hydrocephalus
• Continued bleeding with enlargement of a hematoma
• Hemorrhagic transformation of an infarction
• Recurrent hemorrhage (aneurysms)
• Ischemia
  – Progression of thrombosis
  – Early recurrent embolization
  – Collateral failure
  – Secondary to vasospasm (aneurysms)
• Seizures
• Medical complications

General Management

The general management of patients with recent stroke is multifaceted. Model patient care orders for the first 24 hours are included in **Table 7.2**. Development of inpatient stroke care protocols or pathways may expedite care.[6] Overall management involves the following steps:

- Continuation of therapies begun in the emergency department
- Initiation of interventions to prevent or control medical or neurologic complications
- Treatment of serious comorbid diseases or risk factors for stroke
- Performance of an evaluation to determine the likely cause of stroke
- Develop plans for treatments to prevent recurrent stroke
- Start rehabilitation efforts to maximize recovery from the stroke

- Commence planning for discharge from the hospital and return to the community.

All of these activities take place simultaneously. However, priorities in treatment vary among patients. The patient's neurologic status and overall health affects decisions. In addition, the patient's and family's wishes should be paramount. The most important factor that affects care is the patient's neurologic status. The spectrum of neurologic deficits is broad. The types and severities of neurologic signs reflect the size and location of the brain lesion. In general, patients with hemorrhages are more seriously ill than are those with infarctions. Comatose patients and those with multiple or severe neurologic impairment also have a poor prognosis. In such cases, early care emphasizes efforts to save lives and to prevent or control potentially life-threatening complications. Rehabilitation may be the most important treatment to maximize recovery of a patient with a moderate neurologic deficit. A patient with a mild stroke usually is at low risk for serious complications and rehabilitation may not be needed; thus management focuses on the best prophylaxis for recurrent stroke.

Control and prevention of acute, subacute, and chronic medical or neurologic complications are stressed in general management.[1-7] Potential complications are numerous and generally are the same with either hemorrhagic or ischemic stroke (**Table 7.1** and **Table 7.3**). In addition, management should include therapies for serious comorbid diseases, such as heart disease or diabetes, which may affect outcomes. Symptomatic treatment includes control of complaints, such as pain, headache, nausea, or vomiting (**Table 7.2**).

TABLE 7.2 — Orders for Multidisciplinary Management and Treatment of Acute Stroke: First 24 Hours

Activity
- Bed rest/chair/ambulation with assistance/normal activity

Nursing Care
- Timing of vital signs and neurologic assessments
- Monitor oxygen levels (oximetry):
  - Give supplemental oxygen if hypoxic
- Cardiac monitor:
  - Treat serious cardiac arrhythmias
- Prevention of venous thrombosis in bedridden patients:
  - Anticoagulants
  - Compression stockings and devices
- Bladder care
- Frequent turning or change in posture and skin care
- Range-of-motion exercises

Hydration and Nutrition
- Intravenous fluids
- Swallowing assessment – bedside or fluoroscopic
- Start nasogastric feedings
- Diet as tolerated and to meet nutritional needs
- Assess for future need of enteral feedings

Medications
- Symptomatic medications
- Medications for concomitant diseases
- Continue treatment for stroke

Consultations
- Physical therapy:
  - Difficulty sitting, standing, or walking
  - Need for assistive devices for walking
- Speech pathology:
  - Difficulty swallowing or dysarthria
  - Language impairments

Continued

Consultations (continued)
  • Occupational therapy:
    – Decreased cognitive or upper extremity function
    – Need for adaptive equipment
  • Social services:
    – Discharge planning

Diagnostic Studies
  • Tests to ascertain the cause of stroke
  • Tests to monitor for medical or neurologic complications
  • Information delivery to patient and family:
    – Information about stroke and its complications
    – Treatment of stroke and plans for future care

Level of Activity

7

Most patients are treated with bed rest during the first 24 hours. Thereafter, the decision about level of activity depends upon the patient's status. Patients with mild impairments rapidly return to their prestroke activities. Those with more severe strokes likely will need a prolonged course of treatment to achieve mobilization. A reasonable goal would be to have most patients out of bed within 24 to 48 hours after hospitalization. Mobilization has a number of positive effects. Besides lowering the risk of deep vein thrombosis and pressure sores, it also helps avoid pulmonary complications, such as atelectasis or pneumonia. In addition, increasing activity also improves morale for the patient and family. Mobilization is a first step in rehabilitation and it should be accelerated as the patient's stamina and neurologic status improve. Initiating mobilization should include observation for neurologic worsening or orthostatic drops in blood pressure. If either occurs, the patient should be returned to a recumbent position. Falls also are a potential complication of early mobilization.[8] In particular, a patient with marked limb

TABLE 7.3 — Complications of Stroke

Neurologic
- Brain edema
- Hydrocephalus
- Increased intracranial pressure
- Hemorrhagic transformation of an infarction
- Recurrent hemorrhage
- Recurrent infarction
- Acute delirium
- Depression
- Seizures
- Movement disorders

Pulmonary
- Airway obstruction
- Hypoventilation
- Atelectasis
- Aspiration
- Pneumonia
- Pulmonary embolism

Cardiovascular
- Myocardial infarction
- Cardiac arrhythmias
- Congestive heart failure
- Hypertension
- Hypotension
- Deep vein thrombosis

Nutritional, Metabolic, or Gastrointestinal
- Stress ulcers
- Gastrointestinal bleeding
- Constipation
- Incontinence
- Dehydration
- Electrolyte disturbances
- Malnutrition
- Hyperglycemia
- Hypoglycemia

Continued

Urinary
• Incontinence
• Urinary tract infection

Orthopedic or Dermatologic
• Pressure sores
• Contractures
• Adhesive capsulitis
• Falls with fractures

weakness, incoordination, or poor balance is at high risk for falls with secondary fractures.

Immobilized patients should have passive or active range-of-motion exercises in order to avoid contractures or orthopedic complications. An alternating pressure, air, or water mattress may help prevent pressure sores. Frequent turning is important. Bedridden patients and those with depressed consciousness often need aggressive bronchopulmonary care. Usually vigorous suctioning is avoided in patients with subarachnoid hemorrhage (SAH) if the aneurysm has not been treated or in those with increased intracranial pressure (ICP) because transient rises in arterial or venous pressure may promote recurrent aneurysmal rupture or worsening of intracranial hypertension.

Vital Signs and General Observation

Observation of the vital signs and neurologic assessments should be checked at frequent and regular intervals during the first 24 to 48 hours after admission. The goals are to detect early medical or neurologic complications that may increase morbidity or mortality. If a patient is stable, the intervals between assessments may be extended.

Many patients are dehydrated or have volume depletion during the first hours after stroke. Water and sodium losses secondary to cerebral salt wasting or the syndrome of inappropriate secretion of antidiuretic hormone (SIADH) are especially prominent among patients with hemorrhages. Hypovolemia may result from vomiting or the use of diuretics. Efforts to control brain edema with fluid restriction or the use of mannitol may potentiate contraction of vascular volume. In patients with SAH, strict fluid restriction may increase the risk of ischemia secondary to vasospasm. A shrunken vascular volume may lead to orthostatic hypotension or decreased cerebral perfusion. Most patients initially receive intravenous infusions of fluids, most commonly normal saline, during the first 24 hours. The usual volume is 1.5 to 2 L. Monitoring the fluid status is important throughout the acute illness. The volume of fluids is adjusted to the patient's needs or fluid or electrolyte status. Supplementation of potassium or vitamins may be prescribed in selected cases.

Maintaining nutrition also is important for recovery after stroke.[9] Most patients are not given fluids or food by mouth until their ability to swallow is assessed. Dysphagia is particularly common among patients with brain stem lesions and it is most obvious among patients with dysarthria.[10] Patients with hemisphere stroke usually have less-prominent problems with swallowing. In general, patients with stroke have more difficulty swallowing liquids than solids or soft foods. Choking, nasal regurgitation, and aspiration are common. Thickening of liquids to a soft or pudding consistency is done when restarting swallowing. The diet is liberalized as the patient's condition improves. Patients with severe or persistent dysphagia may require feeding via a nasogastric tube.[11] Care must be exercised to avoid regurgitation of tube feedings with secondary aspiration pneumonia.[12] Those with prolonged dysphagia usually need placement of a percutaneous gastric feeding tube. Most people with stroke do not need intravenous hyperalimentation. The diet should reflect dietary preferences and meet the needs of the particular patient, such as restrictions of cholesterol, glucose, or sodium intake. A clinical trial found that supplementation of the diet with nutritional supplements did not reduce the risk of death or poor outcome after stroke.

The formulas used in nasogastric feedings may induce diarrhea, most probably on an osmolar basis. Reducing the concentration of formula often controls this problem. Patients with lactose intolerance also may not be able to tolerate nasogastric feedings. Some patients may experience constipation and will need stool softeners or laxatives. Fecal incontinence is relatively uncommon.

Bladder Care

Urinary incontinence often is a problem in bedridden patients and in those with depressed consciousness.[13] An indwelling bladder catheter often is inserted to facilitate nursing care and to ease measurement of urinary output. The catheter lessens the likelihood of skin irritation from a wet bed. Unfortunately, an indwelling catheter may promote development of a urinary tract infection. Acidification of the urine may help lower the risk of cystitis, but prophylactic administration of antibiotics is not done. Intermittent catheterization of the bladder may be associated with a lessening in the risk of infection. This strategy is the preferred method for treating incontinent patients. Condom catheters should not be used.

Symptomatic Treatment

Analgesics are prescribed liberally to control pain and headache. In particular, opiate analgesics are administered to patients with SAH and those with pain from arterial dissections. Usually, aspirin is avoided in those patients who have had intracranial bleeding or who have received thrombolytic agents or anticoagulants. Acetaminophen is the most commonly prescribed medication. If acetaminophen does not control pain, more potent analgesics should be prescribed. Ondansetron or other antiemetic agents may be used to treat nausea and vomiting. Agitated or combative patients may be treated with a major tranquilizer.

Treatment of Complications and Concomitant Diseases

Interventions used to control seizures, brain edema, or increased ICP started in the emergency department usually are continued (see Chapter 6 *Emergency Medical Management of Stroke*). Antibiotics, selected on the basis of results of cultures and sensitivities, are prescribed to patients who have infectious complications, most commonly pulmonary or urinary tract in origin. Any of these infections may prolong hospitalization and have a negative effect on outcome after stroke.[14] Those with intracranial bleeding are at greatest risk for stress ulcers, gastritis, or gastrointestinal hemorrhages. Antacids or histamine antagonists usually are administered to patients with recent hemorrhagic stroke. Because cimetidine may depress consciousness, ranitidine usually is prescribed if a histamine antagonist is needed. Sucralfate also may be given.

Control of hyperglycemia or hypoglycemia also should be part of treatment. Because heart disease is a leading cause of death among patients who survive the first few days after stroke, measures to control congestive heart failure or to prevent myocardial ischemia are part of care. As soon as the patient's condition is stabilized, the antihypertensive agents used prior to stroke should be restarted. Medications to treat hypercholesterolemia also are recommended.

Prevention of Deep Vein Thrombosis and Pulmonary Embolism

Pulmonary embolism accounts for approximately 10% of deaths following stroke.[15] Deep vein thrombosis in the lower extremities, which may be found in the paralyzed lower extremity in 20% to 70% of patients, is the usual source of a clot that migrates to the lung.[16] Bedridden patients are at particularly high risk. Prompt mobilization of those patients who can be out of bed is an effective strategy to lessen the risk of deep vein thrombosis. Subcutaneously administered heparin is of proven utility; the usual prophylactic regimen is 5000 units given every 12 hours (Class I Recommendation, Level of Evidence A). Low molecular weight (LMW) heparins also are effective.[17,18] The LMW heparins may be associated with a lower risk of serious bleeding than conventional heparin. Patients with pulmonary embolism or overt deep vein thrombosis usually are treated with an intravenous infusion of an anticoagulant. Oral anticoagulants are given for long-term prophylaxis against deep vein thrombosis and pulmonary embolism. Aspirin has a modest effect in forestalling deep vein thrombosis and it may be given to those patients who cannot tolerate anticoagulants.

Patients who have intracranial hemorrhage usually do not receive anticoagulants. Similarly, heparin should not be administered within 24 hours of thrombolytic treatment. Patients who cannot be treated with anticoagulants may be treated with pressure stockings and alternating pressure devices applied to the legs[19,20] (Class IIb Recommendation, Level of Evidence B). Patients who are at high risk for pulmonary embolism but who cannot receive anticoagulants also may have placation of or insertion of a filter within the inferior vena cava.

Rehabilitation

Initiation of appropriate rehabilitation therapies to assist in recovery from the stroke also is a part of the initial management in the hospital (see Chapter 12, *Rehabilitation After Stroke*). Depending upon the types and severities of neurologic impairments, individual patients should be assessed by speech pathologists, physical therapists, and occupational therapists. The rehabilitation specialists help in efforts to regain swallowing, communication, and mobility. Planning for rehabilitation after discharge from an acute care setting also is appropriate; depending upon the patient's status, this may be done in either an outpatient or inpatient setting. This planning usually involves the assistance of a social worker or another professional to help the patient and family in making decisions about long-term treatment.

REFERENCES

1. van Gijn J, Rinkel GJ. Subarachnoid haemorrhage: diagnosis, causes and management. *Brain.* 2001;124:249-278.
2. van der Worp HB, Kappelle LJ. Complications of acute ischaemic stroke. *Cerebrovasc Dis.* 1998;8:124-132.
3. Solenski NJ, Haley EC Jr, Kassell NF, et al. Medical complications of aneurysmal subarachnoid hemorrhage: a report of the multicenter, cooperative aneurysm study. Participants of the Multicenter Cooperative Aneurysm Study. *Crit Care Med.* 1995;23:1007-1017.
4. Langhorne P, Stott DJ, Robertson L, et al. Medical complications after stroke: a multicenter study. *Stroke.* 2000;31:1223-1229.
5. Roth EJ. The medical complications encountered in stroke rehabilitation. *Phys Med Rehab Clin North Am.* 1991;2:563-578.
6. Awad IA, Fayad P, Abdulrauf SI. Protocols and critical pathways for stroke care. *Clin Neurosurg.* 1999;45:86-100.
7. Kappelle LJ, van der Worp HB. Treatment or prevention of complications of acute ischemic stroke. *Curr Neurol Neurosci Rep.* 2004;4:36-41.
8. Nyberg L, Gustafson Y. Fall prediction index for patients in stroke rehabilitation. *Stroke.* 1997;28:716-721.
9. Gariballa SE, Parker SG, Taub N, Castleden CM. Influence of nutritional status on clinical outcome after acute stroke. *Am J Clin Nutr.* 1998;68:275-281.
10. Paciaroni M, Mazzotta G, Corea F, et al. Dysphagia following stroke. *Eur Neurol.* 2004;51:162-167.
11. Dziewas R, Schilling M, Konrad C, Stogbauer F, Ludemann P. Placing nasogastric tubes in stroke patients with dysphagia: efficiency and tolerability of the reflex placement. *J Neurol Neurosurg Psychiatry.* 2003;74:1429-1431.
12. Dziewas R, Ritter M, Schilling M, et al. Pneumonia in acute stroke patients fed by nasogastric tube. *J Neurol Neurosurg Psychiatry.* 2004;75:852-856.
13. Gariballa SE. Potentially treatable causes of poor outcome in acute stroke patients with urinary incontinence. *Acta Neurol Scand.* 2003;107:336-340.
14. Hilker R, Poetter C, Findeisen N, et al. Nosocomial pneumonia after acute stroke: implications for neurological intensive care medicine. *Stroke.* 2003;34:975-981.
15. Wijdicks EF, Scott JP. Pulmonary embolism associated with acute stroke. *Mayo Clin Proc.* 1997;72:297-300.
16. Gregory PC, Kuhlemeier KV. Prevalence of venous thromboembolism in acute hemorrhagic and thromboembolic stroke. *Am J Phys Med Rehabil.* 2003;82:364-369.
17. Gould MK, Dembitzer AD, Doyle RL, Hastie TJ, Garber AM. Low-molecular-weight heparins compared with unfractionated heparin for treatment of acute deep venous thrombosis. A meta-analysis of randomized, controlled trials. *Ann Intern Med.* 1999;130:800-809.
18. Hillbom M, Erila T, Sotaniemi K, Tatlisumak T, Sarna S, Kaste M. Enoxaparin vs heparin for prevention of deep-vein thrombosis in acute ischaemic stroke: a randomized, double-blind study. *Acta Neurol Scand.* 2002;106:84-92.

7

19. Mazzone C, Chiodo Grandi F, Sandercock P, Miccio M, Salvi R. Physical methods for preventing deep vein thrombosis in stroke. *Cochrane Database Syst Rev.* 2002;CD001922.
20. Kamran SI, Downey D, Ruff RL. Pneumatic sequential compression reduces the risk of deep vein thrombosis in stroke patients. *Neurology.* 1998;50:1683-1688.

8

Treatment of Hemorrhagic Stroke

Approximately 15% to 20% of strokes are secondary to nontraumatic intracranial bleeding[1] (see Chapter 3, *General Measures to Prevent Stroke* for a listing of the potential causes of hemorrhagic stroke). In general, patients with hemorrhagic stroke are more seriously ill than are those persons with acute ischemic stroke. Brain hemorrhage is second to acute myocardial ischemia as a cause of nontraumatic sudden death. The presentations of intraparenchymal hemorrhage and subarachnoid hemorrhage (SAH) are listed in **Table 4.9** and **Table 4.10** (see Chapter 4, *Diagnosis and Evaluation of Patients With Suspected Stroke).

The diagnosis of intracranial hemorrhage is expedited by the use of modern brain imaging studies—in particular, computed tomography (CT) (see Chapter 5, *Imaging of the Brain and Blood Vessels in Stroke*). Besides demonstrating bleeding in the brain or subarachnoid space, CT also visualizes acute complications, including intraventricular hemorrhage, brain edema, or hydrocephalus.[2-4] Occult trauma and cerebral contusion should be suspected if multiple petechial hemorrhages are seen in the white matter–gray matter junction in the frontal and occipital poles or the tips of the temporal lobes. The presence of extensive edema adjacent to a hematoma may point to an underlying tumor. Extensive brain edema and multiple thumbprint hemorrhages aligned along the medial aspects of the cerebral hemispheres point towards thrombosis of the superior sagittal sinus. Multiple hemorrhages may be found with a bleeding disorder. A hemorrhage with a fluid-fluid level may point to prolonged (continued) bleeding, particularly in the setting of hemorrhage complicating the use of an anticoagulant or thrombolytic agent. Occasionally, a patient with an infarction may have a secondary hemorrhagic transformation of all or part of the ischemic lesion. Examination of the cerebrospinal fluid (CSF) usually is restricted to the exceptional patient who has symptoms suggestive of SAH but who has no evidence of bleeding on CT. The utility of magnetic resonance imaging (MRI) to detect intraparenchymal hemorrhage or SAH is described in Chapter 5, *Imaging of the Brain and Blood Vessels in Stroke*.

Both MRI and CT may visualize potential explanations for a hemorrhage. For example, prominent flow voids on MRI may be found in a patient with an aneurysm or vascular malformation. The vascular pathology also may be detected with the use of magnetic resonance angiography (MRA), magnetic resonance venography (MRV), computed tomographic angiography (CTA), or arteriography (see Chapter 5, *Imaging of the Brain and Blood Vessels in Stroke*). Besides detecting an aneurysm or vascular malformation, imaging may provide findings that influence early management, including anatomic relationships or the presence of vasospasm. The latter finding often precludes early surgical treatment of a ruptured aneurysm.

Emergency Management

Many patients with serious intracranial bleeding are unconscious and may have major increases in intracranial pressure (ICP) and blood pressure.[2,5,6] During the first 24 hours, potential lifesaving measures, such as surgical evacuation of a large cerebellar hematoma that is producing a mass effect, may be needed. The blood pressure likely needs to be treated aggressively because of the risk of continued bleeding or recurrent hemorrhage. The level of blood pressure that mandates treatment has not been established but probably is lower than that for patients with ischemic stroke. Caution should be exercised about aggressive lowering of blood pressure in a patient with a massive intracranial hemorrhage with secondary intracranial hypertension.

■ Emergency Administration of Hemostatic Medications

Recently, clinical studies have tested the utility of the emergency administration of recombinant activated Factor VII (r-Factor VIIa) for treatment of patients with acute intracerebral hemorrhages.[7-10] This medication is used to control bleeding in persons with hemorrhages secondary to hemophilia. The goal of early treatment with r-Factor VIIa to stop continued bleeding and growth of the hematoma. The medication should be administered within the first 3 hours after onset of bleeding, a requirement that is similar to that required for using recombinant tissue-type plasminogen activator (rt-PA) for management of acute ischemic stroke. A late phase 2 study testing three different doses of the medication found that the agent was associated with less growth of the hematoma and improvement in the rate of favorable outcomes. The best dose of the agent has not been established. Administration of the r-Factor VIIa may be associated with thrombotic complications, including myocardial or cerebral ischemia. Additional research is under way. Although the therapy seems promising, the preferred situation for the use of this medication would be in the setting of a clinical trial (Class III Recommendation, Level of Evidence B).

■ Surgical Management of Hematomas

A clinical trial testing the utility of surgical evacuation of hemispheric hematomas did not demonstrate efficacy of operative therapy in improving outcomes[11] (see Chapter 6, *Emergency Medical Management of Stroke*).

Management of the Causes of Hemorrhagic Stroke

■ Hypertensive Hemorrhage

Brain hemorrhage complicates either chronic, sustained hypertension or an acute hypertensive crisis. Among the latter cases are women who develop eclampsia following pregnancy. The most common locations for hypertensive hemorrhage are:

- Putamen
- Thalamus
- Lobar white matter of the cerebral hemisphere
- Brain stem (pons in particular)
- Cerebellum.

These locations reflect the vascular territories of short penetrating branches (arterioles) arising from major intracranial arteries.[12-17]

Although an elevated blood pressure is found commonly among patients with acute intracranial hemorrhage, the presence of arterial hypertension alone is not sufficient for the diagnosis of hypertensive hemorrhage. Other evidence of chronic hypertension should be sought. The presence of hypertensive retinopathy, renal insufficiency, or electrocardiographic evidence of left ventricular hypertrophy would help support the diagnosis of hypertensive hemorrhage. In general, patients with strong evidence of hypertension and a hematoma deep in the brain do not need vascular imaging. In particular, hypertensive patients older than 45 years who have deep hemispheric hemorrhages do not need arteriography. The risk of recurrent hemorrhage is relatively low and the likelihood of additional bleeding within the first days after the ictus is even less.[18] Acute management focuses on treatment of the complications of the hemorrhage, including mass effect and increased

ICP. The major emphasis for long-term treatment is control of the elevated blood pressure.

■ Bleeding Diatheses

Acquired or inherited disorders of coagulation are relatively uncommon causes of brain hemorrhage. The use of antiplatelet aggregating agents, anticoagulants, or thrombolytic agents probably is the most common cause of intracranial hemorrhage secondary to a disorder of coagulation[19-26] (**Table 8.1**). Intracranial bleeding should be suspected whenever a patient who is receiving an anticoagulant, antiplatelet agent, or

TABLE 8.1 — Intracranial Hemorrhage Associated With Medications That Affect Hemostasis
Medication-Related Factors Associated With an Increased Risk of Bleeding   • Thrombolytic agents > anticoagulants > antiplatelet agents   • Combination of medications > single medication   • Excessive dose (especially for anticoagulants)   • Excessive prolongation of clotting studies
Clinical Factors That Identify an Increased Risk of Bleeding   • Age >75 years   • Recent major stroke (neurologic impairment/size of lesion on imaging)   • Ischemic stroke > myocardial ischemia > primary prevention   • Markedly elevated blood pressure   • Coexistent deficiency of coagulation factors   • Dementia (Alzheimer's disease/cerebral amyloid angiopathy)   • Poor compliance with use of medications   • Nonavailability of follow-up laboratory assessments   • Concomitant medications   • Alcohol or drug abuse   • Poor balance or incoordination

8

a thrombolytic agent develops new focal neurologic signs, headache, or altered consciousness. Inherited or acquired disorders of coagulation or thrombocytopenia also may cause intracranial hemorrhage.[27,28] These include Factor XIII deficiency, which is notable for a family history of intracranial hemorrhage and oozing from superficial wounds, severe Factor VIII deficiency, or severe Factor IX deficiency. Intracranial bleeding also may complicate leukemia or thrombocytopenia.[29-31]

The prognosis of patients with hemorrhage secondary to bleeding diatheses generally is poorer than that of patients with intracranial bleeding secondary to other causes. Progression of the size of the hematoma and neurologic worsening may occur.[32] However, identification of the hemostatic defect may permit rapid institution of appropriately directed antidotal therapy.

Intracranial hemorrhage is the most frequent fatal complication of the long-term use of oral anticoagulants.[22,23] Both intraparenchymal and subdural hematomas may occur. The risks of bleeding seem to be greatest among elderly patients and those who are taking an anticoagulant to prevent recurrent stroke. Patients with poorly controlled hypertension, poor balance, or poor coordination also have a high risk of bleeding. A major factor predicting hemorrhagic complications is excessive prolongation of the international normalized ratio (INR). The implementation of the INR, which compensates for differences between institutions, has improved the monitoring of the level of anticoagulation and should lessen the risk of major bleeding complications. Long-term prescription of antiplatelet agents in primary or secondary prevention of stroke may be associated with an increased risk of bleeding complications, including intracranial hemorrhage. Overall, the risk of symptomatic intracranial hemorrhage complicating the use of aspirin, clopidogrel, or aspirin/dipyridamole appears to be low and less than that associated with oral anticoagulants.[26] The combination of aspirin and clopidogrel appears to be associated with a higher risk of bleeding than prescription of a single medication.[33]

Symptomatic hemorrhagic transformation of the infarction or primary intracranial hemorrhage is a potential complication of the early administration of heparin or low molecular weight heparins for treatment of acute ischemic stroke.[34-37] Bleeding risks are highest among those patients with large infarctions.[38] The risk of bleeding complications with the administration of aspirin started within 48 hours of acute ischemic stroke is relatively low.[34,35] The potential for an increased risk of bleeding complications is one of the reasons that patients are not prescribed either anticoagulants or antiplatelet agents following thrombolytic treatment.[39,40] The use of thrombolytic agents for management of acute ischemic stroke is accompanied by an increased risk of transformation of the infarction or de novo intracranial hemorrhage.[25,41]

If intracranial hemorrhage is diagnosed, emergency assessment of coagulation studies should be performed; at a minimum, the following tests should be done:

- Prothrombin time/INR
- Activated partial thromboplastin time
- Platelet count.

Additional tests of coagulation may be needed if a bleeding diathesis is suspected to be the cause of hemorrhage. In addition, typing and cross-matching of blood should be performed immediately to allow rapid availability of specific blood products that may be given to ameliorate or reverse coagulopathy. The hemostatic defect should be corrected before invasive procedures, including surgery, are performed.[42] The administration of antidotes is prescribed on the basis of the level of prolongation of the specific coagulation tests (**Table 8.2**). Close observation of the coagulation tests and repeated administration of antidotes, blood

TABLE 8.2 — Treatment of Coagulation Abnormalities Associated With Hemorrhagic Stroke

Oral Anticoagulants
- Stop medication
- Choices for antidote:
  - Intravenously administer 1 to 10 mg vitamin K (administer slowly because of risk of anaphylaxis)
  - Intravenously administer 2 to 3 units fresh frozen plasma or factor concentrates to replace Factors II, VII, IX, X
- The PT will respond to restoration of Factor VII but the effects on Factor II may persist for up to 3 days
- Recheck PT in 6 hours, and if necessary, repeat administration of fresh frozen plasma or factor concentrates
- Monitor patient's cardiopulmonary status during transfusions

Heparin
- Stop medication
- Slow intravenous infusion of 30 mg protamine sulfate
- Monitor aPTT
- Excessive protamine sulfate may cause anticoagulation

Thrombolytic Agents
- Stop medication
- Check hematocrit, PT, aPTT, platelet count, and fibrinogen
- Type and cross-match 4 units blood
- Give 4 to 6 units cryoprecipitate to raise fibrinogen level to >150 mg/dL
- Recheck fibrinogen level every 4 hours
- Transfuse with cryoprecipitate to maintain fibrinogen level to >150 mg/dL

Antiplatelet Agents
- Stop medication
- Give transfusion of platelets

Abbreviations: aPTT, activated partial thromboplastin time; PT, prothrombin time.

products, and/or specific coagulation factors are recommended (Class I Recommendation, Level of Evidence B).

■ Tumors

Intracranial hemorrhage may be the initial manifestation of a primary or metastatic tumor of the brain.[43,44] While bleeding may complicate any brain tumor, those neoplasms that are highly vascular are most prone to bleeding. The primary and metastatic brain tumors that most commonly lead to hemorrhage are:

- Glioblastoma multiforme
- Hemangioblastoma of the cerebellum
- Carcinoma of the lung
- Renal cell carcinoma
- Choriocarcinoma
- Melanoma
- Thyroid carcinoma.

Often patients with neoplastic brain hemorrhages have a history of subtle or progressive neurologic disturbances (eg, personality changes, headache, or gradually appearing/waxing and waning focal neurologic signs) that evolve in the days or weeks before the hemorrhage. The CT finding of prominent edema surrounding a focal hemorrhage, particularly in the gray-white matter junction of the cerebral hemisphere, also points to an underlying brain tumor. Treatment of hemorrhage secondary to a tumor focuses on management of the underlying malignancy.

■ Vasculitis

Isolated central nervous system vasculitis and multisystem vasculitides, especially periarteritis nodosa, are unusual causes of intraparenchymal hemorrhage.[45,46] A vasculitis may be suspected when the patient has other clinical evidence of a multisystem inflammatory vasculopathy or laboratory abnormalities, such as an elevated erythrocyte sedimentation rate or a C-reactive protein. A history of waxing and waning neurologic impairments, cognitive changes, or headache in the weeks before the hemorrhage may provide a clue that a vasculitis is present. Brain imaging may show multifocal lesions that are hemorrhagic or ischemic. Arteriography may reveal segmental areas of narrowing in multiple intracranial arteries in approximately 50% of cases. Often, brain biopsy is required to establish a diagnosis, but the possibility of a false-negative result is high because of the disseminated and segmental nature of the inflammatory vasculopathy. Treatment of patients with hemorrhage secondary to a vasculitis primarily involves the use of corticosteroids and immunosuppressive agents (Class I Recommendation, Level of Evidence B).

■ Drug Abuse

Cocaine, amphetamines, and other stimulants that may be abused have been associated with brain hemorrhage, especially among adolescents and young adults.[47-55] Bleeding may be secondary to an acute hypertensive reaction to these drugs' sympathomimetic effects. Some of these agents may cause a vasculopathy or vasculitis. The acute hypertensive effects of the drugs also may predispose to rupture of an aneurysm or vascular malformation. Bleeding may be associated with single exposure to a drug. Management centers on treatment of the arterial hypertension and avoiding additional exposure to the drug.

Intracranial hemorrhage also has been associated with the use of phenylpropanolamine, a sympathomimetic agent used to relieve associated with upper respiratory tract infections or to suppress the appetite. The risk of bleeding seems to be greatest among young women taking the medication as a weight-loss aid.[56] The medication was removed from the American market because of the potential association with hemorrhagic stroke.

■ Cerebral Amyloid Angiopathy

Cerebral amyloid angiopathy (congophilic angiopathy) is a leading cause of intracerebral hemorrhage in elderly persons, particularly those who have Alzheimer's disease.[57-60] The presence of cerebral amyloid angiopathy may partially explain the high risk of hemorrhage following the use of thrombolytic agents or anticoagulants in persons older than 75 years. There has been a suggestion to screen elderly patients with a gradient-echo MRI to look for small microhemorrhages that are often found in patients with amyloid angiopathy. Patients with several of these lesions would not be treated. The utility of this strategy has not been tested. The most common locations for hemorrhages are at the gray matter–white matter junction in the frontal or parieto-occipital lobes. Hemorrhages in the basal ganglia or thalamus are uncommon. Although rare, cases of hemorrhage in the pons or cerebellum have been attributed to amyloid angiopathy. Patients with cerebral amyloid angiopathy are at high risk for recurrent brain hemorrhages. Although the diagnosis is inferred by the presence of lobar hemorrhages in the cerebral hemisphere in elderly patients, brain biopsy is required for definitive diagnosis. However, because surgery may aggravate the bleeding, it generally is avoided.

■ Venous Thrombosis With Secondary Hemorrhagic Infarction

Venous thrombosis is a relatively uncommon cause of intracranial hemorrhage.[61] Because venous thrombosis often is a less acute illness than acute brain ischemia secondary to arterial occlusion or hemorrhages of other causes, the condition may not be considered. Venous thrombosis most commonly develops in association with one of the following conditions:

- Pregnancy or puerperium
- Dehydration

- Recent surgery
- Sepsis
- Cancer
- Chemotherapy
- Inherited or acquired hypercoagulable disease.

Thrombosis of the superior sagittal sinus or the superficial cortical veins may be associated with brain hemorrhage that results from stagnation of venous blood with secondary rupture of capillaries. The clinical findings, course, and prognosis of venous thrombosis have been the subject of considerable recent study.[62-65] The most common clinical findings include:
- Progressively worsening headaches
- Decreased consciousness
- Encephalopathy
- Seizures
- Papilledema
- Paraparesis or bladder incontinence (superior sagittal sinus)
- Hemiparesis (cortical vein).

While cavernous sinus thrombosis most commonly complicates infections of the face and head, it is a potentially life-threatening disease. It should be suspected if a patient has rapidly evolving ophthalmologic and facial signs including:
- Orbital edema
- Chemosis and proptosis
- Complete external and internal ophthalmoplegia
- Blindness
- Altered alertness.

These signs may be unilateral at first but rapidly become bilateral.

Modern brain imaging has expedited the diagnosis of venous thrombosis; the most common findings are:

- Focal areas of brain edema—particularly in parasagittal locations
- Parasagittal thumbprint hemorrhages
- Clots in the venous sinus (empty delta sign with contrast)
- Absence of flow voids in sinuses or clots detected on MRI.

The best diagnostic study is the MRV.[66,67] The test will demonstrate the clot and an absence of flow in the affected vein. Patients with venous thrombosis should have treatment to local ICP, although dehydration should be avoided. Despite the presence of hemorrhage, anticoagulants are the most prescribed medications[68-70] (Class IIa Recommendation, Level of Evidence B). The goals are to restore venous vascular patency and to prevent propagation of the thrombus. Local administration of thrombolytic agents or endovascular procedures also have been used to treat extensive intravenous thrombosis.[71,72] Experience with these techniques is limited. These interventions usually are not prescribed if the patient has extensive bleeding.

■ **Vascular Malformations**

Vascular malformations may lead to hemorrhage in any location in the brain. The pathologic classification of these lesions includes:
- Arteriovenous malformation
- Venous malformation
- Cavernous malformation
- Telangiectasis.

Intraparenchymal hemorrhage is most commonly associated with an arteriovenous malformation.[73] The risk of bleeding seems to be less with either venous or cavernous malformations, presumably because these lesions do not have an arterial component. A ruptured telangiectasis, which is obliterated at the time of hemorrhage, is a potential cause of an otherwise unexplained intraparenchymal hematoma. Vascular malformations may cause hemorrhage in persons of any age. However, other causes of intraparenchymal hemorrhage are relatively uncommon in children and young adults so as a result, vascular malformations are particularly important in these age groups. Besides hemorrhages, vascular malformations also may cause recurrent, migrainelike headaches or seizures.[74,75] Large, high-flow vascular malformations may produce a cranial or cervical bruit. Occasionally, patients may have progressive worsening of neurologic impairments secondary to ischemia, presumably due to a steal phenomenon. Vascular malformations, other than telangiectasis, often are detected by MRI or contrast-enhanced CT; the finding of serpiginous vessels is highly suggestive of the lesion. MRA, CTA, or arteriography also may be performed to define the vascular malformation, including the size of the lesion and the number and types of feeding arteries and draining veins. Vascular imaging may not visualize the vascular pathology in patients with cavernous or venous malformations that have low flow.

Unless the hematoma is causing signs of increased ICP, surgery usually is delayed.[76] Vascular malformations that are located in eloquent areas of the brain, that are >3 cm in diameter, or that have a large number of feeding or draining vessels usually are not treated operatively.[77] Staging surgical procedures or combining the operation with embolization sometimes is advised when a large malformation is detected.[78,79] Surgical resection of a high-flow vascular malformation may be complicated by hemodynamic disturbances that lead to hyperperfusion syndrome or brain hemorrhage. Some vascular malformations are treated with endovascular procedures.[80] Focused radiation therapy is a potential alternative treatment for management of smaller vascular malformations, especially those located deep in the cerebral hemispheres or brain stem.[81-83] However, focused irradiation does not decrease the risk of hemorrhage during the first 2 years after treatment. This interval corresponds to the presumed sclerosis of the vessels induced by the delayed effects of the irradiation.

■ Nonsaccular Aneurysms

Nonsaccular aneurysms are rare causes of hemorrhage. Fusiform (dolichoectatic) aneurysms usually cause compression of adjacent neurologic structures (most commonly the brain stem or cranial nerves) or brain ischemia. Hemorrhage is uncommon.[84,85] Because a dolichoectatic aneurysm usually is >2.5 cm in diameter and most commonly elongates the basilar artery, both CT and MRI will visualize the vascular lesion. Arteriography usually is not necessary. No specific treatment is available. Surgery may be difficult because of the location and size of the aneurysm and the presence of several penetrating arterioles arising from the diseased segment.

Intracranial aneurysms also may complicate trauma or infective endocarditis.[86,87] Rarely, aneurysms may be secondary to metastatic spread of tumors, such as a left atrial myxoma.[88] These lesions usually are small and located on peripheral (branch cortical) arteries. The risk of bleeding is high. An intracranial aneurysm is especially ominous in a patient with infective endocarditis. Surgical or endovascular treatment of the aneurysm may be necessary and the potential for rupture of these lesions is a reason why anticoagulants are not prescribed to patients with ischemic stroke secondary to infective endocarditis.

Subarachnoid hemorrhage (SAH) also may result from a traumatic or spontaneous dissecting aneurysm of an intracranial artery.[89,90] The most common locations are:

- Distal segment of the vertebral artery
- Proximal segment of the middle cerebral artery
- Basilar artery.

The prognosis for patients with SAH generally is poor. Interventional techniques that lead to the obliteration of the aneurysm may be performed.

■ Saccular Aneurysms and Subarachnoid Hemorrhage

Approximately 75% to 80% of cases of spontaneous SAH are secondary to rupture of a saccular aneurysm. Approximately 30,000 people in North America have a ruptured aneurysm. The natural history of aneurysmal SAH remains poor; approximately 10% of cases die before they may reach medical attention. Overall, approximately 40% of patients with SAH succumb within 3 months and approximately 50% of survivors have neurologic sequelae.[91-93] The leading causes of death and disability after SAH are:

- Effects of the initial hemorrhage
- Recurrent aneurysmal rupture and hemorrhage
- Vasospasm causing ischemic stroke.

The evaluation of patients with suspected SAH is outlined in Chapter 4, *Diagnosis and Evaluation of Patients with Suspected Stroke* and Chapter 5, *Imaging of the Brain and Blood Vessels in Stroke.* CT is the key diagnostic test and CSF examination is reserved for those cases that have a negative CT study. While previously arteriography was the vascular imaging study of choice, now CTA is being used more frequently. Tests to assess for complications, such as hyponatremia, also are ordered. In addition, sequential studies of blood flow, most commonly through the use of transcranial Doppler (TCD) ultrasonography, are done to monitor for the development of vasospasm.[94]

Management of patients with aneurysmal SAH is complex[2,3,95] (**Table 8.3** and **Table 8.4**). Transfer of a patient to a center that has expertise in management of SAH is recommended. In particular, the availability of a neurosurgeon or interventional specialist, who has

TABLE 8.3 — Management of Aneurysmal Subarachnoid Hemorrhage

General and Symptomatic Treatment
- Bed rest in a quiet environment
- Cardiac monitoring and frequent assessment of vital signs
- Soft diet for alert patients
- Nasogastric feedings if consciousness is depressed
- Stool softener
- Analgesics, including opiates, for headache
- Avoid aspirin and nonsteroidal anti-inflammatory agents
- Antiemetics
- Sedatives if agitated
- Anticonvulsants

Treat Increased Intracranial Pressure and Hydrocephalus

Measures to Lessen the Risk of Early Recurrent Hemorrhage
- Antihypertensive medications
- Antifibrinolytic agents
- Surgical clipping of the aneurysm
- Endovascular treatment (coiling/balloons)
- Trapping or wrapping of the aneurysm

experience in operative or endovascular treatment of aneurysms, is paramount.

Prevention of Rebleeding

Rebleeding and ischemia are among the leading causes of neurologic worsening.[96,97] The chance of a second hemorrhage is greatest within the first 24 hours after SAH, when approximately 4% of patients have recurrent rupture.[98,99] Overall, the risk of rebleeding within 10 days is approximately 20%. Recurrent hemorrhage often is fatal. The most effective measures to prevent rebleeding are operative clipping of the aneurysm or endovascular occlusion. Most patients are treated as soon as their condition is stable. Surgery within the first 3 days after SAH often is performed;

TABLE 8.4 — Treatment to Prevent Vasospasm and Ischemic Stroke After Aneurysmal Subarachnoid Hemorrhage

- Treat dehydration and hyponatremia:
  - Avoid fluid restriction
  - Administer intravenous fluids containing sodium
- Nimodipine 60 mg by mouth or nasogastric tube every 4 hours
- Check blood flow with transcranial Doppler ultrasonography every 2 days:
  - If an increase in flow velocity or if ischemic symptoms appear
  - Stop antihypertensive medications
- Hypervolemic hemodilution and induced hypertension:
  - Solutions
    - Plasmanate
    - Albumin
  - Monitor cardiac output:
    - Central venous pressure catheter (<10 mm Hg)
    - Pulmonary artery wedge pressure catheter (<18 to 20 mm Hg)
  - Atropine 1 mg every 3 to 4 hours
  - Vasopressors:
    - Dopamine titrated to increases in arterial pressure
- If no response, consider angioplasty

this recommendation is based on the results of nonrandomized clinical studies.[100-103] However, if the patient does not seek medical attention or if the diagnosis is not made rapidly, this time window may be missed. Surgical clipping of an aneurysm may not be feasible in patients who arrive at the hospital late because of the development of vasospasm and the potential for ischemic complications. In addition, some patients are too unstable neurologically or there are findings that may preclude early operation.

Interventional techniques, including placement of coils or balloons to occlude the aneurysmal lumen of the parent artery, are alternative therapies to prevent rebleeding[104-109] (**Figure 8**.1). A large trial compared the utility of endovascular treatment or operative clipping of a recently ruptured aneurysm.[110] Mortality at 1 year was 23.7% among those having endovascular treatment and 30.6% among patients having operative clipping. While the results of this trial may have some limitations, it does suggest that endovascular treatment has a rapidly enlarging role in the treatment of patients with ruptured aneurysms. In particular, endovascular treatment appears to be the primary treatment option for aneurysms at difficult sites, such as the bifurcation of the basilar artery (Class I Recommendation, Level of Evidence B).

Medical measures aimed at preventing rebleeding, including drug-induced hypotension, largely have been abandoned. While antifibrinolytic agents are effective in lowering the risk for recurrent hemorrhage, these medications do not improve outcomes largely as a result of a high-risk of ischemic stroke.[111,112] Even the concomitant administration of nimodipine does not eliminate the risk of ischemic complications. As a result, antifibrinolytic agents are not recommended for treatment of most patients with recent SAH (Class III Recommendation, Level of Evidence A).

Vasospasm and Secondary Cerebral Ischemia

Approximately 70% of patients may develop vasospasm (a localized or diffuse segmental narrowing of the major arteries at the base of the brain) within 7 to 10 days of SAH.[2,113-116] Approximately one half of these patients will have ischemic symptoms. Vasospasm peaks at approximately 1 week and usually resolves over the next 7 to 14 days.[114,117] Patients with thick focal or diffuse collections of blood found on CT are at highest risk for this complication.[118,119] The cause of vasospasm has not been established; presumably, it is the result of the release of biologically active

FIGURE 8.1 — Digital Subtraction Angiography After Subarachnoid Hemorrhage and the Effect of Coil Embolization

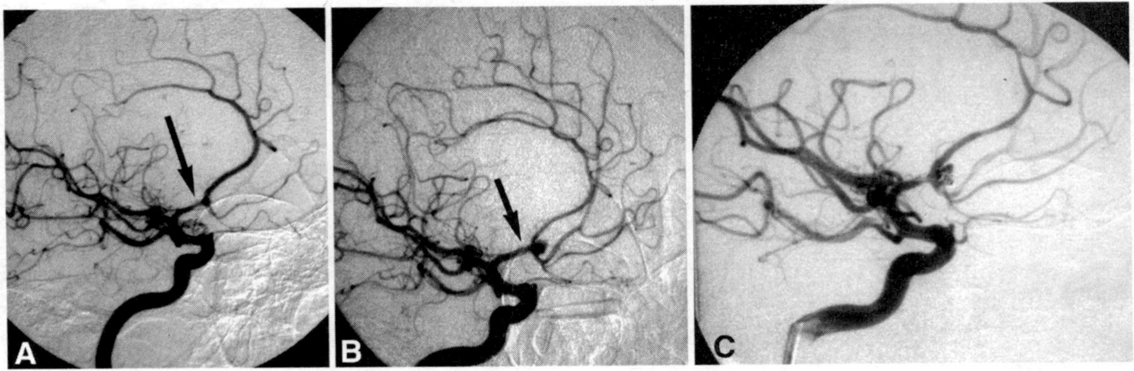

A. Digital subtraction angiography (DSA) (oblique view) after contrast injection into the right internal carotid artery shows a slight vasospasm (*arrow*) of the right A1 segment of the anterior cerebral artery (ACA) 1 day after subarachnoid hemorrhage (SAH). No aneurysm was found.

B. Repetition of DSA 3 days later revealed an aneurysm of the ACA. The vasospasm has disappeared (*arrow*).

C. Treatment of the aneurysm with electrolytically detachable coils. DSA after the detachment of the first coil. Note the guide catheter in the internal carotid artery and the microcatheter passing through the guide with its tip in the aneurysm.

D. DSA after the placement of six coils into the aneurysm. The aneurysm is almost completely occluded.

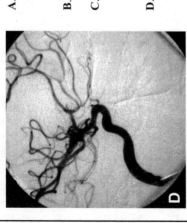

8

209

substances into the subarachnoid space at the time of hemorrhage.[113] The substances induce a sustained arterial contraction and thickening of the arterial wall with constriction of the lumen. The following symptoms usually appear slowly, and they may wax and wane:

- New or increasing headache
- Decline in consciousness
- New or increasing focal neurologic impairment
- Most commonly in territories of anterior or middle cerebral arteries.

The differential diagnosis of vasospasm includes those causes of neurologic worsening that occur during the first 1 to 2 weeks after SAH.[96] The alternative diagnoses include:

- Recurrent hemorrhage
- Brain edema and increased ICP
- Seizures
- Subacute hydrocephalus
- Electrolyte disturbances, most commonly hyponatremia
- Medical complications, such as pneumonia
- Complications of medical therapies
- Complications of surgical or endovascular interventions.

Increases in flow velocities in the major arteries as detected by TCD examination often precede the appearance of the neurologic abnormalities.[94,120] Sequential studies may be used to monitor a patient during the first 2 weeks after SAH, and if changes in flow velocities are detected, more aggressive measures to prevent ischemia may be started.

Treatment involves therapies to prevent or lessen the severity of the vasospasm and therapies to limit brain ischemia[121] (**Table 8.4**). Several interventions have been tested, but very few of these have been successful. Lavage of the subarachnoid space, often with concomitant intrathecal administration of thrombolytic agents, to remove clots at the time of operative clipping has been used, but evidence of effectiveness is lacking. Nimodipine is established as a useful adjunct to prevent ischemia secondary to vasospasm.[121-124] It is recommended for treatment of patients with aneurysmal SAH[2,95] (Class I Recommendation, Level of Evidence A). Nimodipine is started as soon as the diagnosis of SAH is made and is administered in a dose of 60 mg every 6 hours until 14 to 21 days after the ictus.

If signs or symptoms of ischemia appear, hypervolemic hemodilution and induced hypertension (triple-H therapy) often are prescribed to improve blood flow by lowering viscosity and improving perfusion pressure.[121,125-127] This regimen may increase the risk of recurrent hemorrhage if the aneurysm has not been occluded by surgery or coiling. Triple-H therapy is rigorous and requires close observation and cardiovascular monitoring (**Table 8.4**). The most serious potential complications are:

- Acute myocardial ischemia
- Congestive heart failure
- Acute pulmonary edema.

While intra-arterial administration of papaverine showed promise, enthusiasm for this intervention has waned. Patients with refractory vasospasm and increasing ischemic symptoms also may be treated with angioplasty.[128,129] There is a potential risk from the interventional approach, including arterial rupture, but it may be performed if a patient is not responding to other measures.

REFERENCES

1. Qureshi AI, Tuhrim S, Broderick JP, Batjer HH, Hondo H, Hanley DF. Spontaneous intracerebral hemorrhage. *N Engl J Med.* 2001;344:1450-1460.

2. Mayberg MR, Batjer HH, Dacey R, et al. Guidelines for the management of aneurysmal subarachnoid hemorrhage. A statement for healthcare professionals from a special writing group of the Stroke Council, American Heart Association. *Circulation.* 1994;90:2592-2605.

3. van Gijn J, Rinkel GJ. Subarachnoid haemorrhage: diagnosis, causes and management. *Brain.* 2001;124:249-278.

4. Vermeulen M, van Gijn J. The diagnosis of subarachnoid hemorrhage. *J Neurol Neurosurg Psychiatry.* 1990;53:365-372.

5. Broderick JP, Adams HP, Jr, Barsan W, et al. Guidelines for the management of spontaneous intracerebral hemorrhage: A statement for healthcare professionals from a special writing group of the Stroke Council, American Heart Association. *Stroke.* 1999;30:905-915.

6. Broderick JP. Guidelines for medical care and treatment of blood pressure in patients with acute stroke. In: National Institute of Neurological Disorders and Stroke, ed. Proceedings of a National Symposium on Rapid Identification and Treatment of Acute Stroke. Bethesda, Md: 1997:63-68.

7. Mayer SA, Brun NC, Broderick J, et al; Europe/AustralAsia NovoSeven ICH Trial Investigators. Safety and feasibility of recombinant factor VIIa for acute intracerebral hemorrhage. *Stroke.* 2005;36:74-79.

8. Mayer SA, Brun NC, Begtrup K, et al; Recombinant Activated Factor VII Intracerebral Hemorrhage Trial Investigators. Recombinant activated factor VII for acute intracerebral hemorrhage. *N Engl J Med.* 2005;352:777-785.

9. Mayer SA, Brun NC, Broderick J, et al; Europe/AustralAsia NovoSeven ICH Trial Investigators. Safety and feasibility of recombinant factor VIIa for acute intracerebral hemorrhage. *Stroke.* 2005;36:74-79.

10. Kase CS. Hemostatic treatment in the early stage of intracerebral hemorrhage: the recombinant factor VIIa experience. *Stroke.* 2005;36:2321-2322.

11. Mendelow AD, Gregson BA, Fernandes HM, et al; STICH investigators. Early surgery versus initial conservative treatment in patients with spontaneous supratentorial intracerebral haematomas in the International Surgical Trial in Intracerebral Haemorrhage (STICH): a randomised trial. *Lancet.* 2005;365:387-397.

12. St.Louis EK, Wijdicks EF, Li H. Predicting neurologic deterioration in patients with cerebellar hematomas. *Neurology.* 1998;51:1364-1369.

13. Chung CS, Caplan LR, Han W, Pessin MS, Lee KH, Kim JM. Thalamic hemorrhage. *Brain.* 1996;119:1873-1886.

14. Chung CS, Caplan LR, Yamamoto Y, et al. Striatocapsular haemorrhage. *Brain.* 2000;123:1850-1862.

15. Fisher CM, Picard EH, Polak A, Dalal P, Pojemann RG. Acute hypertensive cerebellar hemorrhage: diagnosis and surgical treatment. *J Nerv Ment Dis.* 1965;140:38-57.

16. Kumral E, Evyapan D, Balkir K. Acute caudate vascular lesions. *Stroke.* 1999;30:100-108.

17. Kumral E, Kocaer T, Ertubey NO, Kimral K. Thalamic hemorrhage. A prospective study of 100 patients. *Stroke.* 1995;26:964-970.

18. Bae H, Jeong D, Doh J, Lee K, Yun I, Byun B. Recurrence of bleeding in patients with hypertensive intracerebral hemorrhage. *Cerebrovasc Dis*. 1999;9:102-108.

19. Wong KS, Mok V, Lam WW, et al. Aspirin-associated intracerebral hemorrhage: clinical and radiologic features. *Neurology*. 2000;54:2298-2301.

20. He J, Whelton PK, Vu B, Klag MJ. Aspirin and risk of hemorrhagic stroke: a meta-analysis of randomized controlled trials. *JAMA*. 1998;280:1930-1935.

21. Hart RG, Benavente O, Pearce LA. Increased risk of intracranial hemorrhage when aspirin is combined with warfarin: A meta-analysis and hypothesis. *Cerebrovasc Dis*. 1999;9:215-217.

22. Fihn SD, Callahan CM, Martin DC, McDonell MB, Henikoff JG, White RH. The risk for and severity of bleeding complications in elderly patients treated with warfarin. The National Consortium of Anticoagulation Clinics. *Ann Intern Med*. 1996;124:970-979.

23. Gorter JW. Major bleeding during anticoagulation after cerebral ischemia: patterns and risk factors. Stroke Prevention In Reversible Ischemia Trial (SPIRIT). European Atrial Fibrillation Trial (EAFT) study groups. *Neurology*. 1999;53:1319-1327.

24. Patel SC, Mody A. Cerebral hemorrhagic complications of thrombolytic therapy. *Prog Cardiovasc Dis*. 1999;42:217-233.

25. Intracerebral hemorrhage after intravenous t-PA therapy for ischemic stroke. The NINDS t-PA Stroke Study Group. *Stroke*. 1997;28:2109-2118.

26. Gorelick PB, Weisman SM. Risk of hemorrhagic stroke with aspirin use: an update. *Stroke*. 2005;36:1801-1807.

27. Almaani WS, Awidi AS. Spontaneous intracranial bleeding in hemorrhagic diathesis. *Surg Neurol*. 1982;17:137-140.

28. Cahill MR, Colvin BT. Haemophilia. *Postgrad Med J*. 1997;73:201-206.

29. Lee MS, Kim WC. Intracranial hemorrhage associated with idiopathic thrombocytopenic purpura: report of seven patients and a meta-analysis. *Neurology*. 1998;50:1160-1163.

30. Graus F, Rogers LR, Posner JB. Cerebrovascular complications in patients with cancer. *Medicine*. 1985;64:16-35.

31. Jackson N, Reddy SC, Harun MH, Quah SH, Low HC. Macular haemorrhage in adult acute leukaemia patients at presentation and the risk of subsequent intracranial haemorrhage. *Br J Haematol*. 1997;98:204-209.

32. Yasaka M, Minematsu K, Naritomi H, Sakata T, Yamaguchi T. Predisposing factors for enlargement of intracerebral hemorrhage in patients treated with warfarin. *Thromb Haemost*. 2003;89:278-283.

33. Diener HC, Bogousslavsky J, Brass LM, et al; MATCH investigators. Aspirin and clopidogrel compared with clopidogrel alone after recent ischaemic stroke or transient ischaemic attack in high-risk patients (MATCH): randomised, double-blind, placebo-controlled trial. *Lancet*. 2004;364:331-337.

34. The International Stroke Trial (IST): a randomised trial of aspirin, subcutaneous heparin, both, or neither among 19435 patients with acute ischaemic stroke. International Stroke Trial Collaborative Group. *Lancet*. 1997;349:1569-1581.

35. CAST: randomised placebo-controlled trial of early aspirin use in 20,000 patients with acute ischaemic stroke. CAST (Chinese Acute Stroke Trial) Collaborative Group. *Lancet*. 1997;349:1641-1649.

8

36. Adams HP Jr, Bendixen BH, Leira E, et al. Antithrombotic treatment of ischemic stroke among patients with occlusion or severe stenosis of the internal carotid artery: a report of the Trial of Org 10172 in Acute Stroke Treatment (TOAST). *Neurology*. 1999;53:122-125.

37. Bath P. Anticoagulants and antiplatelet agents in acute ischaemic stroke. *Lancet Neurol*. 2002;1:405.

38. Low molecular weight heparinoid, ORG 10172 (danaparoid), and outcome after acute ischemic stroke: a randomized controlled trial. The Publications Committee for the Trial of ORG 10172 in Acute Stroke Treatment (TOAST) Investigators. *JAMA*. 1998;279:1265-1272.

39. Adams HP Jr, Adams RJ, Brott T, et al. Guidelines for the early management of patients with ischemic stroke. A scientific statement from the Stroke Council of the American Stroke Association. *Stroke*. 2003;34:1056-1083.

40. Adams H, Adams R, del Zoppo G, Goldstein LB; Stroke Council of the American Heart Association; American Stroke Association. Guidelines for the early management of patients with ischemic stroke: 2005 guidelines update a scientific statement from the Stroke Council of the American Heart Association/American Stroke Association. *Stroke*. 2005;36:916-923.

41. Thrombolytic therapy with streptokinase in acute ischemic stroke. The Multicenter Acute Stroke Trial–Europe Study Group. *N Engl J Med*. 1996;335:145-150.

42. Mayer SA. Ultra-early hemostatic therapy for intracerebral hemorrhage. *Stroke*. 2003;34:224-229.

43. Wakai S, Yamakawa K, Manaka S, Takakura K. Spontaneous intracranial hemorrhage caused by brain tumor: its incidence and clinical significance. *Neurosurgery*. 1982;10:437-444.

44. Mandybur TI. Intracranial hemorrhage caused by metastatic tumors. *Neurology*. 1977;27:650-655.

45. Biller J, Loftus CM, Moore SA, Schelper RL, Danks KR, Cornell SH. Isolated central nervous system angiitis first presenting as spontaneous intracranial hemorrhage. *Neurosurgery*. 1987;20:310-315.

46. Liou HH, Liu HM, Chiang IP, Yeh TS, Chen RC. Churg-Strauss syndrome presented as multiple intracerebral hemorrhage. *Lupus*. 1997;6:279-282.

47. Perez JA Jr, Arsura EL, Strategos S. Methamphetamine-related stroke: four cases. *J Emerg Med*. 1999;17:469-471.

48. Karch SB. Use of Ephedra-containing products and risk for hemorrhagic stroke. *Neurology*. 2003;61:724-725.

49. Karch SB, Stephens BG, Ho CH. Methamphetamine-related deaths in San Francisco: demographic, pathologic, and toxicologic profiles. *J Forensic Sci*. 1999;44:359-368.

50. Fessler RD, Esshaki CM, Stankewitz RC, Johnson RR, Diaz FG. The neurovascular complications of cocaine. *Surg Neurol*. 1997;47:339-345.

51. Aggarwal SK, Williams V, Levine SR, Cassin BJ, Garcia JH. Cocaine-associated intracranial hemorrhage: absence of vasculitis in 14 cases. *Neurology*. 1996;46:1741-1743.

52. Levine SR, Brust JC, Futrell N, et al. A comparative study of the cerebrovascular complications of cocaine: alkaloidal versus hydrochloride–a review. *Neurology*. 1991;41:1173-1177.

53. Levine SR, Brust JC, Futrell N, et al. Cerebrovascular complications of the use of the "crack" form of alkaloidal cocaine. *N Engl J Med*. 1990;323:699-704.

54. Morgenstern LB, Viscoli CM, Kernan WN, et al. Use of Ephedra-containing products and risk for hemorrhagic stroke. *Neurology*. 2003;60:132-135.

55. Feldmann E, Broderick JP, Kernan WN, et al. Major risk factors for intracerebral hemorrhage in the young are modifiable. *Stroke*. 2005;36:1881-1885.

56. Kernan WN, Viscoli CM, Brass LM, et al. Phenylpropanolamine and the risk of hemorrhagic stroke. *N Engl J Med*. 2000;343:1826-1832.

57. Yamada M, Itoh Y, Otomo E, Hayakawa M, Miyatake T. Subarachnoid haemorrhage in the elderly: a necropsy study of the association with cerebral amyloid angiopathy. *J Neurol Neurosurg Psychiatry*. 1993;56:543-547.

58. Yamada M. Cerebral amyloid angiopathy: an overview. *Neuropathology*. 2000;20:8-22.

59. Greenberg SM. Cerebral amyloid angiopathy and vessel dysfunction. *Cerebrovasc Dis*. 2002;13(suppl 2):42-47.

60. Greenberg SM. Cerebral amyloid angiopathy and dementia: two amyloids are worse than one. *Neurology*. 2002;58:1587-1588.

61. Fink JN, McAuley DL. Cerebral venous sinus thrombosis: a diagnostic challenge. *Intern Med J*. 2001;31:384-390.

62. Bergui M, Bradac GB. Clinical picture of patients with cerebral venous thrombosis and patterns of dural sinus involvement. *Cerebrovasc Dis*. 2003;16:211-216.

63. Breteau G, Mounier-Vehier F, Godefroy O, et al. Cerebral venous thrombosis 3-year clinical outcome in 55 consecutive patients. *J Neurol*. 2003;250:29-35.

64. Ferro JM, Canhao P, Stam J, Bousser MG, Barinagarrementeria F; ISCVT Investigators. Prognosis of cerebral vein and dural sinus thrombosis: results of the International Study on Cerebral Vein and Dural Sinus Thrombosis (ISCVT). *Stroke*. 2004;35:664-670.

65. Buccino G, Scoditti U, Patteri I, Bertolino C, Mancia D. Neurological and cognitive long-term outcome in patients with cerebral venous sinus thrombosis. *Acta Neurol Scand*. 2003;107:330-335.

66. Lee SK, terBrugge KG. Cerebral venous thrombosis in adults: the role of imaging evaluation and management. *Neuroimaging Clin North Am*. 2003;13:139-152.

67. Yuh WT, Simonson TM, Wang AM, et al. Venous sinus occlusive disease: MR findings. *AJNR Am J Neuroradiol*. 1994;15:309-316.

68. Einhaupl KM, Villringer A, Meister W, et al. Heparin treatment in sinus venous thrombosis. *Lancet*. 1991;338:597-600.

69. Brucker AB, Vollert-Rogenhofer H, Wagner M, et al. Heparin treatment in acute cerebral sinus venous thrombosis: a retrospective clinical and MR analysis of 42 cases. *Cerebrovasc Dis*. 1998;8:331-337.

70. Stam J, De Bruijn SF, DeVeber G. Anticoagulation for cerebral sinus thrombosis. *Cochrane Database Syst Rev*. 2002;CD002005.

71. Canhao P, Falcao F, Ferro JH. Thrombolytics for cerebral sinus thrombosis: a systematic review. *Cerebrovasc Dis*. 2003;15:159-166.

72. Philips MF, Bagley LJ, Sinson GP, et al. Endovascular thrombolysis for symptomatic cerebral venous thrombosis. *J Neurosurg*. 1999;90:65-71.

73. Hartmann A, Mast H, Mohr JP, et al. Morbidity of intracranial hemorrhage in patients with cerebral arteriovenous malformation. *Stroke*. 1998;29:931-934.

8

74. Al-Shahi R, Bhattacharya JJ, Currie DG, et al; Scottish Intracranial Vascular Malformation Study Collaborators. Prospective, population-based detection of intracranial vascular malformations in adults: the Scottish Intracranial Vascular Malformation Study (SIVMS). *Stroke.* 2003;34:1163-1169.

75. Hofmeister C, Stapf C, Hartmann A, et al. Demographic, morphological, and clinical characteristics of 1289 patients with brain arteriovenous malformation. *Stroke.* 2000;31:1307-1310.

76. Ogilvy CS, Stieg PE, Awad I, et al; Stroke Council, American Stroke Association. Recommendations for the management of intracranial arteriovenous malformations: a statement for healthcare professionals from a special writing group of the Stroke Council, American Stroke Association. *Circulation.* 2001;103:2644-2657.

77. Spetzler RF, Martin NA. A proposed grading system for arteriovenous malformations. *J Neurosurg.* 1986;65:476-483.

78. Kinouchi H, Mizoi K, Takahashi A, Ezura M, Yoshimoto T. Combined embolization and microsurgery for cerebral arteriovenous malformation. *Neurol Med Chir.* 2002;42:372-378.

79. Hartmann A, Mast H, Mohr JP, et al. Determinants of staged endovascular and surgical treatment outcome of brain arteriovenous malformations. *Stroke.* 2005;36:2431-2435.

80. Liu HM, Wang YH, Chen YF, Tu YK, Huang KM. Endovascular treatment of brain-stem arteriovenous malformations: safety and efficacy. *Neuroradiology.* 2003;45:644-649.

81. Yamamoto M, Jimbo M, Hara M, Saito I, Mori K. Gamma knife radiosurgery for arteriovenous malformations: long-term follow-up results focusing on complications occurring more than 5 years after irradiation. *Neurosurgery.* 1996;38:906-914.

82. Pollock BE, Meyer FB. Radiosurgery for arteriovenous malformations. *J Neurosurg.* 2004;101:390-392.

83. Pollock BE, Gorman DA, Brown PD. Radiosurgery for arteriovenous malformations of the basal ganglia, thalamus, and brainstem. *J Neurosurg.* 2004;100:210-214.

84. Anson JA, Lawton MT, Spetzler RF. Characteristics and surgical treatment of dolichoectatic and fusiform aneurysms. *J Neurosurg.* 1996;84:185-193.

85. Rabb CH, Barnwell SL. Catastrophic subarachnoid hemorrhage resulting from ruptured vertebrobasilar dolichoectasia: case report. *Neurosurgery.* 1998;42:379-382.

86. Bohmfalk GL, Story JL, Wissinger JP, Brown WE Jr. Bacterial intracranial aneurysm. *J Neurosurg.* 1978;48:369-382.

87. Bakshi R, Wright PD, Kinkel PR, et al. Cranial magnetic resonance imaging findings in bacterial endocarditis: the neuroimaging spectrum of septic brain embolization demonstrated in twelve patients. *J Neuroimaging.* 1999;9:78-84.

88. Branch CL Jr, Laster DW, Kelly DL Jr. Left atrial myxoma with cerebral emboli. *Neurosurgery.* 1985;16:675-680.

89. Hosoda K, Fujita S, Kawaguchi T, et al. Spontaneous dissecting aneurysms of the basilar artery presenting with a subarachnoid hemorrhage. Report of two cases. *J Neurosurg.* 1991;75:628-633.

90. Kaplan SS, Ogilvy CS, Gonzalez R, Gress D, Pile-Spellman J. Extracranial vertebral artery pseudoaneurysm presenting as subarachnoid hemorrhage. *Stroke.* 1993;24:1397-1399.

91. Hop JW, Rinkel GJ, Algra A, van Gijn J. Case-fatality rates and functional outcome after subarachnoid hemorrhage: a systematic review. *Stroke*. 1997;28:660-664.

92. Wong KS. Risk factors for early death in acute ischemic stroke and intracerebral hemorrhage: a prospective hospital-based study in Asia. Asian Acute Stroke Advisory Panel. *Stroke*. 1999;30:2326-2330.

93. Baptista MV, vanMelle G, Bogousslavsky J. Prediction of in-hospital mortality after first-ever stroke: the Lausanne Stroke Registry. *J Neurol Sci*. 1999;166:107-114.

94. Vora YY, Suarez-Almazor M, Steinke DE, Martin ML, Findlay JM. Role of transcranial Doppler monitoring in the diagnosis of cerebral vasospasm after subarachnoid hemorrhage. *Neurosurgery*. 1999;44:1237-1248.

95. Findlay JM. Current management of aneurysmal subarachnoid hemorrhage guidelines from the Canadian Neurosurgical Society. *Can J Neurol Sci*. 1997;24:161-170.

96. Vermeulen M, van Gijn J, Hijdra A, van Crevel H. Causes of acute deterioration in patients with a ruptured intracranial aneurysm. A prospective study with serial CT scanning. *J Neurosurg*. 1984;60:935-939.

97. Naidech AM, Janjua N, Kreiter KT, et al. Predictors and impact of aneurysm rebleeding after subarachnoid hemorrhage. *Arch Neurol*. 2005;62:410-416.

98. Torner JC, Kassell NF, Wallace RB, Adams HP Jr. Preoperative prognostic factors for rebleeding and survival in aneurysm patients receiving antifibrinolytic therapy: report of the Cooperative Aneurysm Study. *Neurosurgery*. 1981;9:506-513.

99. Brilstra EH, Rinkel GJ, Algra A, van Gijn J. Rebleeding, secondary ischemia, and timing of operation in patients with subarachnoid hemorrhage. *Neurology*. 2000;55:1656-1660.

100. Kassell NF, Torner JC, Haley EC Jr, Jane JA, Adams HP, Kongable GL. The International Cooperative Study on the Timing of Aneurysm Surgery. Part 1: Overall management results. *J Neurosurg*. 1990;73:18-36.

101. Kassell NF, Torner JC, Jane JA, Haley EC Jr, Adams HP. The International Cooperative Study on the Timing of Aneurysm Surgery. Part 2: Surgical results. *J Neurosurg*. 1990;73:37-47.

102. de Gans K, Nieuwkamp DJ, Rinkel GJ, Algra A. Timing of aneurysm surgery in subarachnoid hemorrhage: a systematic review of the literature. *Neurosurgery*. 2002;50:336-340.

103. Ross N, Hutchinson PJ, Seeley H, Kirkpatrick PJ. Timing of surgery for supratentorial aneurysmal subarachnoid haemorrhage: report of a prospective study. *J Neurol Neurosurg Psychiatry*. 2002;72:480-484.

104. Guglielmi G, Vinuela F, Duckwiler G, et al. Endovascular treatment of posterior circulation aneurysms by electrothrombosis using electrically detachable coils. *J Neurosurg*. 1992;77:515-524.

105. Murayama Y, Viñuela F, Duckwiler GR, Gobin YP, Guglielmi G. Embolization of incidental cerebral aneurysms by using the Guglielmi detachable coil system. *J Neurosurg*. 1999;90:207-214.

106. Eskridge JM, Song JK. Endovascular embolization of 150 basilar tip aneurysms with Guglielmi detachable coils: results of the Food and Drug Administration multicenter clinical trial. *J Neurosurg*. 1998;89:81-86.

107. van den Berg R, Rinkel GJ, Vandertop WP. Treatment of ruptured intracranial aneurysms: implications of the ISAT on clipping versus coiling. *Eur J Radiol*. 2003;46:172-177.

8

108. Lozier AP, Connolly ES Jr, Lavine SD, Solomon RA. Guglielmi detachable coil embolization of posterior circulation aneurysms: a systematic review of the literature. *Stroke*. 2002;33:2509-2518.

109. Qureshi AI, Suri MF, Khan J, et al. Endovascular treatment of intracranial aneurysms by using Guglielmi detachable coils in awake patients: safety and feasibility. *J Neurosurg*. 2001;94:880-885.

110. Molyneux A, Kerr R, Stratton I, et al; International Subarachnoid Aneurysm Trial (ISAT) Collaborative Group. International Subarachnoid Aneurysm Trial (ISAT) of neurosurgical clipping versus endovascular coiling in 2143 patients with ruptured intracranial aneurysms: a randomised trial. *Lancet*. 2002;360:1267-1274.

111. Roos YB, Vermeulen M, Rinkel GJ, Algra A, van Gijn J, Algra A. Systematic review of antifibrinolytic treatment in aneurysmal subarachnoid haemorrhage. *J Neurol Neurosurg Psychiatry*. 1998;65:942-943.

112. Roos YB, Rinkel GJ, Vermeulen M, Algra A, van Gijn J. Antifibrinolytic therapy for aneurysmal subarachnoid haemorrhage. *Cochrane Database Syst Rev*. 2003;CD001245.

113. Weir B, Macdonald RL, Stoodley M. Etiology of cerebral vasospasm. *Acta Neurochir*. 1999;72(suppl):27-46.

114. Weir B, Grace M, Hansen J, Rothberg C. Time course of vasospasm in man. *J Neurosurg*. 1978;48:173-178.

115. Janjua N, Mayer SA. Cerebral vasospasm after subarachnoid hemorrhage. *Curr Opin Crit Care*. 2003;9:113-119.

116. Dumont AS, Chow M, Kassell NF. Vasospasm. *J Neurosurg*. 2002; 96:985-986.

117. Dumont AS, Dumont RJ, Chow MM, et al. Cerebral vasospasm after subarachnoid hemorrhage: putative role of inflammation. *Neurosurgery*. 2003;53:123-133.

118. Qureshi AI, Sung GY, Razumovsky AY, Lane K, Straw RN, Ulatowski JA. Early identification of patients at risk for symptomatic vasospasm after aneurysmal subarachnoid hemorrhage. *Crit Care Med*. 2000;28:984-990.

119. Charpentier C, Audibert G, Guillemin F, et al. Multivariate analysis of predictors of cerebral vasospasm occurrence after aneurysmal subarachnoid hemorrhage. *Stroke*. 1999;30:1402-1408.

120. Lindegaard KF. The role of transcranial Doppler in the management of patients with subarachnoid haemorrhage–a review. *Acta Neurochir*. 1999;72(suppl):59-71.

121. Egge A, Waterloo K, Sjoholm H, Solberg T, Ingebrigtsen T, Romner B. Systematic review of the prevention of delayed ischemic neurological deficits with hypertension, hypervolemia, and hemodilution therapy following subarachnoid hemorrhage. *J Neurosurg*. 2004;100:359-360.

122. Pickard JD, Murray GD, Illingworth R, et al. Effect of oral nimodipine on cerebral infarction and outcome after subarachnoid haemorrhage: British aneurysm nimodipine trial. *BMJ*. 1989;298:636-642.

123. Barker FG 2nd, Ogilvy CS. Efficacy of prophylactic nimodipine for delayed ischemic deficit after subarachnoid hemorrhage: a metaanalysis. *J Neurosurg*. 1996;84:405-414.

124. Feigin VL, Rinkel GJ, Algra A, Vermeulen M, van Gijn J. Calcium antagonists for aneurysmal subarachnoid haemorrhage. *Cochrane Database Syst Rev*. 2000;CD000277.

125. Tseng MY, Al-Rawi PG, Pickard JD, Rasulo FA, Kirkpatrick PJ. Effect of hypertonic saline on cerebral blood flow in poor-grade patients with subarachnoid hemorrhage. *Stroke*. 2003;34:1389-1396.

218

126. Egge A, Waterloo K, Sjoholm H, Solberg T, Ingebrigtsen T, Romner B. Prophylactic hyperdynamic postoperative fluid therapy after aneurysmal subarachnoid hemorrhage: a clinical, prospective, randomized, controlled study. *Neurosurgery*. 2001;49:593-605.
127. Sen J, Belli A, Albon H, Morgan L, Petzold A, Kitchen N. Triple-H therapy in the management of aneurysmal subarachnoid haemorrhage. *Lancet Neurol*. 2003;2:614-621.
128. Bejjani GK, Bank WO, Olan WJ, Sekhar LN. The efficacy and safety of angioplasty for cerebral vasospasm after subarachnoid hemorrhage. *Neurosurgery*. 1998;42:979-986.
129. Andaluz N, Tomsick TA, Tew JM Jr, van Loveren HR, Yeh HS, Zuccarello M. Indications for endovascular therapy for refractory vasospasm after aneurysmal subarachnoid hemorrhage: experience at the University of Cincinnati. *Surg Neurol*. 2002;58:131-138.

8

9

Acute Treatment of Ischemic Stroke: Blood Supply to the Brain

Because most ischemic strokes are due to thromboembolic occlusion of an artery supplying the brain, measures to restore or improve blood supply are the most commonly prescribed interventions. A number of strategies have been attempted, but unfortunately, not all of these treatments have proven successful (**Table 9.1**). The most widely prescribed medical therapies are agents that affect coagulation or promote lysis of the clot. These agents include:

- Plasminogen activators (PAs)
- Anticoagulants
- Antiplatelet aggregating agents.

Intravenous and intra-arterial administration of thrombolytic agents can achieve recanalization and improve outcome in carefully selected patients experiencing acute ischemic stroke.[1-5] Still, the number of patients who can be treated is disappointingly small. While long-term administration of anticoagulants is effective in reducing the frequency of embolic events in patients with high-risk cardiac disease leading to embolic stroke, their value is not established for treatment of patients with acute stroke. Recent clinical trials have not been able to demonstrate a benefit from early use of anticoagulation.[6-11] Platelet antiaggregating agents are effective in reducing the risk of stroke in high-risk patients with arterial disease, such as atherosclerosis, but their role in acute management is not clear.[8,12] All antithrombotic agents increase the risk of symptomatic ischemia-related hemorrhage, with fibri-

TABLE 9.1 — Interventions to Restore or Improve Blood Flow to the Brain During Acute Ischemic Stroke

- Thrombolytic agents:
  - Recombinant tissue-type plasminogen activator (rt-PA)
  - Streptokinase
  - Urokinase
  - Prourokinase
  - Single-chain urokinase plasminogen activator (scu-PA)
  - Tenecteplase
  - Desmoteplase
  - Reteplase
- Fibrinogen-depleting agent:
  - Ancrod
- Anticoagulants:
  - Heparin
  - Low molecular weight heparins
  - Danaparoid
- Direct thrombin inhibitor:
  - Argatroban
- Antiplatelet agents:
  - Aspirin
  - Glycoprotein IIb/IIIa receptor blockers
- Inhibitors of leukocyte-endothelial cell adhesion receptors
- Hemodilution and hypervolemia:
  - Low molecular weight dextran
- Vasopressors/vasoconstrictors
- Vasodilators
- Endovascular treatment:
  - Clot extraction
  - Angioplasty and stenting
- Transcranial Doppler ultrasonography
- Operative procedures:
  - Carotid endarterectomy
  - Extracranial-intracranial arterial anastomosis

nolytic agents associated with the highest frequency and antiplatelet agents the lowest. A recent report of the combination of a PA with abciximab demonstrated significant risk.[13]

Volume expansion and viscosity-altering agents have been used to maintain or enhance the cerebral circulation in the event of focal brain ischemia in some centers. While success has been shown in the setting of vasospasm after subarachnoid hemorrhage (SAH), these agents have not been effective in the management of other acute forms of stroke.[14-17] Operative procedures can be effective in removing an arterial occlusion and restoring flow, but the clinical safety and efficacy of these approaches, including the innovative intra-arterial endovascular procedures, have not been tested in comparison to pharmacologic thrombolysis.

Although several promising therapies are available, currently only intravenous administration of recombinant tissue plasminogen activator (rt-PA) is established as effective in improving outcomes after acute ischemic stroke. Recombinant tissue PA is approved in the United States, Canada, parts of South America, Europe, and Australia.

Pharmacologic Thrombolysis

■ Intravenous Administration of Thrombolytic Agents
Efficacy of rt-PA and Other PAs

The thrombolytic agents are obligate PAs that convert plasminogen to plasmin, which, in turn cleaves fibrinogen and the fibrin network of a thrombus. Several agents have been examined, but to date, only intravenous administration of rt-PA is approved for the acute treatment of patients with acute ischemic stroke.[18] Only rt-PA has so far been shown to have potential benefit in improving outcome to justify its use in comparison to the risk of serious bleeding complications. Three trials of intravenously administered streptokinase were terminated because of increased mortality with treatment—largely as the result of massive brain hemorrhage.[19-21] Potential contributors to the hazards included severe strokes in one trial and the high doses of streptokinase (equivalent to that used for treatment of acute myocardial infarction) administered in all three studies. Pending the availability of data that show that it has an acceptable safety profile, streptokinase should not be used to treat patients with acute ischemic stroke under these conditions (Class III Recommendation, Level of Evidence A).

While acute intravenous thrombolytic treatment within the first 3 hours of ischemic stroke is emphasized, the potential for serious complications, especially intracranial hemorrhages, means that thrombolytic therapy should not be given until computed tomography (CT) has excluded hemorrhage as the cause of the acute neurologic symptoms.[1]

Three nonarteriographically based trials underscore the utility of acutely administered intravenous rt-PA for acute management of ischemic stroke. In the National Institutes of Neurological Disorders and Stroke (NINDS) studies, rt-PA was given within 3 hours of onset of symptoms.[18] It was associated with an 11% to 13% absolute increase in the number of people who had minimal or no disability, but there was no major overall change in mortality at 90 days after stroke (**Table 9.2** and **Table 9.3**). The investigators used four rating instruments to assess outcomes:

- National Institutes of Health Stroke Scale (NIHSS) score
- Glasgow Outcome Scale score
- Modified Rankin Scale (mRS) score
- Barthel Index score.

TABLE 9.2 — Favorable Outcomes at 3 Months in Patients Treated <90 Minutes After Onset of Acute Ischemic Stroke

	rt-PA n = 157 (%)	Placebo n = 145 (%)	Odds Ratio	Relative Risk (95% CI)	P Value
Barthel Index	53	38	1.8	1.4 (1.1–1.8)	0.010
Modified Rankin Scale	40	28	1.7	1.4 (1.0–1.9)	0.035
Glasgow Outcome Scale	43	32	1.6	1.3 (1.0–1.8)	0.057
NIH Stroke Scale	34	20	2.0	1.7 (1.1–2.5)	0.008

Abbreviations: CI, confidence interval; NIH, National Institutes of Health; rt-PA, recombinant tissue-type plasminogen activator.

The National Institute of Neurological Disorders and Stroke rt-PA Stroke Study Group. *N Engl J Med.* 1995;333:1581-1587.

TABLE 9.3 — Favorable Outcomes at 3 Months in Patients Treated 91 to 180 Minutes After Onset of Acute Ischemic Stroke

	rt-PA n = 155 (%)	Placebo n = 167 (%)	Odds Ratio	Relative Risk (95% CI)	P Value
Barthel Index	51	38	1.6	1.3 (1.0–1.7)	0.026
Modified Rankin Scale	45	25	2.4	1.8 (1.3–2.4)	<0.001
Glasgow Outcome Scale	47	30	2.0	1.6 (1.2–2.1)	0.002
NIH Stroke Scale	34	21	2.0	1.6 (1.1–2.3)	0.008

Abbreviations: CI, confidence interval; NIH, National Institutes of Health; rt-PA, recombinant tissue-type plasminogen activator.

The National Institute of Neurological Disorders and Stroke rt-PA Stroke Study Group. *N Engl J Med.* 1995;333:1581-1587.

These clinically based scales assess different components of outcome, including neurologic impairment, disability, and global functioning. In the NINDS-sponsored trial, benefits with rt-PA treatment were noted in all four measures (**Table 9.2** and **Table 9.3**). Approximately 50% of the patients were treated within 90 minutes. Based on that trial, the approved dose of rt-PA is 0.9 mg/kg (maximum, 90 mg) given over 1 hour, with 10% of the dose given rapidly within the first few minutes. It is the first and, to date, the only intervention to be approved for the acute treatment of patients with this condition.

Two separate trials of intravenous rt-PA given within 6 hours of onset of stroke displayed no substantial benefit according to prespecified criteria.[22] The European Cooperative Acute Stroke Study (ECASS) suggested that patients with evidence of major ischemic injury on initial CT have increased mortality and an unacceptably high rate of brain hemorrhage when treated with rt-PA (**Table 9.4**). Subsequent analyses that excluded those patients indicated rates of improvement that were similar to those reported by the NINDS trials.[23] ECASS-2 gave rt-PA within 6 hours of symptom onset to carefully selected stroke patients using stringent CT criteria to exclude patients with early signs of ischemia.[5] Favorable outcomes (mRS 0-2) were noted in 40.3% of patients treated with rt-PA and in 36.6% of the control patients, but those results were not statistically significant. Another trial, (Alteplase Thrombolysis for Acute Noninterventional Therapy in Ischemic Stroke [ATLANTIS]), performed in the United States, focused on treating patients 3 to 5 hours after stroke.[24,25] No net benefit from treatment was found in that incomplete trial. Those negative trials imply that the time window and patient selection are important elements in beneficial outcome with rt-PA. Post-therapy analysis of pooled data has indicated that benefit is greatest with treatment

TABLE 9.4 — Hemorrhagic Events Noted in Patients Treated in the European Cooperative Acute Stroke Study-I

	Hemorrhagic Infarction			Parenchymal Hematoma		
	n	%	95% CI	*n*	%	95% CI
Intention-to-Treat Population						
rt-PA (*n* = 313)	72	23	18.5–28.1	62	19.8	15.6–24.8
Placebo (*n* = 307)	93	30.3	24.3–35.8	20	6.5	4.1–10.0
Target Population						
rt-PA (*n* = 247)	60	24.3	19.3–30.1	48	19.4	14.8–25.0
Placebo (*n* = 264)	79	29.9	24.5–35.9	18	6.8	4.2–10.7

Abbreviations: CI, confidence interval; rt-PA, recombinant tissue-type plasminogen activator.

Hacke W, et al. *JAMA*. 1995;274:1017-1025.

within 90 minutes, and that baseline severity affects responses to treatment.

Safety of Plasminogen Activators

These trials also show that the administration of rt-PA within a few hours of onset of ischemic stroke is associated with the risk of symptomatic intracranial hemorrhage. In the NINDS trials, the risk was approximately 10 times that seen in the patients in the control group (**Table 9.5**).[26] While the use of rt-PA was not associated with an increased likelihood of dying, mortality was increased among the treated patients in the ECASS and the ATLANTIS study.[22,24] Those trials also confirm that while hemorrhagic transformation of the infarction that causes no neurologic symptoms is commonly found in patients with large infarctions, the

TABLE 9.5 — Mortality and Intracranial Hemorrhages in Patients Enrolled in the NINDS rt-PA Trial		
	rt-PA ($n = 312$)	Placebo ($n = 312$)
Deaths <30 days	30	49
Deaths <90 days	54	64
Hemorrhages <36 hours		
Symptomatic	20	2
Fatal	9	1
Nonfatal	11	1
Asymptomatic	14	9
Serious nonneurologic bleeding	2	0

Abbreviations: NINDS, National Institute of Neurological Disorders and Stroke; rt-PA, recombinant tissue-type plasminogen activator.

The National Institute of Neurological Disorders and Stroke rt-PA Stroke Study Group. *N Engl J Med.* 1995;333:1581-1587.

presence of the thrombolytic agent is associated with the development of parenchymal hematomas that can be associated with neurologic worsening.

Several factors appear to influence the chances of having a symptomatic brain hemorrhage following treatment:

- The longer the interval from onset of stroke until treatment
- The presence of diastolic hypertension
- The relative dose of rt-PA
- Advanced age
- Severity of stroke as judged by the initial neurologic assessment
- Early signs of ischemia (>30% of hemisphere) as demonstrated by the changes on the initial CT scan.

Since the approval of rt-PA for treatment of stroke, several groups have reported on their experience in administering rt-PA in a general clinical environment.[27-32] The rates of favorable outcomes, symptomatic hemorrhage, and mortality have varied widely (**Table 9.6**). In one particular study, there was an unacceptably high frequency of symptomatic hemorrhage (15.7%), with a large percentage of stroke patients seen >3 hours after symptom onset.[33] Conversely, other studies show that rt-PA can be administered successfully in rural settings as well as in metropolitan areas. Coordinated regional stroke care systems have increased the number of patients who can be treated. The differences between the studies may reflect a number of variables, including the severity of the patients' strokes, their ages, and the presence of concomitant diseases. Thus comparisons between those studies should not be made. Further studies have provided some insights about these factors that could contribute to responses to intravenous delivery of rt-PA. On the other hand, they point out

TABLE 9.6 — Community Experience: Emergency Administration of rt-PA in the Treatment of Acute Ischemic Stroke				
Study	Number Treated	Symptomatic Hemorrhage (%)	Mortality (%)	Favorable Outcomes (%)
Grond et al	100	5	12	53
Tanne et al	189	6	9.5	46
Egan et al	33	9.1	18.2	36.4
Wang et al	57	5	9	47
Albers et al	389	3.3	13	35
Katzan et al	70	15.7	15.7	28.6

that thrombolytic therapy is potentially dangerous. A protocol for administration of rt-PA, which is modeled on the methods used in the NINDS trials, has been developed.[1] Adherence to the protocol improves the safety of the treatment.

In summary, the current data support the intravenous administration of rt-PA for treatment of carefully selected patients with acute ischemic stroke who can receive the medication within 3 hours of onset of symptoms (Class I Recommendation, Level of Evidence A). Because of the concerns about the safety of the use of streptokinase, it should not be considered as a substitute for rt-PA. Other PAs are in clinical trials.

Recommendations for Patient Selection

Guidelines, based on the criteria developed for the NINDS trials, can assist in selection of patients and their treatment.[1] **Figure 9.1** provides an algorithm to use when assessing a patient for possible treatment with rt-PA. Because the time window is short, the steps to assess the patient should be performed quickly and simultaneously. A goal should be to complete the evaluation and start treatment with rt-PA within 1 hour of the patient's arrival in the emergency department. Still, the sequence is important. For example, if the patient does not meet the first criterion (interval since stroke <3 hours), the remainder of the algorithm becomes moot because the patient cannot be treated.

The treatment regimen for use of rt-PA described in **Table 9.7** conforms to the licensed regimen based on that used by the NINDS investigators. The approach for controlling elevated blood pressure after treatment with rt-PA is outlined in **Table 6.4**. Ancillary care is critical for successful use of rt-PA in the acute treatment of stroke. In particular, patients should not receive anticoagulants or antiplatelet agents within 24 hours after the use of rt-PA (**Table 9.7**).

Recent clinical and experimental observations have suggested other factors that could contribute to poor outcomes with use of rt-PA. These include:

- Elevated blood glucose levels
- Cortical involvement of the ischemic injury
- Disturbances in consciousness
- Advanced age.

These factors seem to affect the brain's response to ischemic injury or reflect large areas of injury that could be less susceptible to recovery and more susceptible to hemorrhage.

Thrombolytic agents cannot be given with impunity; potentially life-threatening bleeding, including intracranial hemorrhages, can complicate the use of these medications. Patients and families should be apprised of this risk. Based on prospective trial experience, hemorrhage is expected to occur in at least one of 16 patients with stroke who are treated with rt-PA.[3] The NINDS investigators reported that patients with a NIHSS score >20 and those with CT findings of a large stroke were at markedly increased risk for hemorrhage.[18] Assessing the presence of early signs of ischemia is an important element of reducing the risk of intracranial bleeding. Features of early ischemia include regional decreases in x-ray attenuation and evidence of mass effect. Regions of hypoattenuation exceeding 50% of the territory of the middle cerebral artery (MCA) are associated with a mortality of approximately 85% (see Chapter 5, *Imaging of the Brain and Blood Vessels in Stroke*). Therefore, patients with early CT findings of a major ischemic stroke (parenchymal hypoattenuation exceeding 33% of the territory of the MCA) should not be treated. In order to reduce the likelihood of bleeding, patients with prolonged prothrombin time (PT) (international normalized ratio [INR] >1.5) or activated partial thromboplastin time (aPTT), or who are currently

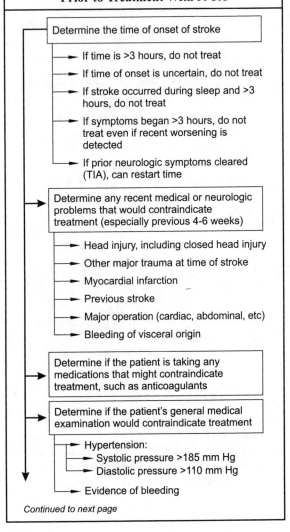

FIGURE 9.1 — Algorithm for Mandatory Baseline Assessment Prior to Treatment With rt-PA

Determine the time of onset of stroke

- If time is >3 hours, do not treat
- If time of onset is uncertain, do not treat
- If stroke occurred during sleep and >3 hours, do not treat
- If symptoms began >3 hours, do not treat even if recent worsening is detected
- If prior neurologic symptoms cleared (TIA), can restart time

Determine any recent medical or neurologic problems that would contraindicate treatment (especially previous 4-6 weeks)

- Head injury, including closed head injury
- Other major trauma at time of stroke
- Myocardial infarction
- Previous stroke
- Major operation (cardiac, abdominal, etc)
- Bleeding of visceral origin

Determine if the patient is taking any medications that might contraindicate treatment, such as anticoagulants

Determine if the patient's general medical examination would contraindicate treatment

- Hypertension:
  - Systolic pressure >185 mm Hg
  - Diastolic pressure >110 mm Hg
- Evidence of bleeding

Continued to next page

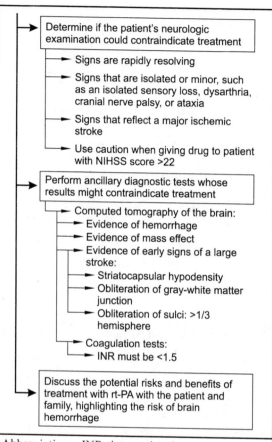

Determine if the patient's neurologic examination could contraindicate treatment

→ Signs are rapidly resolving

→ Signs that are isolated or minor, such as an isolated sensory loss, dysarthria, cranial nerve palsy, or ataxia

→ Signs that reflect a major ischemic stroke

→ Use caution when giving drug to patient with NIHSS score >22

Perform ancillary diagnostic tests whose results might contraindicate treatment

→ Computed tomography of the brain:
→ Evidence of hemorrhage
→ Evidence of mass effect
→ Evidence of early signs of a large stroke:
→ Striatocapsular hypodensity
→ Obliteration of gray-white matter junction
→ Obliteration of sulci: >1/3 hemisphere
→ Coagulation tests:
→ INR must be <1.5

Discuss the potential risks and benefits of treatment with rt-PA with the patient and family, highlighting the risk of brain hemorrhage

9

Abbreviations: INR, international normalized ratio; NIHSS, National Institutes of Health Stroke Scale; rt-PA, recombinant tissue-type plasminogen activator; TIA, transient ischemic attack.

receiving heparin or warfarin should not be treated. In addition, withholding treatment with rt-PA for patients whose strokes are older than 3 hours or who have severe hypertension also is aimed at improving safety. Vigorous control of arterial hypertension, close observation, and careful attention to other components

TABLE 9.7 — Regimen for Treatment With rt-PA: Acute Ischemic Stroke

Dose of rt-PA
- 0.9 mg/kg – up to a maximum dose of 90 mg

Administration
- 10 % of the total dose given as an intravenous bolus
- Remainder infused over 1 hour

Ancillary Antithrombotic Medications
- No anticoagulants (warfarin or heparin) for 24 hours
- No antiplatelet agents (including aspirin) for 24 hours

Ancillary Medical Management
- Admit to a skilled care unit (stroke unit)
- Close observation of neurologic status and vital signs
- Frequent measurements of blood pressure
- Aggressively treat elevated blood pressure*
- Delay placement of indwelling bladder catheter, nasogastric tube, or intra-arterial catheter for several hours

Abbreviation: rt-PA, recombinant tissue plasminogen activator.

* See **Table 6.4** for levels of blood pressure to treat and medications.

of ancillary care also endeavor to reduce the likelihood of bleeding complications (**Table 9.7**) (see Chapter 6, *Emergency Medical Management of Stroke*). The management of intracranial hemorrhage following the use of rt-PA or other antithrombotic agents is outlined in Chapter 8, *Treatment of Hemorrhagic Stroke*.

■ Intra-arterial Administration of Thrombolytic Agents

Local, direct delivery (intra-arterial administration) of a PA has several potential advantages. In general, the PA would only be given to those patients who have occlusions demonstrated by the arteriography. It could permit administration of a dosage of medication at a local concentration higher than that achieved by a related systemic dose (and also thereby producing a lower systemic dose). The catheter is placed directly into the thrombus (mechanical devices might be used in conjunction with the treatment in study settings). As a result, intra-arterial therapy could be more effective than intravenous administration in dissolving large thrombi. On the other hand, the resources, including physician expertise, to administer thrombolytic agents intra-arterially are not widely available. Because time is critical for success with thrombolytic therapy, there are concerns that the minutes or hours consumed by transferring patients and mobilizing hospital resources may lessen the efficacy of an intra-arterial approach. Also, the safety and efficacy of intra-arterial treatment have not been rigorously tested.

Efficacy of Intra-arterial Administration of Thrombolytic Agents

Several trials have used recanalization as the marker of success for intra-arterial administration of thrombolytic agents.[34-38] Uncontrolled studies of intra-arterial delivery of streptokinase, urokinase, or rt-PA have demonstrated the feasibility of recanalization of occlusions in the carotid circulation.[39-41] Overall, recanalization can be achieved in approximately 40% to 70% of patients. The lowest frequencies of recanalization are seen in patients with occlusion of the internal carotid artery.[42] Several groups have reported successful recanalization of the basilar artery with the use of intra-arterial thrombolytic agents.[43-45]

Two clinical trials have tested the usefulness of intra-arterial administration of prourokinase in treatment of patients with acute stroke secondary to an occlusion of the proximal middle cerebral artery.[46,47] No prospective controlled trials of intra-arterial delivery of urokinase or rt-PA have been undertaken, however, Prolyse in Acute Cerebral Thromboembolism (PROACT), a prospective placebo-controlled phase-2

9

study, demonstrated that prourokinase with heparin significantly increased recanalization but also increased hemorrhage. In PROACT II, patients received 9 mg prourokinase intra-arterially and heparin, or heparin alone intravenously within 6 hours of onset of stroke. While the frequency of symptomatic hemorrhage was higher in the patients who received prourokinase than in the control group, favorable outcomes were more common in the treated group (**Table 9.8**). Although the experience was small, patients with a baseline NIHSS score of 10 to 20 seemed to benefit most from treatment. The prognosis of patients with milder strokes (in this case NIHSS score <10) was generally good. Conversely, patients with a major stroke (NIHSS score >20) presented a prognosis that, regardless of treatment, was generally poor. This group also has a high risk for intracerebral hemorrhage following treatment of carotid territory occlusions.

A very small randomized trial of intra-arterial urokinase applied to posterior circulation occlusion suggested relative benefit in patients receiving urokinase compared with controls.[48,49] A retrospective series suggested similar outcomes between intravenous rt-PA and endovascular procedures in the treatment of basilar thrombosis.[50] These studies demand appropriately sized prospective-controlled trials of thrombolysis for posterior circulation thrombosis.[48]

While intra-arterial thrombolytic therapy holds promise for the treatment of patients with acute ischemic stroke, it is not known to be either more effective or safer than intravenous treatment. Because there are no head-to-head comparisons between the utility of intravenous and that of intra-arterial thrombolysis, withholding intravenous treatment in order to provide intra-arterial is not appropriate. The use of this approach should be in the context of an appropriately designed and ethically approved prospective clinical

TABLE 9.8 — Results of Trial of Intra-arterial Prourokinase in the Treatment of Acute Ischemic Stroke

Outcome	Prourokinase and Heparin (n = 121)		Heparin (n = 59)	
	n	%	n	%
Symptomatic hemorrhage	11/121	10.1	1/54	1.8
Mortality	30	25	16	27
Favorable outcome	31	26	10	17

Furlan A, et al. *JAMA.* 1999;282:2003-2011.

trial. The patient and family must know that this form of treatment remains experimental.

PAs Under Clinical Trial

Pilot, dose-escalation studies have evaluated the utility of desmoteplase or tenecteplase (TNK).[51,52] The early use of desmoteplase by intravenous delivery employing MRI in patient selection is under study. Excessive doses of desmoteplase were associated with symptomatic intracerebral hemorrhage in initial safety studies. When the agent was administered in a weight-based regimen, desmoteplase appeared to be relatively safe and a trial testing the efficacy is under way. Another study tested several doses of TNK when the agent was given in a relatively short time period.[53] The highest dose of medication was associated with an increase in hemorrhage frequency. TNK is being tested in a clinical trial. Uchino and colleagues[54] tested a lower dose of rt-PA (0.6 mg/kg) when the agent was given at time periods longer than 3 hours. The agent appeared to be safe. Those results are provisional and do not support the use of these agents outside the setting of a clinical study (Class III Recommendation, Level of Evidence B). Another strategy has been to treat patients within the 3-hour window with intravenous rt-PA and if subsequent arteriography demonstrates an occlusion, then additional rt-PA would be given by local intra-arterial infusion.[55-58] The feasibility of that approach has been shown, as well as the potential safety. However, no comparison with intravenous or intra-arterial PA delivery alone has been made. This strategy for treatment is not recommended outside the setting of clinical trials (Class III Recommendation, Level of Evidence B).

Parenteral administration of rapidly acting anti-coagulants, including heparin, has been a mainstay in the treatment of patients with acute ischemic stroke despite the lack of any definitive data about efficacy of heparin or similar compounds. The rationale for early anticoagulation includes:

- Halting propagation of a thrombus
- Preventing recurrent embolism
- Helping maintain blood flow to the ischemic region via collaterals.

Despite their widespread use, uncertainties about the utility of acute anticoagulation agents persist.[11,59-62] In part, the controversies might be a consequence of confusion between the data obtained from trials testing long-term anticoagulation for prevention of stroke and the early (>24-hour intervention)-treatment trials. While anticoagulants are effective in preventing cerebral and systemic embolization in patients with high-risk cardiac lesions, including mechanical values and nonvalvular atrial fibrillation (AF), the data from the recent clinical trials of early stroke intervention are largely negative. Currently, there are no data establishing the efficacy of acute anticoagulation in patients with ischemic stroke. Conversely, the trials do demonstrate the risk of major hemorrhagic complications.

■ Heparin

The International Stroke Trial (IST) tested two different subcutaneously administered doses of heparin (5,000 or 25,000 units/day) alone or in combination with aspirin.[8] Heparin lessened the risk of early recurrent stroke but the benefit was negated by an increased risk of serious intracranial hemorrhage, particularly with the higher dose (**Table 9.9**). The rate of early

TABLE 9.9 — Rates of Symptomatic Hemorrhage Trials of Emergency Anticoagulation: Acute Ischemic Stroke

Trial	Agent	Dosage	Active		Control	
			n	%	n	%
IST*	Heparin	5000 IU/d	35/4681	0.7	41/9718	0.4
		25000 IU/d	85/4856	1.8		
FISS	Nadroparin	4100 IU/d	0/101	0	1/105	1.0
		8200 IU/d	0/100	0		
TOAST	Danaparoid	Adjusted	10/638	1.5	3/628	0.4
FISS-bis	Nadroparin	Low dose‡	10/271	3.7	7/250	2.8
		High dose‡	15/245	6.1		
HAEST†	Dalteparin	200 IU/kg/d	6/224	2.7	4/225	1.8
TOPAS	Certoparin	3000 U/d	2/99	2.0	NC	
		6000 U/d	1/102	1.0		
		10000 U/d	2/103	1.9		

242

		16000 U/d						
TAIST[†]	Tinzaparin	Low dose[§]	4/100	4.0	3/507	0.6	1/491	0.2
		High dose[§]	7/486	1.4				
RAPID[†]	Heparin	Adjusted	2/32	6.3	3/35	8.6		
Camerlingo	Heparin	Adjusted	13/208	6.2	3/210	1.4		

Abbreviations: d, day; FISS, Fraxiparine Ischemic Stroke Study; FISS-bis, second Fraxiparin Ischemic Stroke Study; HAEST, Heparin Aspirin Ischemic Stroke Study; IST, International Stroke Trial; IU, international units; NC, no control; RAPID, Rapid Anticoagulation Prevents Ischemic Damage; TAIST, Tinzaparin in Acute Ischaemic Stroke Trial; TOAST, Trial of ORG 10172 in Acute Stroke Treatment; TOPAS, Therapy of Patients With Acute Stroke.

* Some patients in treatment and control groups also received aspirin.
† Control patients received aspirin.
‡ Low dose 85 anti-Xa units/kg/day and high dose 85 anti-Xa units/kg/bid.
§ Low dose 100 anti-Xa units/kg/day and high dose .175 anti-Xa units/kg/day.

International Stroke Trial Collaborative Group. *Lancet*. 1997;349:1569-1581; Kay R, et al. *N Engl J Med*. 1995;333:1588-1593; The Publications Committee for the Trial of ORG 10172 in Acute Stroke Treatment (TOAST) Investigators. *JAMA*. 1998;279:1265-1272; Chamorro A. *Cerebrovasc Dis*. 1999;9(suppl 3):16-23; Berge E, et al. *Lancet*. 2000;355:1205-1210; Diener HC, et al. *Stroke*. 2001;32:22-29; Bath PM, et al. *Lancet*. 2001;358:683-684; Chamorro A, et al. *Cerebrovasc Dis*. 2005;19:402-404; Camerlingo M, et al. *Stroke*. 2005;36:2415-2420.

9

recurrent embolization was higher in patients who had atrial fibrillation than in those with sinus rhythm but the benefit from anticoagulation was not seen in that group. No net effect in improving outcomes was noted with the use of heparin (**Table 9.10**). That very practical trial can be criticized for a number of reasons: concerns related to uncertain targets, the route of administration, the lack of effect monitoring, and especially the relatively long interval from stroke onset to treatment (up to 48 hours). It is possible that a fixed dose of medication resulted in some patients being excessively treated, with the risk of hemorrhage, while others were undertreated. In addition, IST did not test intravenously administered heparin, which is the common strategy for giving the medication to acutely ill patients with ischemic stroke.

One recent trial compared intravenous administration of heparin, including a bolus dose to start treatment or aspirin in patients with recent nonlacunar stroke.[63] No differences in outcomes were noted, although the trial recruited a very small number of patients. Another trial found that adjusted-dose intravenous heparin started within 3 hours of onset of stroke was associated with an increased rate of favorable outcomes and an increased chance of symptomatic hemorrhage.[64] Emergency administration of heparin for treatment of most patients with acute ischemic stroke is not recommended (Class III Recommendation, Level of Evidence A).

■ **Low Molecular Weight Heparin**

Two trials tested nadroparin, a low molecular weight heparin (LMWH). The first trial (Fraxiparine in Stroke Study [FISS]) tested two doses given subcutaneously, when the medication was started <48 hours of stroke (**Table 9.9** and **Table 9.10**).[7] At 6 months after stroke, the frequency of favorable outcomes was significantly higher in patients given the higher dose of nadroparin than in the patients treated with placebo. However, the success of treatment was not evident at either 10 days (end of acute-treatment period) or at 3 months. A subsequent trial of nadroparin did not confirm efficacy and found high rates of intracranial and systemic bleeding with the anticoagulant.[11] Another LMWH, dalteparin, was tested in a trial that enrolled patients with atrial fibrillation (**Table 9.9** and **Table 9.10**).[9] The ability of the anticoagulant to prevent early recurrent embolism was compared with that of aspirin. Symptomatic intracranial hemorrhage was more common in the patients given dalteparin. Surprisingly, the rate of early recurrent stroke was higher with the anticoagulant than with aspirin. Another LMWH trial tested four different doses of certoparin in early treatment of ischemic stroke.[10] No differences in favorable outcomes were noted among the four groups, but the rate of serious hemorrhage was highest in the patients who received the highest dose.

A prospective controlled trial tested the usefulness of danaparoid (an LMWH) in improving outcomes following acute ischemic stroke.[6] The agent was given intravenously within 24 hours of the onset of an ischemic stroke and continued for 1 week. Dosage adjustments were made in response to levels of antifactor Xa activity. An increase in the risk of symptomatic intracranial bleeding or serious systemic hemorrhage was found with treatment. No reduction in the rate of neurologic worsening and no decline in the rate of early recurrent embolization were found, including in patients with cardioembolism. A trend toward an increase in favorable outcomes at the end of the 7-day treatment period was found, but the treatment effects were not sustained at 3 months. The subgroup of patients with stroke secondary to large-artery atherosclerosis seemed to have an advantage from treatment at 3 months, but patients with cardioembolic stroke were not helped.

TABLE 9.10 — Favorable Outcomes: Trials of Emergency Anticoagulation in Acute Ischemic Stroke

Trial	Agent	Dosage	Active		Control	
			n	%	n	%
IST*	Heparin	5000 IU/d	1776/4681	36.9	3582/9718	37.1
		25000 IU/d	1802/4856	37.4		
FISS	Nadroparin	4100 IU/d	47/101	47	35/105	36
		8200 IU/d	54/100	54		
TOAST	Danaparoid	Adjusted dose	482/641	75.2	467/634	73.7
FISS-bis	Nadroparin	Low dose‡	155/271	57.2	142/250	56.8
		High dose‡	145/245	59.2		
HAEST†	Dalteparin	200 IU/kg/d	51/224	22.8	48/225	21.3
TOPAS	Certoparin	3000 U/d	59/96	61.5	NC	
		6000 U/d	59/97	60.8		
		10000 U/d	62/98	63.3		

246

		16000 U/d						
TAIST†	Tinzaparin	Low dose§	54/96	56.3	188/507	38.3	206/491	42.5
		High dose§			181/486	38.4		
RAPID†	Heparin	Adjusted	13/32	40.6			19/35	54.3
Camerlingo	Heparin	Adjusted	81/208	38.9			60/210	28.6

Abbreviations: FISS, Fraxiparine Ischemic Stroke Study; FISS-bis, second Fraxiparin Ischemic Stroke Study; HAEST, Heparin Aspirin Ischemic Stroke Trial; IST, International Stroke Trial; NC, no control; RAPID, Rapid Anticoagulation Prevents Ischemic Damage; TAIST, Tinzaparin in Acute Ischemic Stroke Trial; TOAST, Trial of ORG 10172 in Acute Stroke Treatment; TOPAS, Therapy of Patients With Acute Stroke.

* Some patients in treatment and control groups also received aspirin.
† Control patients received aspirin.
‡ Low dose 85 anti-Xa units/kg/day and high dose 85 anti-Xa units/kg/bid.
§ Low dose 100 anti-Xa units/kg/day and high dose 175 anti-Xa units/kg/day.

International Stroke Trial Collaborative Group. *Lancet.* 1997;349:1569-1581; Kay R, et al. *N Engl J Med.* 1995;333:1588-1593; The Publications Committee for the Trial of ORG 10172 in Acute Stroke Treatment (TOAST) Investigators. *JAMA.* 1998;279:1265-1272; Chamorro A. *Cerebrovasc Dis.* 1999;9(suppl 3):16-23; Berge E, et al. *Lancet.* 2000;355:1205-1210; Diener HC, et al. *Stroke.* 2001;32:22-29; Bath PM, et al. *Lancet.* 2001;358:683-684; Chamorro A, et al. *Cerebrovasc Dis.* 2005;19:402-404; Camerlingo M, et al. *Stroke.* 2005;36:2415-2420.

9

Those recent clinical trials confirm that the early administration of anticoagulants is associated with an increased risk of serious bleeding complications.[6,8-11] Although the incidence of symptomatic hemorrhagic transformation can be increased, the recently completed WARSS trial demonstrated that the incidence of symptomatic intracerebral hemorrhage could be no different than control if anticoagulation levels (warfarin) were tightly managed. Unfortunately, that recent clinical trial did not provide evidence for efficacy in preventing early recurrent stroke, halting neurologic worsening, or improving neurologic outcomes. Future trials might be able to establish the efficacy of acute or early anticoagulant treatment, but until such data become available, anticoagulants should be considered only in limited circumstances (Class III Recommendation, Level of Evidence A).

■ Adjunctive Anticoagulation

Heparin has been used as an adjunct in intra-arterial delivery of thrombolytic agents to prevent catheter-related thrombosis. Experience is limited. Two trials of prourokinase included heparin as an adjunct to the PA, which in PROACT, resulted in a heparin dose-dependent increase in symptomatic hemorrhage together with an increase in recanalization frequency.[46]

Small, uncontrolled studies show a reasonable degree of safety with adjunctive heparin treatment with intravenous rt-PA, but the efficacy of this strategy has not been established.[65,66] Current guidelines recommend that no anticoagulant be given within 24 hours of treatment with rt-PA.[1] At that point, a CT scan also should be performed to screen for a hemorrhagic transformation of the infarction. The medication could be started subsequently if the CT is negative. This recommendation is aimed primarily at maintaining safety. Until data confirming the safety and efficacy of adjunctive anticoagulation become available, the most prudent approach is to withhold heparin for the first 24 hours after treatment with rt-PA.

Despite the lack of supporting data, physicians continue to administer anticoagulants to some patients with recent stroke, such as those with recent cardioembolic events. If anticoagulants are prescribed, several steps probably should be followed (**Table 9.11**). These medications should not be given unless a CT scan excludes the presence of a hemorrhage. Patients with clinical signs of severe stroke or CT evidence of a multilobar infarction should not be given anticoagulants because of the high risk of brain hemorrhage. A plan for the administration of heparin is outlined in **Table 9.11**. Monitoring the level of anticoagulation with adjustments in the doses in response to the laboratory studies should be done to improve safety. Although a continuous intravenous infusion appears to be safer than intermittent injections of heparin, the safety and

9

TABLE 9.11 — Administration of Heparin Following Acute Ischemic Stroke

Baseline Assessment of Patient
- Do not treat if baseline NIHSS score is >15
- Do not treat if CT shows evidence of bleeding
- Do not treat if CT shows evidence of major ischemic stroke
- Do not treat if aPTT, INR, or platelet count is abnormal

Administration of Heparin
- Use a weight-based nomogram*
- Give as a continuous intravenous infusion
- Monitor level of anticoagulation with aPTT
- Adjust doses of heparin in response to aPTT

Abbreviations: aPTT, activated partial thromboplastin time; CT, computed tomography; INR, international normalized ratio; NIHSS, National Institutes of Health Stroke Scale.

* Weight-based nomograms: Raschke RA, et al. *Ann Intern Med.* 1993;119:874-881; Brill-Edwards P, et al. *Ann Intern Med.* 1993;119:104-109.

efficacy of starting treatment with a bolus dose have not been established. The current weight-based nomograms for the use of heparin do include a bolus dose to initiate therapy.[67,68]

■ Coumarins

While oral anticoagulants are effective in prophylaxis against ischemic stroke, their delayed pharmacologic actions prevent them from being effective in the initial management of the acute neurologic event. However, these agents should be started following stroke with the goal of anticoagulation for long-term prophylaxis against recurrent stroke in patients with high-risk cardiac lesions.

■ Direct Thrombin Inhibitors

A pilot study of the direct thrombin inhibitor argatroban showed a modest increase in hemorrhage with treatment.[69] No improvement in outcomes was noted.

Antiplatelet Agents

Agents that inhibit platelet aggregation are of established utility for the prevention of ischemic stroke in high-risk patients (see Chapter 11, *Prevention of Ischemic Stroke or Recurrent Ischemic Stroke*).

■ Aspirin

Because aspirin affects platelet function almost immediately, it may have a role in acute treatment, but the timing of initiation of treatment after stroke is not clear. Two large trials tested the safety and efficacy of aspirin (160 mg to 300 mg) given within 48 hours of onset of stroke.[8,12] Aspirin produced modest reductions in mortality and recurrent stroke and a minimal reduction in neurologic morbidity. As a result, guidelines recommend that most patients with stroke should receive aspirin within 48 hours of their event (Class 1

Recommendation, Level of Evidence A). Although the risks of hemorrhage were small, the usefulness of acute administration of aspirin in ameliorating the effects of acute ischemic stroke has not been established.

Overall, the benefit of aspirin in ameliorating the effects of ischemic stroke in the acute setting has not been established. The administration of aspirin should not be considered as "definitive" therapy for acute treatment of ischemic stroke. It should not be given as an alternative to treatment with rt-PA to an otherwise eligible patient. Rather, the results of these trials suggest that starting aspirin (as part of long-term stroke prophylaxis) can be accomplished safely within the first hours after stroke. One trial that tested the concomitant use of aspirin and streptokinase found an extraordinarily high rate of serious intracranial hemorrhage, suggesting that in some circumstances, aspirin might augment the bleeding risk of thrombolytic therapy.[20] Current guidelines recommend that no aspirin be given within 24 hours after treatment with rt-PA[1] (Class III Recommendation, Level of Evidence A). On the other hand, 50% of patients who receive rt-PA are already taking aspirin, without ill effects (eg, hemorrhage).

■ **Clopidogrel**

Some groups have prescribed clopidogrel to achieve immediate inhibition of platelet function in the setting of acute cardiovascular procedures, such as coronary artery angioplasty.[70,71] Although the administration of clopidogrel shows promise, this regimen has not been tested in the setting of treatment of acute ischemic stroke. Its use for acute treatment of ischemic stroke is not recommended. Furthermore, the recently reported Clopidogrel for High Atherothrombotic Risk and Ischemic Stabilization, Management, and Avoidance (CHARISMA) trial does not support combination antiplatelet treatment with aspirin plus clopidogrel in stroke patients.

■ **Aspirin and Dipyridamole**

The combination of low-dose aspirin with extended-release dipyridamole has demonstrated efficacy in preventing recurrent strokes in patients presenting with transient ischemic attacks (TIAs) and completed stroke.[72]

■ **GPIIb/IIIa Inhibitors**

The glycoprotein IIb/IIIa receptor antagonists are used as adjuncts to angioplasty or low doses of thrombolytic agents to treat patients with acute myocardial ischemia. These agents do not yet have a role in acute management of ischemic stroke. Pilot studies demonstrated that abciximab could be given with relative safety to a broad spectrum of patients with ischemic stroke. However, in combination with rt-PA, significant safety concerns arose that led to the termination of a phase 3 trial.[13] Eckert and colleagues[73] gave the combination of abciximab and low-dose intra-arterial rt-PA to 47 patients, and the outcomes of this group were compared with those of 41 patients who received thrombolysis alone. Additional testing of the agent is under way. Currently, abciximab is not established as useful in treating patients with acute ischemic stroke, either alone or when given in combination with thrombolytic agents (Class III Recommendation, Level of Evidence B).

Fibrinogen-Depleting Agent

Studies of the fibrinogen-depleting agent ancrod have indicated benefit when outcome was adjusted to baseline stroke severity in a North American Study.[74] The European parallel study was inconclusive.[75] The final report of the latter study is expected. A phase 3 trial is in preparation.

Volume Expansion and Induced Hypertension

Considerable research has focused on the maintenance of cerebral blood flow by methods to increase flow by expanding the circulating volume or changing viscosity. These approaches have been based on the observation that the vascular bed in an ischemic region loses autoregulation and that flow becomes pressure dependent. In addition, changes in viscosity have a major impact on flow, especially in small-caliber vessels. Dilution of blood viscosity to levels that do not compromise arterial oxygen content might increase blood flow without changing brain oxygenation. Both isovolemic and hypervolemic hemodilution paradigms have been tested. In the latter, colloid volume expanders, such as hydroxyethyl starch or LMW dextran, and crystalloids, such as saline, are given. In the isovolemic setting, the medications are supplemented by varying degrees of phlebotomy. Reducing viscosity through hypervolemic hemodilution is used as part of the regimen to prevent ischemic stroke secondary to vasospasm following SAH. However, the studies of the use of hemorheologic agents or volume expanders in acute or early treatment of ischemic stroke are discouraging.[76-80] While anecdotal reports suggest that some patients might be helped, the results of large clinical trials are negative. Besides a lack of efficacy in ischemic stroke per se, side effects, including congestive heart failure, myocardial ischemia, or worsening of brain edema, limit the role of hemodilution, especially in elderly patients. Current guidelines recommend that hemodilution not be used in the management of acute ischemic stroke. Volume expansion has therefore been abandoned.

Maintenance of vascular perfusion is central to limiting ischemic injury and thus vasoactive compounds might be helpful. Vasoconstrictors (vasopressors) can improve blood flow in the ischemic region by increasing perfusion pressure in areas of the brain where autoregulation has been lost. Blood is shunted from relatively normal areas of the brain to those regions with ischemia. While vasopressors are an important part of management of vasospasm-related ischemia after SAH, their utility in other stroke settings is not known. Trials of induced hypertension will be necessary because a population of elderly patients with a high prevalence of ischemic heart disease might be at risk for major cardiovascular complications from the administration of vasopressors. Thus, although increasing blood pressure usually is not attempted unless the patient with ischemic stroke is hypotensive, an aggressive stance toward rapidly lowering the blood pressure also is avoided (see Chapter 6, *Emergency Medical Management of Stroke*). Vasodilators have been abandoned because they can aggravate increased intracranial pressure and may shunt blood from the ischemic locus to areas of the brain with relatively normal perfusion. In addition, these agents can cause arterial hypotension, an effect that could worsen perfusion and ischemia.

Other Pharmacologic Strategies

Other interventions that may alter the development of the ischemic lesion include medications that might block activation of an inflammatory reaction or processes at the vascular-parenchymal interface or manipulate cerebral vasodynamics. Leukocyte adhesion and transmigration are initiated by local ischemia and their secondary effects may contribute to the evolution of an infarction. Unfortunately, trials testing the potential utility of blockers of white blood cell receptors have so far not been successful in the setting of acute ischemic stroke.

Nonpharmacologic Surgical and Endovascular Measures to Restore Perfusion

Several nonpharmacologic endovascular interventions, including lasers, clot-extraction devices, microsnares, angioplasty, stenting, and ultrasonography, have been used to facilitate removal of thrombi and to improve perfusion to the brain.[86-91] (**Figure 9.2**). These devices have been tested alone or in combination with the use of PAs or other antithrombotic agents. Clinical experience with many of these innovative devices is limited. Alexandrov[92] tested the usefulness of transcranial Doppler ultrasonography as an adjunct to intravenous administration of rt-PA. Nedelmann and colleagues[93] found that thrombus lysis was most successful with low-frequency ultrasound. Preliminary data suggest that this approach could help improve early recanalization, but experience is thus far limited.

■ Endovascular Extraction of a Thrombus

The Mechanical Embolus Removal in Cerebral Ischemia (MERCI) trial tested the utility of a clot-extraction device in restoring circulation in patients with intracranial arterial occlusions.[94] This nonrandomized trial enrolled 151 patients; recanalization was achieved in 69 (46%). This recanalization frequency was compared with the control group of patients enrolled in the trial of intra-arterial administration of prourokinase. When compared with patients who did not display recanalization, favorable outcomes were higher (46% vs 10%) and mortality was lower (32% vs 54%) in patients demonstrating recanalization. Symptomatic hemorrhages occurred in 7.8% of the treated patients. The device was approved for use for removal of intracranial arterial thrombi but not by efficacy. Nonetheless, the role of the clot-extraction

FIGURE 9.2 — Restoration of Cerebral Blood Flow in Progressing Stroke by Stenting the Internal Carotid Artery

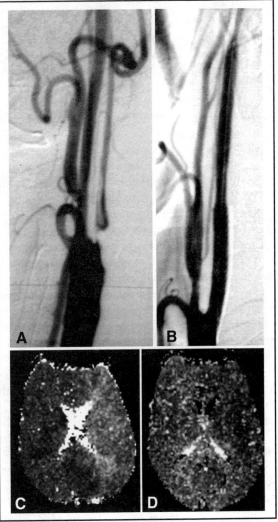

Continued

A. Digital subtraction angiography (DSA) of the left carotid artery shows a tight stenosis (pseudoocclusion) in a 51-year-old man with progressive paresis of his right arm. The patient had cardiomyopathy with a reduced ejection fraction and additional stenoses of the right internal carotid artery (ICA) and of both vertebral arteries. The left ICA stenosis was diagnosed as occlusion by duplex ultrasound.

B. DSA after stent placement and subsequent balloon dilatation.

C. Perfusion imaging with magnetic resonance image (MRI): the time-to-peak (TTP) parameter image shows a prolongation of the time until contrast peak within the entire middle cerebral artery territory indicated by relatively high signal.

D. TTP parameter image immediately after stent placement shows normalization of flow disturbance. The patient reported a complete recovery of his arm's weakness.

device in management of patients with stroke is not established[95] (Class IIb Recommendation, Level of Evidence B). Another assessment of the clinical role of this device and efficacy comparatively is required.

■ **Other Surgical Procedures**

Surgical procedures, such as embolectomy or carotid endarterectomy, have been explored to restore perfusion in patients with acute stroke.[96-100] These interventions have not been subjected to clinical trials and experience is limited. The most common scenario for emergency surgery is immediate arterial occlusion and infarction following a carotid endarterectomy. In this situation, surgical exploration has been performed to remove a fresh thrombus at the operative site. However, surgical procedures to remove distal emboli are generally severely debilitating and no longer studied.

REFERENCES

1. Adams HP, Brott TG, Furlan AJ, et al. Guidelines for thrombolytic therapy for acute stroke: a supplement to the guidelines for the management of patients with acute ischemic stroke. A statement for healthcare professionals from a Special Writing Group of the Stroke Council, American Heart Association. *Circulation*. 1996;94:1167-1174.

2. Practice advisory: thrombolytic therapy for acute ischemic stroke—summary statement. Report of the Quality Standards Subcommittee of the American Academy of Neurology. *Neurology*. 1996;47:835-839.

3. The National Institute of Neurological Disorders and Stroke rt-PA Stroke Study Group. Tissue plasminogen activator for acute ischemic stroke. *N Engl J Med*. 1995;333:1581-1587.

4. Norris JW, Buchan A, Cote R, et al. Canadian guidelines for intravenous thrombolytic treatment in acute stroke. A consensus statement of the Canadian Stroke Consortium. *Can J Neurol Sci*. 1998;25:259.

5. Norris JW, Buchan A, Cote R, et al. Canadian guidelines for intravenous thrombolytic treatment in acute stroke. A consensus statement of the Canadian Stroke Consortium. *Can J Neurol Sci*. 1998;25:257-259.

6. The Publications Committee for the Trial of ORG 10172 in Acute Stroke Treatment (TOAST) Investigators. Low molecular weight heparinoid, ORG 10172 (danaparoid), and outcome after acute ischemic stroke: a randomized controlled trial. *JAMA*. 1998;279:1265-1272.

7. Kay R, Wong KS, Yu YL, et al. Low-molecular-weight heparin for the treatment of acute ischemic stroke. *N Engl J Med*. 1995;333:1588-1593.

8. International Stroke Trial Collaborative Group. The International Stroke Trial (IST): a randomised trial of aspirin, subcutaneous heparin, both, or neither among 19435 patients with acute ischaemic stroke. *Lancet*. 1997;349:1569-1581.

9. Berge E, Abdelnoor M, Nakstad PH, Sandset PM. Low molecular-weight heparin versus aspirin in patients with acute ischaemic stroke and atrial fibrillation: a double-blind randomised study. HAEST Study Group. Heparin in Acute Embolic Stroke Trial. *Lancet*. 2000;355:1205-1210.

10. Diener HC, Ringelstein EB, von Kummer R, et al. Treatment of acute ischemic stroke with the low-molecular-weight heparin certoparin: results of the TOPAS trial. Therapy of Patients With Acute Stroke (TOPAS) Investigators. *Stroke*. 2001;32:22-29.

11. Chamorro A. Heparin in acute ischemic stroke: the case for a new clinical trial. *Cerebrovasc Dis*. 1999;9(suppl 3):16-23.

12. CAST (Chinese Acute Stroke Trial) Collaborative Group. CAST: randomised placebo-controlled trial of early aspirin use in 20,000 patients with acute ischaemic stroke. *Lancet*. 1997;349:1641-1649.

13. Reuters. News Release: J & J, Lilly halt trial of Reopro for stroke. Reuters Health. October 29, 2005.

14. Feigin VL, Rinkel GJ, Algra A, van Gijn J. Circulatory volume expansion for aneurysmal subarachnoid hemorrhage. *Cochrane Database Syst Rev*. 2000;CD000483.

15. Miller JA, Dacey RG, Diringer MN. Safety of hypertensive hypervolemic therapy with phenylephrine in the treatment of delayed ischemic deficits after subarachnoid hemorrhage. *Stroke*. 1995;26:2260-2266.

16. Mori T, Katayama Y, Kawamata T, Hirayama T. Improved efficiency of hypervolemic therapy with inhibition of natriuresis by fludrocortisone in patients with aneurysmal subarachnoid hemorrhage. *J Neurosurg*. 1999; 91:947-952.

17. Mayberg MR, Batjer HH, Dacey R, et al. Guidelines for the management of aneurysmal subarachnoid hemorrhage. A statement for healthcare professionals from a special writing group of the Stroke Council, American Heart Association. *Circulation*. 1994;90:2592-2605.

18. Generalized efficacy of t-PA for acute stroke. Subgroup analysis of the NINDS t-PA Stroke Trial. *Stroke*. 1997;28:2119-2125.

19. Donnan GA, Davis SM, Chambers BR, et al. Streptokinase for acute ischemic stroke with relationship to time of administration: Australian Streptokinase (ASK) Trial Study Group. *JAMA*. 1996;276:961-966.

20. Multicentre Acute Stroke Trial—Italy (MAST-I) Group. Randomised controlled trial of streptokinase, aspirin, and combination of both in treatment of acute ischaemic stroke. *Lancet*. 1995;346:1509-1514.

21. The Multicenter Acute Stroke Trial—Europe Study Group. Thrombolytic therapy with streptokinase in acute ischemic stroke. *N Engl J Med*. 1996;335:145-150.

22. Hacke W, Kaste M, Fieschi C, et al. Intravenous thrombolysis with recombinant tissue plasminogen activator for acute hemispheric stroke. The European Cooperative Acute Stroke Study (ECASS). *JAMA*. 1995;274:1017-1025.

23. Steiner T, Bluhmki E, Kaste M, et al. The ECASS 3-hour cohort. Secondary analysis of ECASS data by time stratification. ECASS Study Group. European Cooperative Acute Stroke Study. *Cerebrovasc Dis*. 1998;8:198-203.

24. Clark WM, Albers GW, for the ATLANTIS Stroke Study Investigators. The ATLANTIS rt-PA (alteplase) Acute Stroke Trial. Final results. *Stroke*. 1999;30:234

25. Clark WM, Albers GW, Madden KP, Hamilton S. The rtPA (alteplase) 0- to 6-hour acute stroke trial, part A (A0276g): results of a double-blind, placebo-controlled, multicenter study. Thromblytic therapy in acute ischemic stroke study investigators. *Stroke*. 2000;31:811-816.

26. The NINDS t-PA Stroke Study Group. Intracerebral hemorrhage after intravenous t-PA therapy for ischemic stroke. *Stroke*. 1997;28:2109-2118.

27. Chiu D, Krieger D, Villar-Cordova C, et al. Intravenous tissue plasminogen activator for acute ischemic stroke: feasibility, safety, and efficacy in the first year of clinical practice. *Stroke*. 1998;29:18-22.

28. Osborn TM, La Monte MP, Gaasch WR. Intravenous thrombolytic therapy for stroke: a review of recent studies and controversies. *Ann Emerg Med*. 1999;34:244-255.

29. Tanne D, Bates VE, Verro P, et al. Initial clinical experience with IV tissue plasminogen activator for acute ischemic stroke: a multicenter survey. The t-PA Stroke Survey Group. *Neurology*. 1999;53:424-427.

30. Egan R, Lutsep HL, Clark WM, et al. Open label tissue plasminogen activator for stroke: the Oregon experience. *J Stroke Cerebrovasc Dis*. 1999;8:287-290.

31. Wirkowski E, Gottesman MH, Mazer C, Brody GM, Manzella SM. Tissue plasminogen activator for acute stroke in everyday clinical practice. *J Stroke Cerebrovasc Dis*. 1999;8:291-294.

9

32. Wang DZ, Rose JA, Honings DS, Garwacki DJ, Milbrandt JC. Treating acute stroke patients with intravenous tPA. The OSF stroke network experience. *Stroke*. 2000;31:77-81.

33. Katzan IL, Furlan AJ, Lloyd LE, et al. Use of tissue-type plasminogen activator for acute ischemic stroke: the Cleveland area experience. *JAMA*. 2000;283:1151-1158.

34. Sasaki O, Takeuchi S, Koike T, Koizumi T, Tanaka R. Fibrinolytic therapy for acute embolic stroke: intravenous, intracarotid, and intra-arterial local approaches. *Neurosurgery*. 1995;36:246-253.

35. Urbach H, Ries F, Ostertun B, Solymosi L. Local intra-arterial fibrinolysis in thromboembolic "T" occlusions of the internal carotid artery. *Neuroradiology*. 1997;39:105-110.

36. Endo S, Kuwayama N, Hirashima Y, Akai T, Nishijima M, Takaku A. Results of urgent thrombolysis in patients with major stroke and athero-thrombotic occlusion of the cervical internal carotid artery. *AJNR Am J Neuroradiol*. 1998;19:1169-1175.

37. Zeumer H, Freitag HJ, Zanella F, Thie A, Arning C. Local intra-arterial fibrinolytic therapy in patients with stroke: urokinase versus recombinant tissue plasminogen activator (r-TPA). *Neuroradiology*. 1993;35:159-162.

38. Casto L, Caverni L, Camerlingo M, et al. Intra-arterial thrombolysis in acute ischaemic stroke: experience with a superselective catheter embedded in the clot. *J Neurol Neurosurg Psychiatry*. 1996;60:667-670.

39. Gonner F, Remonda L, Mattle H, et al. Local intra-arterial thrombolysis in acute ischemic stroke. *Stroke*. 1998;29:1894-1900.

40. Jahan R, Duckwiler GR, Kidwell CS, et al. Intraarterial thrombolysis for treatment of acute stroke: experience in 26 patients with long-term follow-up. *AJNR Am J Neuroradiol*. 1999;20:1291-1299.

41. Suarez JI, Sunshine JL, Tarr R, et al. Predictors of clinical improvement, angiographic recanalization, and intracranial hemorrhage after intra-arterial thrombolysis for acute ischemic stroke. *Stroke*. 1999;30:2094-2100.

42. del Zoppo GJ, Poeck K, Pessin MS, et al. Recombinant tissue plasminogen activator in acute thrombotic and embolic stroke. *Ann Neurol*. 1992;32:78-86.

43. Huemer M, Niederwieser V, Ladurner G. Thrombolytic treatment for acute occlusion of the basilar artery. *J Neurol Neurosurg Psychiatry*. 1995;58:227-228.

44. Brandt T, von Kummer R, Muller-Kuppers M, Hacke W. Thrombolytic therapy of acute basilar artery occlusion. Variables affecting recanalization and outcome. *Stroke*. 1996;27:875-881.

45. Wijdicks EF, Nichols DA, Thielen KR, et al. Intra-arterial thrombolysis in acute basilar artery thromboembolism: the initial Mayo Clinic experience. *Mayo Clin Proc*. 1997;72:1005-1013.

46. del Zoppo GJ, Higashida RT, Furlan AJ, Pessin MS, Rowley HA, Gent M. PROACT: a phase II randomized trial of recombinant pro-urokinase by direct arterial delivery in acute middle cerebral artery stroke. PROACT Investigators. Prolyse in Acute Cerebral Thromboembolism. *Stroke*. 1998;29:4-11.

47. Furlan A, Higashida R, Wechsler L, et al. Intra-arterial prourokinase for acute ischemic stroke. The PROACT II study: a randomized controlled trial. Prolyse in Acute Cerebral Thromboembolism. *JAMA*. 1999;282:2003-2011.

48. Hacke W, Zeumer H, Ferbert A, Bruckmann H, del Zoppo GJ. Intra-arterial thrombolytic therapy improves outcome in patients with acute vertebrobasilar occlusive disease. *Stroke*. 1988;19:1216-1222.

49. Macleod MR, Davis SM, Mitchell PJ, et al. Results of a multicentre, randomised controlled trial of intra-arterial urokinase in the treatment of acute posterior circulation ischaemic stroke. *Cerebrovasc Dis*. 2005;20:12-17.

50. Ezaki Y, Tsutsumi K, Onizuka M, et al. Retrospective analysis of neurological outcome after intra-arterial thrombolysis in basilar artery occlusion. *Surg Neurol*. 2003;60:423-429; discussion 429-430.

51. Hacke W, Albers G, Al-Rawi Y, et al. The desmoteplase in acute ischemic stroke trial (DIAS). A phase II MRI-based 9-hour window acute stroke thrombolysis trial with intravenous desmoteplase. *Stroke*. 2005;36:66-73.

52. Haley EC Jr, Kassell NF, Torner JC. A randomized, controlled trial of high-dose intravenous nicardipine in aneurysmal subarachnoid hemorrhage: a report of the Cooperative Aneurysm Study. *J Neurosurg*. 1993;78:537-547.

53. Haley EC, Lyden PD, Johnston KC, Hemmen TM; the TNK in Stroke Investigators. A pilot dose escalation safety study of tenecteplase in acute ischemic stroke. *Stroke*. 2005;36:607-612.

54. Uchino K, Alexandrov AV, Garami Z, El-Mitwalli A, Morgenstern LB, Grotta JC. Safety and feasibility of a lower dose intravenous TPA therapy for ischemic stroke beyound the first three hours. *Cerebrovasc Dis*. 2005;19:260-266.

55. Suarez JI, Zaidat OO, Sunshine JL, Tarr R, Selman WR, Landis DM. Endovascular administration after intravenous infusion of thrombolytic agents for the treatment of patients with acute ischemic strokes. *Neurosurgery*. 2002;50:251-260.

56. Zaidat OO, Suarez JI, Santillan C, et al. Response to intra-arterial and combined intravenous and intra-arterial therapy in patients with distal internal carotid artery occlusion. *Stroke*. 2002;33:1821-1827.

57. Hill MD, Barber PA, Demchuk AM, et al. Acute intravenous intra-arterial revascularization therapy for severe ischemic stroke. *Stroke*. 2002;33:279-282.

58. The IMS Study Investigators. Combined intravenous and intra-arterial recanalization for acute ischemic stroke: the interventional management of stroke study. *Stroke*. 2004;35:904-912.

59. Marsh EE, Adams HP, Biller J, et al. Use of antithrombotic drugs in the treatment of acute ischemic stroke: a survey of neurologists in practice in the United States. *Neurology*. 1989;39:1631-1634.

60. Caplan LR. When should heparin be given to patients with atrial fibrillation-related embolic brain infarcts? *Arch Neurol*. 1999;56:1059-1060.

61. Sandercock P. Is there still a role for intravenous heparin in acute stroke? No. *Arch Neurol*. 1999;56:1160-1161.

62. Grau AJ, Hacke W. Is there still a role for intravenous heparin in acute stroke? Yes. *Arch Neurol*. 1999;56:1159-1160.

63. Chamorro A, Busse O, Obach V, et al. The rapid anticoagulation prevents ischemic damage study in acute stroke — final results from the writing committee. *Cerebrovasc Dis*. 2005;19:402-404.

64. Camerlingo M, Salvi P, Belloni G, Gamba T, Cesana BM, Mamoli A. Intravenous heparin started within the first 3 hours after onset of symptoms as a treatment for acute nonlacunar hemispheric cerebral infarctions. *Stroke*. 2005;36:2415-2420.

9

65. Trouillas P, Nighoghossian N, Getenet JC, et al. Open trial of intravenous tissue plasminogen activator in acute carotid territory stroke. Correlations of outcome with clinical and radiological data. *Stroke.* 1996;27:882-890.

66. Grond M, Rudolf J, Neveling M, Stenzel C, Heiss WD. Risk of immediate heparin after rt-PA therapy in acute ischemic stroke. *Cerebrovasc Dis.* 1997;7:318-323.

67. Raschke RA, Reilly BM, Guidry JR, Fontana JR, Srinivas S. The weight-based heparin dosing nomogram compared with a "standard care" nomogram. A randomized controlled trial. *Ann Intern Med.* 1993;119:874-881.

68. Brill-Edwards P, Ginsberg JS, Johnston M, Hirsh J. Establishing a therapeutic range for heparin therapy. *Ann Intern Med.* 1993;119:104-109.

69. LaMonte MP, Nash ML, Wang DZ, et al. Argatroban anticoagulation in patients with acute ischemic stroke (ARGIS-1). A randomized, placebo-controlled safety study. *Stroke.* 2004;35:1677-1682.

70. The Clopidogrel in Unstable Angina to Prevent Recurrent Events Trial Investigators. Effects of clopidogrel in addition to aspirin in patients with acute coronary syndromes without ST-segment elevation. *N Engl J Med.* 2001;345:494-502.

71. Mehta SR, Yusuf S, Peters RJ, et al. Effects of pretreatment with clopidogrel and aspirin followed by long-term therapy in patients undergoing percutaneous coronary intervention: the PCI-CURE study. *Lancet.* 2001;358:527-533.

72. Diener H, Cunha L, Forbes C, Sivenius J, Smets P, Lowenthal A. European Stroke Prevention Study 2. Dipyridamole and acetylsalicylic acid in the secondary prevention of stroke. *J Neurol Sci.* 1996;143:1-13.

73. Eckert B, Koch C, Thomalla G, et al. Aggressive therapy with intravenous abciximab and intra-arterial rtPA and additional PTA/stenting improves clinical outcome in acute vertebrobasilar occlusion: combined local fibrinolysis and intravenous abciximab in acute vertebrobasilar stroke treatment (FAST): results of a multicenter study. *Stroke.* 2005;36:1160-1165.

74. Sherman DG, Atkinson RP, Cheppendale T, et al. Intravenous ancrod for treatment of acute ischemic stroke: the STAT study: a randomized controlled trial. Stroke Treatment With Ancrod Trial. *JAMA.* 2000;283:2395-2403.

75. Sherman DG, for the STAT Writers Group. Defibrinogenation with Viprinex (ancrod) for the treatment of acute ischemic stroke. *Stroke.* 1999;30:234.

76. The Hemodilution in Stroke Study Group. Hypervolemic hemodilution treatment of acute stroke. Results of a randomized multicenter trial using pentastarch. *Stroke.* 1989;20:317-323.

77. Scandinavian Stroke Study Group. Multicenter trial of hemodilution in acute ischemic stroke. Results of subgroup analyses. *Stroke.* 1988;19:464-471.

78. Berrouschot J, Barthel H, Scheel C, Koster J, Schneider D. Extracorporeal membrane differential filtration—a new and safe method to optimize hemorheology in acute ischemic stroke. *Acta Neurol Scand.* 1998;97:126-130.

79. Berrouschot J, Barthel H, Koster J, et al. Extracorporeal rheopheresis in the treatment of acute ischemic stroke: a randomized pilot study. *Stroke.* 1999;30:787-792.

80. Frazee JG, Luo X, Luan G, et al. Retrograde transvenous neuroperfusion: a back door treatment for stroke. *Stroke*. 1998;29:1912-1916.

81. Rordorf G, Koroshetz WJ, Ezzeddine MA, Segal AZ, Buonanna FS. A pilot study of drug-induced hypertension for treatment of acute stroke. *Neurology*. 2001;56:1210-1213.

82. Rordorf G, Cramer SC, Efird JT, Schwamm LH, Buonanno F, Koroshetz WJ. Pharmacological elevation of blood pressure in acute stroke. Clinical effects and safety. *Stroke*. 1997;28:2133-2138.

83. Hillis AE, Ulatowski JA, Barker PB, et al. A pilot randomized trial of induced blood pressure elevation: effects on function and focal perfusion in acute and subacute stroke. *Cerebrovasc Dis*. 2003;16:236-246.

84. Hillis AE, Wityk RJ, Barker PB, Ulatowski JA, Jacobs MA. Change in perfusion in acute nondominant hemisphere stroke may be better estimated by tests of hemispatial neglects than by the National Institute of Health Stroke Scale. *Stroke*. 2003;34:2392-2396.

85. Marzan AS, Hungerbühler HJ, Studer A, Baumgartner RW, Georgiadis AL. Feasibility and safety of norepinephrine-induced arterial hypertension in acute ischemic stroke. *Neurology*. 2004;62:1193-1195.

86. Molina CA, Saver JL. Extending reperfusion therapy for acute ischemic stroke: Emerging pharmacological, mechanical, and imaging strategies. *Stroke*. 2005;36:2311-2320.

87. Leary MC, Saver JL, Gobin YP, et. al. Beyond tissue plasminogen activator: mechanical intervention in acute stroke. *Ann Emerg Med*. 2003;41:838-846.

88. Ringer AJ, Qureshi AI, Fessler RD, Guterman LR, Hopkins LN. Angioplasty of intracranial occlusion resistant to thrombolysis in acute ischemic stroke. *Neurosurgery*. 2001;48:1282-1288.

89. Qureshi AI, Siddiqui AM, Suri MFK, et al. Aggressive mechanical clot disruption and low-dose intra-arterial third-generation thrombolytic agent for ischemic stroke: a prospective study. *Neurosurgery*. 2002;51:1319-1329.

90. Lutsep HL, Clark WM, Nesbit GM, Kuether TA, Barnwell SL. Intra-arterial suction thrombectomy in acute stroke. *Am J Neuroradiol*. 2002;23:783-786.

91. Daffertshofer M, Gass A, Ringleb P, et al. Transcranial low-frequency ultrasound-mediated thrombolysis in brain ischemia: increased risk of hemorrhage with combined ultrasound and tissue plasminogen activator: results of a phase II clinical trial. *Stroke*. 2005;36:1441-1446.

92. Alexandrov AV. Ultrasound identification and lysis of clots. *Stroke*. 2004;35(suppl 1):2722-2725.

93. Nedelmann M, Brandt C, Schneider F, et al. Ultrasound-induce blood clot dissolution without a thrombolytic drug is more effective with lower frequencies. *Cerebrovasc Dis*. 2005;20:18-22.

94. Smith WS, Sung G, Starkman S, et al. Safety and efficacy of mechanical embolectomy in acute ischemic stroke: results of the MERCI trial. *Stroke*. 2005;36:1432-1438.

95. Becker K, Brott T. Approval of the MERCI clot retriever. A critical view. *Stroke*. 2005;36:400-403.

96. Meyer FB, Sundt TMJ, Piepgras DG, Sandok BA, Forbes G. Emergency carotid endarterectomy for patients with acute carotid occlusion and profound neurological deficits. *Ann Surg*. 1986;203:82-89.

97. Meyer FB, Piepgras DG, Sundt TMJ. Emergency embolectomy for acute occlusion of the middle cerebral artery. *J Neurosurg*. 1985;62:639-647.

98. Huber R, Muller BT, Seitz RJ, Siebler M, Modder U, Sandmann W. Carotid surgery in acute symptomatic patients. *Eur J Vasc Endovasc Surg*. 2003;25:60-67.

99. Eckstein HH, Schumacher H, Klemm K, et al. Emergency carotid endarterectomy. *Cerebrovasc Dis*. 1999;9:270-281.

100. Eckstein HH, Ringleb P, Dorfler A, et al. The Carotid Surgery for Ischemic Stroke Trial: a prospective observational study on carotid endarterectomy in the early period after ischemic stroke. *J Vasc Surg*. 2002;36:997-1004.

101. Bath PM, Lindenstrom E, Boysen G, et al. Tinzaparin in acute ischaemic stroke (TAIST): a randomised aspirin-controlled trial. *Lancet*. 2001;358:683-684.

10

Acute Treatment of Ischemic Stroke: Neuroprotection

Occlusion of a cerebral artery initiates a complex series of cellular and metabolic events that affect the functions and structure of neurons, glia, and endothelial cells. In addition, changes also occur in the extracellular space. But these events cannot be taken out of the context of the vascular responses (which include endothelial cells and astrocytes) and the need for adequate sustained blood flow. These effects on brain cell function are considered primarily in the setting of acute ischemic stroke, but patients with intracranial hemorrhage may also have secondary ischemia in adjacent tissues within the brain. The relevance of ischemia to the local effects of hemorrhage in the brain is under study in experimental systems. But some agents with channel-related activity have been used in the setting of cerebral hemorrhage.

Neuron and astrocyte homeostasis is dependent upon membrane stability, which in part involves the ability of ion pumps to regulate fluxes of sodium (Na^+) and potassium (K^+) and to keep calcium (Ca^{++}) from entering the cell. Ca^{++} entry mediates cell injury and is controlled by Ca^{++}–dependent receptor-mediated processes. Reduction of blood flow below a critical level initiates receptor-mediated Ca^{++} entry and neurogeneration.[1] Ca^{++} influx is regulated through two types of membrane channels:

- Voltage-sensitive Ca^{++} channels (VSCC) and
- Receptor-operated Ca^{++} channels.

Experimental studies show that the receptor-mediated events rapidly lead to loss of neuronal function. Stimulation of the VSCC increases Ca^{++} at presynaptic sites, causing an excessive release of excitatory amino acids, such as glutamate, from presynaptic terminals. Among the membrane sites that affect Ca^{++} channels are both inotropic and metabotropic glutamate receptors. Overstimulation of the inotropic glutamate receptors (N-methyl-D-aspartate [NMDA] and alpha-3-hydroxy-5-methy-4-isooxazoloproprionic acid [AMPA/kainate] types) produces an abnormal elevation of Ca^{++} within neurons. In contrast, activation of metabotropic receptors promotes the production of inositol-1,4,5-triphosphate and stimulates release of Ca^{++} from intracellular stores. Ca^{++} entry results in membrane depolarization and significant shifts in ions, inducing an intracellular accumulation of water. Swelling of neurons and glia results. These events coincide with the loss in blood-brain barrier and microvascular integrity. Inhibitors of the various Ca^{++} channel–associated receptors, including postsynaptic VSCC antagonists and antagonists of the glutamate receptors, have been evaluated as potential therapies. In addition, inhibition of presynaptic glutamate release may reduce postsynaptic neuronal injury.

Neuroprotective agents are most successful in lessening the consequences of neuronal ischemia in experimental models when they are administered prior to the onset of ischemia. However, the experience with these agents in clinical trials has been extremely disappointing to date. Potential roles for neuroprotective agents have been thought to be as prophylactic interventions in situations that carry a high risk for ischemia, such as major cardiovascular or cerebrovascular operations or as an adjunct to interventions that restore or augment perfusion to the brain. So far, none of these agents has demonstrated the ability to safely reduce the volume of infarction or improve clinical outcomes in patients with stroke who are treated acutely or soon after the onset of neurologic symptoms.

Blocking the Ca⁺⁺ Channels

L-glutamate and related excitatory amino acids play pivotal roles in triggering neurotoxic events by activating Ca^{++} influx through agonist-operated channels. Of the six identified subtypes of VSCC, the L-type VSCC modulators, some of which are used in hypertension and ischemic heart disease, have demonstrated limited usefulness in the setting of stroke because of their vasodepressor effects.

Nimodipine was tested in several stroke trials. Nimodipine is of proven usefulness in improving outcomes after subarachnoid hemorrhage (SAH) by lessening the ischemic consequences of vasospasm.[2,3] The results of trials of nimodipine delivered within 6 hours of ischemic stroke are largely negative, and in some cases treated patients had poorer outcomes than did the controls.[4-8] One retrospective analysis suggested that patients treated earliest fared better. But two meta-analyses did not show any net improvement in outcomes with nimodipine treatment.[7-9] Nimodipine is not recommended for the acute treatment of patients with ischemic stroke[10] (Class III Recommendation, Level of Evidence A). Importantly, many patients with ischemic stroke are volume depleted, and administration of this medication may further reduce cerebral blood flow by its hypotensive effects.

S-emopamil, an L-type Ca^{++} channel blocker, is reported to reduce neuronal injury in experimental models of brain ischemia. Several N-type VSCC blockers, possibly affecting presynaptic release neurotransmitters, and T-type VSCC blockers may reduce tissue injury after experimental focal ischemia. Data are not available from clinical studies.

10

Gamma-aminobutyric acid (GABA), an inhibitory neurotransmitter, blocks voltage-gated Ca^{++} influx associated with glutamate release and may protect neurons from ischemic damage. The GABA agonist muscimol is effective in experimental models. Clomethiazole, which is neuroprotective in experimental brain ischemia, was tested in clinical trials, but the results were negative.[11,12]

Four adenosine receptor subtypes (A1, A2a, A2b, and A3) have been identified. Adenosine blocks release of excitatory amino acids by acting on central nervous system presynaptic A1 receptors to reduce influx of Ca^{++}.[13] Activation of the A2 receptor potentially increases microvascular flow by inducing tonic relaxation of smooth muscle in microvessels, inhibiting platelet aggregation, and blocking leukocyte adherence to endothelial cells and subsequent microvascular plugging.[14,15] Experimental studies report the potential efficacy of adenosine receptor agonists and adenosine-regulating agents in brain ischemia but clinical studies have not been performed.

Inhibitors of Glutamate Release

Several Na^+ channel-blocking agents inhibit release of glutamate from presynaptic terminals. In experimental studies, these agents reduce infarct size when given before or after the onset of ischemia. Lubeluzole normalizes excitability in the peri-infarct region by decreasing extracellular concentrations of glutamate; a nitric oxide mechanism also was reported. Unfortunately, clinical trials of lubeluzole were unable to demonstrate any benefit from treatment.[16-18] A recent test of the concept that a neuroprotectant medication can enhance the benefits of thrombolysis, a trial of rt-PA and lubeluzole, failed to demonstrate a significant outcome in favor of the two medications.

NMDA or AMPA Antagonists

To date, no antagonist of the NMDA receptor has been shown to be clinically efficacious. Common side effects of this class of compounds include:

- Sedation
- Changes in blood pressure
- Cardiac conduction disturbances
- Respiratory depression
- Agitation, confusion, or delirium
- Ataxia
- Nystagmus
- Dysphoria or hallucinations
- Memory disturbances
- Psychosis.

Aptiganel, a noncompetitive NMDA antagonist, is no longer being studied clinically and several other agents also were tested without success.[12,19-23] At higher doses, dextrorphan was found to produce hypotension, respiratory failure, or coma.[24] Eliprodil, an antagonist of the polyamine modulatory site of the NMDA receptor complex, demonstrated a dose-dependent prolongation of the QT interval.[25] Selfotel was found to be ineffective in patients at a dose shown to be effective in animal models. A trend to increased early mortality was observed.[19] While remacemide may help prevent poor neurological outcomes following major cardiac operations, the medication has not improved outcomes after stroke.[26,27] High rates of adverse experiences also were reported with the use of licostinel or eliprodil.[28-30] The AMPA antagonist ZK200775 was found to worsen the neurologic status of patients with acute ischemic stroke, in part due to its sedative effects.[31] Despite these setbacks, other agents of the NMDA/AMPA antagonist class that might have neuroprotective activity continue to be studied. These currently include memantine, CGS 19755, GPI 3000, CNS 5161A, CGP-40116, 4a-phenanthrenamine derivatives acting at the phencyclidine binding site AR-R15896AR and others.

Magnesium (Mg^{++}) blocks the NMDA ion channel in a voltage-dependent fashion. Preliminary trials of intravenous infusions of magnesium sulfate ($MgSO_4$) given to patients within 24 hours of onset of stroke have been shown to be safe.[32,33] Large clinical trials are testing the agent.

Several AMPA/kainate antagonists have reduced the volume of brain injury in experimental models. The AMPA/kainate antagonists have fewer behavioral effects than do the NMDS antagonists. In high doses, these agents severely depress glucose utilization. Antagonizing the AMPA/kainate channel alone or in combination with other Ca^{++} channels may be a potential cytoprotective strategy for management of stroke. The role of these medications remains uncertain.

Membrane-Active Agents

Systemic administration of choline and cytidine promote phosphatidylcholine synthesis and the generation of cell membranes. Preclinical and clinical studies suggest that cytidine diphosphocholine (citicoline) may be effective in improving outcomes after stroke.[34] While citicoline is available for treatment of patients with stroke in Europe and Japan, subsequent clinical trials were unable to confirm the efficacy of this therapy.[34,35]

Neurotrophic Factors

In experimental models, basic fibroblast growth factor (basic FGF) and transforming growth factor-β (TGF-β) significantly reduced volumes of infarctions.[36,37] However, clinical studies of basic FGF were not completed because of a lack of efficacy.

Nitric Oxide Modulation

Nitric oxide (NO) mediates endothelial cell–dependent vasodilation as endothelium-derived relaxing factor (EDRF) and promotes ischemic neuron damage by stimulating glutamate-mediated processes and forming highly toxic peroxynitrate radicals. Therefore, inhibitors of NO synthase may provide a potentially useful treatment to reduce ischemic brain injury. In experimental studies, low doses of NO synthase inhibitors reduced evidence of brain damage, while high doses increased histologic evidence of brain damage.[38-42]

Hypothermia

Hypothermia reduces ischemic injury in animal models. In nonischemic brain tissue, the cerebral metabolic rate of oxygen ($CMRO_2$) consumption decreases 7% for every 1°C reduction in temperature.[43] Hypothermic conditions decrease metabolic demands of both viable and ischemic tissue. Hypothermia also may affect inflammatory cell reactivity and cytokine synthesis and release directly or indirectly. Rapid induction of mild hypothermia currently is not practical for the acute management of most patients with acute ischemic stroke but some pharmacologic interventions may reduce brain temperature.

Hypothermia has been successful in limiting the neurologic consequences of cardiac arrest and global ischemia.[44,45] There are uncertainties about the use of induced hypothermia in treatment of patients with stroke. It is not a benign therapy; hypotension, cardiac arrhythmias, and infections are potential complications.[46,47] These complications seem to be associated with lower temperatures and prolonged periods of treatment. Pilot studies suggest that cooling with the use of external cooling devices or endovascular interventions may be safe and feasible.[48-51] However, a recent review could find no evidence that either physical or pharmacologic cooling improved outcomes after stroke.[52] In addition, a trial of induced hypothermia to protect the brain during surgical treatment of ruptured aneurysms did not show improvement in outcomes in patients treated with modest reductions in body temperature.[53] While induced lowering of temperature holds promise, currently there is insufficient evidence to support the use of hypothermia to treat patients with acute ischemic or hemorrhagic stroke (Class IIb Recommendation, Level of Evidence B).

Other Interventions

A number of novel, but so far unsuccessful, interventions have been used. High doses of barbiturates lower cellular metabolism and reduce brain injury in experimental paradigms. Unfortunately, the use of barbiturates has not been successful in a clinical setting and this approach has been limited to nonacute situations. Tirilazad mesylate, a 21-aminosteroid with nonglucocorticoid properties, was effective in experimental models under conditions of cerebral arterial occlusion and reperfusion but clinical trials in acute stroke were negative.[54,55] Although experimental models suggested a potential benefit, monosialoganglioside (GM1), an agent with both neuroprotective and neurotrophic properties in experimental models, had no significant clinical therapeutic effects.[56] Clinical trials of naloxone, a nonagonist opiate receptor antagonist, did not show a benefit of treatment (Class III Recommendation, Level of Evidence B).

Free-Radical Scavenger

A recently reported prospective trial of 1700 ischemic stroke patients of the free-radical scavenger NXY-059 within 6 hours of stroke onset suggested a modest benefit to patients treated with this compound compared with placebo.[65,66] A second prospective trial is underway.

Combination of Neuroprotectants With Reperfusion

Often clinical trials of acute intervention face the potential issue of including patients who are appropriate candidates for the delivery of rt-PA. Additionally, limited experimental work supports the notion that protection of neurons and glial cells in the ischemic territory requires maintenance or reinstitution of flow. Hence, some have proposed that only combination treatments make sense. Two combination trials have been disappointing.

Lubeluzole was tested alone or in combination with rt-PA in a series of trials.[57,58] A review of all the data concluded that there was no evidence of efficacy of the medication.[59] Clomethiazole was tested alone or in combination with rt-PA to treat patients with ischemic stroke or as an intervention for hemorrhagic stroke.[60,61] Large trials did not demonstrate efficacy of the medication.[20,62-64]

Subarachnoid Hemorrhage From Aneurysmal Rupture

Despite its lack of proven efficacy in clinical ischemic stroke, nimodipine is the first medication demonstrated as effective in improving outcomes after any form of acute cerebrovascular disease. In clinical trials, nimodipine has been demonstrated as effective in lessening morbidity and mortality (from brain ischemia) following SAH.[3] It is recommended as an important adjunct for treatment of patients with recently ruptured aneurysms[2] (Class I Recommendation, Level of Evidence A).

Window of Treatment and Conclusions

An important, unresolved issue concerning the salvage of ischemic brain tissue is the timing and duration of the therapeutic window. Hypothermia and agents that mildly lower brain temperature have been proposed to extend the window of time for treatment of acute ischemic stroke. Blockade of postsynaptic Ca^{++} channels and inhibition of release of excitatory amino acids are potential targets in experimental neuroprotection that may exceed the window of time for reperfusion. Limited experimental studies have suggested that the addition of an NMDA receptor antagonist to a thrombolytic agent may reduce the volume of an ischemic stroke. However, the concept is yet to be confirmed in clinical studies.

To date, there is reason to believe that none of the trials of neuroprotectants have adequately tested their underlying hypotheses.[67-69] Therefore, most of the trials should not be taken as showing unequivocal evidence that refutes the hypothesis that these medications could modulate injury or alter specific functions in the clinical setting. Limitations of those trials variously include the lack of adherence to preclinical testing paradigms, inadequate power to differentiate active from inactive stroke subtypes, and the curtailment of recruitment because of serious dose-limiting side effects, such as stupor or hypotension. In addition, some of the trials have failed because of inadequate or inappropriate dosing, flawed clinical trial design, differences in responses between species to specific agents, thresholding of outcome events, and other issues. Attention to many of these issues offers the promise that future studies of agents with neuroprotectant properties may be successful.

REFERENCES

1. Pulsinelli W. Pathophysiology of acute ischaemic stroke. *Lancet.* 1992;339:533-536.
2. Mayberg MR, Batjer HH, Dacey R, et al. Guidelines for the management of aneurysmal subarachnoid hemorrhage. A statement for healthcare professionals from a special writing group of the Stroke Council, American Heart Association. *Stroke.* 1994;25:2315-2328.
3. Pickard JD, Murray GD, Illingworth R, et al. Effect of oral nimodipine on cerebral infarction and outcome after subarachnoid haemorrhage: British aneurysm nimodipine trial. *BMJ.* 1989;298:636-642.
4. The American Nimodipine Study Group. Clinical trial of nimodipine in acute ischemic stroke. *Stroke.* 1992;23:3-8.
5. Kaste M, Fogelholm R, Erila T, et al. A randomized, double-blind, placebo-controlled trial of nimodipine in acute ischemic hemispheric stroke. *Stroke.* 1994;25:1348-1353.
6. Wahlgren NG, MacMahon DG, DeKeyser J, Indredavik B, Ryman T. Intravenous Nimodipine West European Stroke Trial (INWEST) of nimodipine in the treatment of acute ischaemic stroke. *Cerebrovasc Dis.* 1994;4:204-210.
7. Mohr JP, Orgogozo JM, Harrison MJG, et al. Meta-analysis of oral nimodipine trials in acute ischemic stroke. *Cerebrovasc Dis.* 1999;4:197-203.
8. Infeld B, Davis SM, Donnan GA, et al. Nimodipine and perfusion changes after stroke. *Stroke.* 1999;30:1417-1423.
9. Leys D, Hommel M, Woimant F, Pruvo JP. Treatment of cerebral ischemia in its acute phase and prospectives. *Rev Med Intern.* 1994;15:350-356.
10. Adams HP, Brott TG, Crowell RM, et al. Guidelines for the management of patients with acute ischemic stroke. A statement for healthcare professionals from a special writing group of the Stroke Council, American Heart Association. *Circulation.* 1994;90:1588-1601.
11. Wahlgren NG; The Clomethiazole Acute Stroke Study Collaborative Group. The clomethiazole acute stroke study (CLASS): results of a randomised controlled study of clomethiazole versus placebo in 1360 acute stroke patients. *Cerebrovasc Dis.* 1997;7(suppl 4):24-30.
12. Wahlgren NG, Ranasinha KW, Rosolacci T, et al. Clomethiazole acute stroke study (CLASS): results of a randomized, controlled trial of clomethiazole versus placebo in 1360 acute stroke patients. *Stroke.* 1999;30:21-28.
13. Simpson RE, O'Regan MH, Perkins LM, Phillis JW. Excitatory transmitter amino acid release from the ischemic rat cerebral cortex: effects of adenosine receptor agonists and antagonists. *J Neurochem.* 1992;58:1683-1690.

14. Phillis JW. Adenosine in the control of the cerebral circulation. *Cerebrovasc Brain Metab Rev.* 1989;1:26-54.

15. Cronstein BN. Adenosine, an endogenous anti-inflammatory agent. *J Appl Physiol.* 1994;76:5-13.

16. Diener HC, Hacke W, Hennerici M, Radberg J, Hantson L, De Keyser J. Lubeluzole in acute ischemic stroke. A double-blind, placebo-controlled phase II trial. Lubeluzole International Study Group. *Stroke.* 1996;27:76-81.

17. Grotta J. Lubeluzole treatment of acute ischemic stroke. The US and Canadian Lubeluzole Ischemic Stroke Study Group. *Stroke.* 1997;28:2338-2346.

18. Hacke W, Lees KR, Timmerhuis T, et al. Cardiovascular safety of lubeluzole (Prosynap(R)) in patients with ischemic stroke. *Cerebrovasc Dis.* 1998;8:247-254.

19. Davis SM, Lees KR, Albers GW, et al. Selfotel in acute ischemic stroke: possible neurotoxic effects of an NMDA antagonist. *Stroke.* 2000;31:347-354.

20. Wester P, Strand T, Wahlgren NG, Ashwood T, Osswald G. An open study of clomethiazole in patients with acute cerebral infarction. *Cerebrovasc Dis.* 1998;8:188-190.

21. Lees KR, Asplund K, Carolei A, et al. Glycine antagonist (gavestinel) in neuroprotection (GAIN International) in patients with acute stroke: a randomised controlled trial. GAIN International Investigators. *Lancet.* 2000;355:1949-1954.

22. Sacco RL, De Rosa JT, Haley EC, et al. Glycine antagonist in neuroprotection for patients with acute stroke: GAIN Americas: a randomized controlled trial. *JAMA.* 2001;285:1719-1728.

23. Dyker AG, Edwards KR, Fayad PB, Hormes JT, Lees KR. Safety and tolerability study of aptiganel hydrochloride in patients with an acute ischemic stroke. *Stroke.* 1999;30:2038-2042.

24. Albers GW, Atkinson RP, Kelley RE, Rosenbaum DM. Safety, tolerability, and pharmacokinetics of the N-methyl-D-aspartate antagonist dextrorphan in patients with acute stroke. Dextrorphan Study Group. *Stroke.* 1995;26:254-258.

25. Dyker AG, Muir KW, Lees KR. A double-blind, randomized, placebo-controlled, dose-escalation study of remacemide in patients with acute stroke. *Stroke.* 1997;28:233.

26. Arrowsmith JE, Harrison MJ, Newman SP, Stygall J, Timberlake N, Pugsley WB. Neuroprotection of the brain during cardiopulmonary bypass: a randomized trial of remacemide during coronary artery bypass in 171 patients. *Stroke.* 1998;29:2357-2362.

27. Dyker AG, Lees KR. Remacemide hydrochloride: a double-blind, placebo-controlled, safety and tolerability study in patients with acute ischemic stroke. *Stroke.* 1999;30:1796-1801.

28. Albers GW, Clark WM, Atkinson RP, Madden K, Data JL, Whitehouse MJ. Dose escalation study of the NMDA glycine-site antagonist licostinel in acute ischemic stroke. *Stroke.* 1999;30:508-513.

29. Dyker AG, Lees KR. Safety and tolerability of GV150526 (a glycine site antagonist at the N-methyl-D-aspartate receptor) in patients with acute stroke. *Stroke.* 1999;30:986-992.

30. Lees KR. Cerestat and other NMDA antagonists in ischemic stroke. *Neurology.* 1997;49(suppl 4):S66-S69.

31. Walters MR, Kaste M, Lees KR, et al. The AMPA antagonist ZK 200775 in patients with acute ischaemic stroke: a double-blind, multicentre, placebo-controlled safety and tolerability study. *Cerebrovas Dis.* 2005;20:304-309.

32. Muir KW, Lees KR. A randomized, double-blind, placebo-controlled pilot trial of intravenous magnesium sulfate in acute stroke. *Stroke*. 1995;26:1183-1188.

33. Muir KW, Lees KR. Dose optimization of intravenous magnesium sulfate after acute stroke. *Stroke*. 1998;29:918-923.

34. Clark WM, Warach SJ, Pettigrew LC, Gammans RE, Sabounjian LA. A randomized dose-response trial of citicoline in acute ischemic stroke patients. Citicoline Stroke Study Group. *Neurology*. 1997;49:671-678.

35. Clark WM, Williams BJ, Selzer KA, Zweifler RM, Sabounjian LA, Gammans RE. A randomized efficacy trial of citicoline in patients with acute ischemic stroke. *Stroke*. 1999;30:2592-2597.

36. Fisher M, Meadows ME, Do T, et al. Delayed treatment with intravenous basic fibroblast growth factor reduces infarct size following permanent focal cerebral ischemia in rats. *J Cereb Blood Flow Metab*. 1995;15:953-959.

37. Koketsu N, Berlove DJ, Moskowitz MA, Kowall NW, Caday CG, Finklestein SP. Pretreatment with intraventricular basic fibroblast growth factor decreases infarct size following focal cerebral ischemia in rats. *Ann Neurol*. 1994;35:451-457.

38. Buisson A, Plotkine M, Boulu RG. The neuroprotective effect of a nitric oxide inhibitor in a rat model of focal cerebral ischaemia. *Br J Pharmacol*. 1992;106:766-767.

39. Nagafuji T, Matsui T, Koide T, Asano T. Blockade of nitric oxide formation by N omega-nitro-L-arginine mitigates ischemic brain edema and subsequent cerebral infarction in rats. *Neurosci Lett*. 1992;147:159-162.

40. Nishikawa T, Kirsch JR, Koehler RC, Bredt DS, Snyder SH, Traystman RJ. Effect of nitric oxide synthase inhibition on cerebral blood flow and injury volume during focal ischemia in cats. *Stroke*. 1993;24:1717-1724.

41. Dawson DA, Kusumoto K, Graham DI, McCulloch J, Macrae IM. Inhibition of nitric oxide synthesis does not reduce infarct volume in a rat model of focal cerebral ischaemia. *Neurosci Lett*. 1992;142:151-154.

42. Yamamoto S, Golanov EV, Berger SB, Reis DJ. Inhibition of nitric oxide synthesis increases focal ischemic infarction in rat. *J Cereb Blood Flow Metab*. 1992;12:717-726.

43. Rosomoff HL, Holaday DA. Cerebral blood flow and cerebral oxygen consumption during hypothermia. *Am J Physiol*. 1954;179:85-88.

44. Bernard SA, Buist M. Induced hypothermia in critical care medicine: a review. *Crit Care Med*. 2003;31:2041-2051.

45. Bernard SA, Gray TW, Buist M, et al. Treatment of comatose survivors of out-of-hospital cardiac arrest with induced hypothermia. *N Engl J Med*. 2002;346:557-563.

46. Olsen TS, Weber UJ, Kammersgaard LP. Therapeutic hypothermia for acute stroke. *Lancet Neurol*. 2003;2:410-416.

47. Feigin VL, Anderson CS, Rodgers A, Anderson NE, Gunn AJ. The emerging role of induced hypothermia in the management of acute stroke. *J Clin Neurosci*. 2002;9:502-507.

48. Georgiadis D, Schwarz S, Kollmar R, Schwab S. Endovascular cooling for moderate hypothermia in patients with acute stroke: first results of a novel approach. *Stroke*. 2001;32:2550-2553.

49. Keller E, Imhof HG, Gasser S, Terzic A, Yonekawa Y. Endovascular cooling with heat exchange catheters: a new method to induce and maintain hypothermia. *Intensive Care Med*. 2003;29:939-943.

10

50. Slotboom J, Kiefer C, Brekenfeld C, et al. Locally induced hypothermia for treatment of acute ischaemic stroke: a physical feasibility study. *Neuroradiology*. 2004;46:923-934.

51. Krieger D, De Georgia M, Abou-Chebl A, et al. Cooling for acute ischemic brain damage (cool aid): an open pilot study of induced hypothermia in acute ischemic stroke. *Stroke*. 2002;32:1847-1854.

52. Correia M, Silva M, Veloso M. Cooling therapy for acute stroke. *Cochrane Database Syst Rev*. 2000;CD001247.

53. Todd MM, Hindman BJ, Clarke WR, Torner JC; Intraoperative Hypothermia for Aneurysm Surgery Tiral (IHAST) Investigators. Mild intraoperative hypothermia during surgery for intracranial aneurysm. *N Engl J Med*. 2005;352:135-145.

54. The RANTTAS Investigators. A randomized trial of tirilazad mesylate in patients with acute stroke (RANTTAS). *Stroke*. 1996;27:1453-1458.

55. Tirilazad International Steering Committee. Tirilazad mesylate in acute ischemic stroke: a systematic review. *Stroke*. 2000;31:2257-2265.

56. The SASS Trial. Ganglioside GM1 in acute ischemic stroke. *Stroke*. 1994;25:1141-1148.

57. Grotta J; The Combination Therapy Stroke Trial Investigators. Combination Therapy Stroke Trial: recombinant tissue-type plasminogen activator with/without lubeluzole. *Cerebrovasc Dis*. 2001;12:258-263.

58. Diener HC, Cortens M, Ford G, et al. Lubeluzole in acute ischemic stroke treatment: a double-blind study with an 8-hour inclusion window comparing a 10-mg daily dose of lubeluzole with placebo. *Stroke*. 2000;31:2543-2551.

59. Gandolfo C, Sandercock P, Conti M. Lubeluzole for acute ischaemic stroke. *Cochrane Database Syst Rev*. 2002;CD001924.

60. Lyden P, Jacoby M, Schim J, et al. The Clomethiazole Acute Stroke Study in tissue-type plaminogen activator-treated stroke (CLASS-T): final results. *Neurology*. 2001;57:1199-1205.

61. Wahlgren NG, Diez-Tejedor E, Teitelbaum JK. Results in 95 hemorrhagic stroke patients included in CLASS, a controlled trial of clomethiazole versus placebo in acute stroke patients. *Stroke*. 2000;31:82-85.

62. Wahlgren NG, The Clomethiazole Acute Stroke Study Collaborative Group. The clomethiazole acute stroke study (CLASS): results of a randomised controlled study of clomethiazole versus placebo in 1360 acute stroke patients. *Cerebrovasc Dis*. 1997;7(suppl 4):24-30.

63. Zingmark PH, Ekblom M, Odergren T, et al. Population pharmacokinetics of clomethiazole and its effect on the natural course of sedation in acute stroke patients. *Br J Clin Pharmacol*. 2003;56:173-183.

64. Lyden P, Shuaib A, Ng K, et al. Clomethiazole acute stroke study in ischemic stroke (CLASS-I): final results. *Stroke*. 2002;33:122-128.

65. Lees KR, Zivin JA, Ashwood T, et al; Stroke-Acute Ischemic NXY-Treatment (SAINT I) Trial Investigators. NXY-059 for acute ischemic stroke. *N Engl J Med*. 2006;354:588-600.

66. del Zoppo GJ. Stroke and neurovascular protection. *N Engl J Med*. 2006;354:553-555.

67. Muir KW, Grosset DG. Neuroprotection for acute stroke: making clinical trials work. *Stroke*. 1999;30:180-182.

68. Lees KR. Does neuroprotection improve stroke outcome? *Lancet*. 1998;351:1447-1448.

69. Zivin JA. Neuroprotective therapies in stroke. *Drugs*. 1997;54(suppl 3):83-89.

Prevention of Ischemic Stroke or Recurrent Ischemic Stroke

Therapies of proven usefulness can lower the risk of ischemic stroke (primary prevention) or recurrent ischemic stroke (secondary prevention). Because many patients with a transient ischemic attack (TIA), amaurosis fugax, or ischemic stroke also are at high risk for myocardial infarction (MI) and vascular death, prophylactic measures should include interventions to prevent or treat ischemic heart disease. Fortunately, most of the medications that are effective in lowering the risk of ischemic stroke also lower the risk of MI. Still, one must remember that none of the measures intended to prevent stroke or other ischemic events is uniformly successful. Rather, these interventions help lower the risk. Additional therapies and research are needed. Both patients and physicians need other interventions that, in the future, will further reduce the likelihood of ischemic stroke.

General Measures

Some of the most effective interventions to prevent stroke are aimed at slowing the course of atherosclerosis, preventing rupture of an atherosclerotic plaque, and stabilizing the vascular endothelium.[1] Many medications are aimed at controlling risk factors or conditions that promote the development of advanced atherosclerosis. Attention to these risk factors also is critical when making decisions about the secondary prevention of ischemic stroke. For example, efforts to stop smoking may be very cost-effective because the risk of stroke drops dramatically within 2 years of halt-ing the use of cigarettes. The role of the management of these risk factors is described in more detail in Chapter 3, *General Measures to Prevent Stroke*.

Medications to Prevent Thromboembolism

Several therapies that prevent thromboembolism are of proven usefulness in preventing stroke in high-risk patients[2,3] (**Table 11.1**). Decisions about the prescription of medications to prevent thromboembolic events are based on several factors, including:

- Likely cause of the ischemic symptoms
- Previous use of medications or prior surgical therapy
- Contraindications for a specific medication
- Potential indications for a surgical or endovas-cular procedure
- Wishes of the patient.

The affected vascular territory, as reflected by the patient's neurologic symptoms, influences decisions

TABLE 11.1 — Therapies to Prevent Thromboembolic Stroke
Long-Term Anticoagulants   • Warfarin
Antiplatelet Agents   • Aspirin   • Aspirin and dipyridamole   • Clopidogrel   • Ticlopidine
Surgical Interventions   • Carotid endarterectomy   • Extracranial-intracranial arterial anastomoses   • Other reconstructive operations   • Endovascular procedures

about the recommendation for vascular operations, including carotid endarterectomy (CEA) or endovascular procedures. Patients having these vascular interventions usually receive antiplatelet agents as part of their management in order to prevent post-operative thromboembolism.

The presumed cause of stroke greatly affects decisions about selecting antithrombotic medications.[1] An algorithm based on the cause of stroke and other clinical variables, such as the prior use of medications or intolerance for specific therapies, is outlined in **Figure 11.1**. Patients with nonatherosclerotic vascular diseases may need specific treatments; for example, corticosteroids or cyclophosphamide may be required to treat a patient with stroke secondary to a vasculitis. Differentiating events due to cardioembolism from a high-risk cardiac lesion from emboli of arterial origin greatly affects plans for long-term medical prophylaxis to prevent recurrent ischemic stroke.[2,4] Anticoagulants usually are the first choice for patients with cardioembolic stroke, while antiplatelet agents are preferred for most patients with ischemia secondary to arterial diseases.

Oral Anticoagulants

Warfarin is the oral anticoagulant most commonly prescribed in the United States and compounds with similar actions are administered in other countries. The coumarins are antagonists of vitamin K–dependent γ-carboxylation of terminal glutamic acid residues of specific coagulation factors.[5] As a result, plasma levels of active factors II, VII, IX, X, and proteins C and S are reduced. Oral anticoagulants are of proven utility for prevention of deep vein thrombosis and cardioembolic stroke. Patients with heart disease associated with a high risk of thromboembolism usually are treated with long-term oral anticoagulant therapy unless a specific contraindication exists[2,6] (**Table 11.2**).

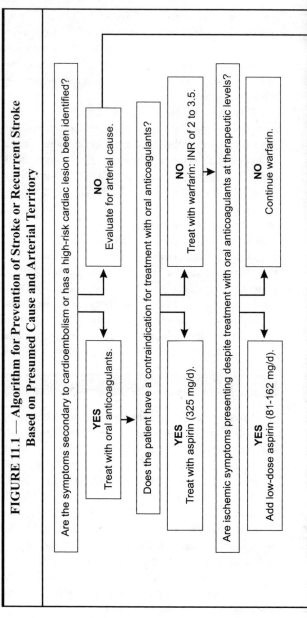

FIGURE 11.1 — Algorithm for Prevention of Stroke or Recurrent Stroke Based on Presumed Cause and Arterial Territory

Are the symptoms secondary to cardioembolism or has a high-risk cardiac lesion been identified?

YES
Treat with oral anticoagulants.

NO
Evaluate for arterial cause.

Does the patient have a contraindication for treatment with oral anticoagulants?

YES
Treat with aspirin (325 mg/d).

NO
Treat with warfarin: INR of 2 to 3.5.

Are ischemic symptoms presenting despite treatment with oral anticoagulants at therapeutic levels?

YES
Add low-dose aspirin (81-162 mg/d).

NO
Continue warfarin.

Are symptoms presenting in the circulation of a severely stenotic extracranial internal carotid artery, is the patient a reasonable candidate for surgical intervention, and is a skilled surgeon available?

YES

Consider carotid endarterectomy combined with low-dose aspirin (50-325 mg/d), aspirin/extended-release dipyridamole (50 mg/400 mg/d) combination, clopidogrel (75 mg/d), or ticlopidine (500 mg/d).

NO

Medical treatment with low-dose aspirin (50-325 mg/d), aspirin/extended-release dipyridamole (50 mg/400 mg/d) combination, clopidogrel (75 mg/d), or ticlopidine (500 mg/d).

Does the patient have recurrent ischemic symptoms despite treatment with aspirin?

NO
Continue aspirin

YES

Does the patient have an allergy or major gastrointestinal intolerance to aspirin?

NO
Continue aspirin

YES
Treat with clopidogrel (75 mg/d) or ticlopidine (500 mg/d).

YES
Treat with aspirin/extended-release dipyridamole (50 mg/400 mg/d) combination, clopidogrel (75 mg/d), or ticlopidine (500 mg/d).

Abbreviation: INR, international normalized ratio.

11

283

TABLE 11.2 — Cardiac Conditions Associated With the Highest Risk for Thromboembolism

- Recent myocardial infarction:
  – Anterior wall myocardial infarction
  – Akinetic segment
  – Intraventricular thrombus
- Mechanical prosthetic valve, especially the mitral valve
- Bioprosthetic valve, especially the mitral valve
- Rheumatic mitral stenosis, especially with AF
- Dilated cardiomyopathy, especially with AF
- Atrial fibrillation not associated with valvular heart disease:
  – Age >75 years
  – Women
  – Hypertension
  – Prior neurologic symptoms
  – Left atrial enlargement

Abbreviation: AF, atrial fibrillation.

■ Prevention of Cardioembolic Stroke

Several clinical trials have established the utility of oral anticoagulants in the primary prevention of stroke among patients with nonvalvular atrial fibrillation (AF).[7] Overall, oral anticoagulants reduce the risk of cardioembolic stroke by approximately 68%. Recent guidelines provide additional information about the use of oral anticoagulants among patients with heart disease; these agents are strongly recommended[1,2,8] (Class I Recommendation, Level of Evidence A) (**Table 11.3**). The usual target international normalized ratio (INR) is 2 to 3. The exception to the recommendation for oral anticoagulants in the setting of AF is the patient under the age of 60 who does not have structural heart disease (lone AF) because the risk of stroke is low.[9,10] In this situation, aspirin often is given. Aspirin (325 mg/day) may also be given in patients with AF who cannot tolerate anticoagulants[1] (Class I Recommendation, Level of Evidence A).

TABLE 11.3 — Desired Levels of Anticoagulation	
Indications	**INR**
Recent myocardial infarction	2-3
Rheumatic mitral stenosis	2-3.5
Mechanical prosthetic mitral valve	2.5-3.5
Biologic prosthetic mitral valve	2-3
Dilated cardiomyopathy	2-3
Atrial fibrillation	2-3
Abbreviation: INR, international normalized ratio.	

Oral anticoagulants also are recommended for prevention of cardioembolic stroke among patients with heart conditions, such as mechanical prosthetic valves or a recent anterior wall MI[1,11-14] (Class IIa Recommendation, Level of Evidence A). The goal is an INR of 2 to 3.

For patients with dilated cardiomyopathy, warfarin often is recommended[1] (Class IIb Recommendation, Level of Evidence B).

The utility of warfarin was compared with that of aspirin for preventing recurrent thromboembolic events among patients with a patent foramen ovale (PFO) and previous stroke in a multicenter trial; the two medications had equal efficacy.[8] Pending additional data that refute these findings, warfarin should not be recommended for most patients with stroke and PFO[1] (Class IIa Recommendation, Level of Evidence B). Although, with evidence of a venous thrombotic source and a PFO, oral anticoagulation is indicated. The role of PFO closure devices for ischemic stroke is not proven by appropriate clinical trials.

There are insufficient data to provide guidance about the use of warfarin among patients with other cardiac lesions that are associated with a low or uncertain risk for thromboembolism. However, an ongoing trial, Warfarin versus Aspirin in patients with Reduced Cardiac Ejection Fraction (WARCEF), tests the relative efficacy of warfarin or aspirin to prevent ischemic stroke in patients with low ejection fractions (congestive heart failure).

In many settings of coronary artery disease, aspirin is also recommended[1] (Class IIa Recommendation, Level of Evidence A). For instance, aspirin (and, in some cases, clopidogrel) is indicated in the acute management of non–ST-elevation acute coronary syndromes (NSTE ACS) and in patients with ACS with and without ST-segment elevation. These antiplatelet agents have also been used in patients with congestive heart failure with and without coronary artery disease.

■ **Disorders of Coagulation**

Oral anticoagulants often are given to patients with acquired or inherited disorders of coagulation who have demonstrated a related risk for arterial or venous occlusions.[15-17] But in general, the medications have not been tested in these situations and definitive data are not available. Although the factor V Leiden mutation is relatively common in some small stroke series, its presence does not dictate the use of antithrombotic agents prophylactically.

The usefulness of warfarin was compared with aspirin in treatment of patients with antiphospholipid antibodies; the two agents were equally effective.[18] However, this study generally enrolled older patients and it is not clear if warfarin is not superior to aspirin in preventing thromboembolic events in younger patients with antiphospholipid antibody syndrome. A role for oral anticoagulants may still be present. Oral anticoagulants are standard care in treatment of arterial or venous thrombosis in the setting of antiphospholipid antibodies of high titer.

■ Arterial Diseases

The role of oral anticoagulants for prevention of stroke among patients with noncardioembolic causes of cerebral ischemia appears to be limited. While oral anticoagulants have been given to patients with intracranial stenoses, posterior circulation disease, arterial dissections, or recurrent symptoms despite treatment with antiplatelet agents, the utility of the medications in these situations has not been established. A European trial testing oral anticoagulants with a relatively high INR was halted because of an unacceptably high rate of hemorrhagic complications.[19] A North American trial testing warfarin at a lower INR level found the medication to be safe, but the oral anticoagulant was not superior to aspirin in preventing recurrent stroke.[20]

Another study tested the usefulness of oral anticoagulants or aspirin among patients with symptomatic intracranial stenoses. No benefit in reduction in ischemic stroke was noted and adverse effects, including vascular deaths and hemorrhage, were significantly higher among the patients treated with warfarin.[21] No data are available about the efficacy and safety of oral anticoagulants in preventing recurrent ischemic symptoms among patients with extracranial arterial dissections.[22,23] Based on the aggregate, largely negative data, there appears little reason to prescribe anticoagulants to most patients with arterial disease causing stroke[1] (Class III Recommendation, Level of Evidence A). Additional research is testing the utility of oral anticoagulants in patients with atherosclerotic disease, including aortic disease.

■ Potential Complications

Maintaining patient safety is essential in the administration of oral anticoagulants, and assuring accuracy in the assessment of the level of anticoagulation is critical. Problems with interlaboratory differences in measurement of the prothrombin time secondary to variations in potency of reagents led to the use of the INR by institutions around the world.[24] This methodology is lessening the differences in laboratory follow-up measurements and is improving the ability to maintain proper levels of anticoagulation. Excessively high levels are associated with marked increases in the risk of serious bleeding complications, including potentially life-threatening intracranial hemorrhages. On the other hand, inadequate levels of anticoagulation lower the therapeutic efficacy of oral anticoagulants. For most indications, the desired level of anticoagulation is a target INR between 2 and 3 (**Table 11.3**).

A number of interactions with other medications, foods, and beverages add to the complexity of the administration of warfarin (**Table 11.4**). Frequent assessment of the level of anticoagulation and adjustments in doses are required. Contraindications for the use of oral anticoagulants are few but the factors that may limit their safety and potential efficacy are important to recognize (**Table 11.4**). In particular, physicians should review the potential interactions between warfarin and another medication that is started, adjusted, or discontinued. Many medications may prolong or shorten the INR.[25] Special attention should be paid to the concomitant use of antibiotics. Patients should receive instruction about the foods that contain large amounts of vitamin K. Although the consumption of these foods and beverages is not prohibited, patients should be advised to use moderation or to include these foods in the diet regularly so the dosage of warfarin may be adjusted accordingly. Multivitamins that do not contain vitamin K are available. Long-term administration of oral anticoagulants may lead to demineralization of bone or osteopenia because of their effects on vitamin K-dependent formation of the bone matrix.[26,27] Patients with hepatic or bowel disease may have problems with vitamin K absorption or metabolism and have problems with anticoagulation.

TABLE 11.4 — Potential Contraindications and Cautions for Treatment of Patients Taking Oral Anticoagulants

Contraindications
- Intolerance or allergy to oral anticoagulants
- Dementia
- High fall risk
- Laboratory follow-up not available
- Liver disease or malnutrition
- Recent head injury
- Pregnancy

Cautions
- Age >75 years, especially >80 years
- Alcohol or drug abuse
- Poor balance
- Past history of stroke or neurologic disease
- Concomitant medications that might affect coagulation:
  - Antiplatelet agents
  - Nonsteroidal anti-inflammatory agents
  - Antibiotics
  - Minor or major tranquilizers
- Concomitant illnesses that might affect coagulation:
  - Poor diet
  - Diet with foods high in vitamin K
  - Malabsorption
  - Use of vitamin K

Oral anticoagulants should not be prescribed to patients who have problems following the treatment regimen or for whom no laboratory follow-up is available. Patients who are at high risk for falls or cranial trauma, in particular elderly patients, should not receive warfarin. Because of the relatively high risk of teratogenicity associated with oral anticoagulants, the use of these medications during pregnancy is contra-indicated.[28,29] A young woman who is at high risk for embolic events should be treated with appropriate daily dosing of low molecular weight heparin for prophylaxis during pregnancy, depending upon the risk.

Hemorrhage is the most frequent complication from administration of oral anticoagulants; the leading fatal adverse experience is intracranial hemorrhage[30] (see Chapter 8, *Treatment of Hemorrhagic Stroke*). A subdural hematoma is a particularly dangerous complication that can follow relatively trivial head trauma. The "purple toe syndrome" and skin necrosis are rare complications that can appear during the initiation of oral anticoagulant therapy; these adverse experiences are secondary to the early inhibitory effects on levels of proteins C and S that may lead to a transient hypercoagulable state and ischemia. This complication is largely restricted to those patients who already have deficiencies of protein C or S. Concurrent administration of heparin during the initiation of treatment with warfarin may be used to avoid this complication.

Starting therapy with warfarin sometimes is achieved with doses that are higher than that required for maintenance of anticoagulation. An alternative strategy is to start maintenance doses of warfarin to achieve gradual anticoagulation without some of the attendant risk of bleeding or the frequent adjustments in dose that are associated with the former regimen.[31,32] The gradual approach also may lower the likelihood of a transient prothrombotic state. Once the desired level of anticoagulation is achieved, the INR should be measured at regular intervals and the dosage of medication should be adjusted in response to the results of the blood tests.

■ Direct Thrombin Inhibitors

The direct thrombin inhibitor ximelagatran has been tested for prevention of stroke among patients with AF. Potential advantages are the lack of necessity of coagulation monitoring and dosage adjustments. The trials demonstrated that ximelagatran and warfarin were approximately equal in forestalling new ischemic events.[33,34] However, the use of ximelagatran was associated with the elevation of liver enzymes in some patients. The medication has no antidote and there is no test to monitor adequacy of treatment. The medication has not been approved for prevention of stroke. Other antithrombotics, including lepirudin and argatroban, are not indicated for stroke.

Antiplatelet Agents

Antiplatelet agents are the usual medications to prevent stroke among high-risk patients. Large clinical trials and meta-analyses provide strong evidence that this class of medications is effective in lowering the risk of recurrent ischemic events.[35] These medications are effective among older and younger persons, women and men, those with diabetes and nondiabetics, and those with or without hypertension. Although antiplatelet agents are less effective than oral anticoagulants in preventing cardioembolic stroke, they are an alternative intervention for patients who cannot tolerate warfarin. The role of antiplatelet agents in preventing thromboembolic events among patients with most inherited or acquired hypercoagulable states has not been tested extensively. The only data are from the trial comparing warfarin and aspirin in preventing embolic events among patients with antiphospholipid antibodies.[18] In that trial, the two agents were found to be relatively similar in efficacy.

■ Aspirin

Aspirin interferes with platelet function and production of thromboxane A_2 by irreversible acetylation and inactivation of cyclooxygenase.[36] It has little action on platelet adhesion or aggregation at high shear stress. Aspirin is the most commonly prescribed medication for the primary or secondary prevention of ischemic stroke or other arterial diseases that lead to ischemia (**Figure 11.1** and **Table 11.5**).

TABLE 11.5 — Ranges of Effective Doses and Most Common Adverse Experiences With Antiplatelet Agents

- Aspirin 30-1300 mg/day:
  - Gastritis
  - Peptic ulcer disease
  - Gastrointestinal hemorrhage
  - Other bleeding
  - Allergic reactions
- Dipyridamole 400 mg/day:
  - Headache
- Ticlopidine 500 mg/day:
  - Skin eruptions, allergic reactions
  - Epigastric distress and diarrhea
  - Neutropenia (agranulocytosis)
  - Thrombotic thrombocytopenia purpura
- Clopidogrel 75 mg/day:
  - Skin eruptions, allergic reactions
  - Epigastric distress and diarrhea
  - Thrombotic thrombocytopenia purpura

Several clinical trials and meta-analyses show that aspirin is effective in lowering the risk of stroke, MI, and vascular death among high-risk men and women, regardless of age.[2,35] The medication also is used in primary prevention. Aspirin also is used as an alternative to oral anticoagulants for those persons with cardiac sources of thromboembolism, such as AF, who cannot take warfarin[1,37,38] (Class I Recommendation, Level of Evidence A). Aspirin may be started safely within the first 48 hours after stroke[39,40] (Class I Recommendation, Level of Evidence A).

Aspirin has several advantages. It is inexpensive and easy to administer. Its potential side effects are well known. Allergy to aspirin is reported by a sizable number of people. Bleeding, including intracranial hemorrhage, is a potential complication that may occur with a wide range of doses.[41] The most common side effects of aspirin, which are strongly related to the dose, are gastrointestinal (GI) complications, including:

- Gastritis
- Peptic ulcer disease
- GI hemorrhage.

Low doses of aspirin (<100 mg/day) are much less likely to be complicated by major GI adverse experiences than larger doses (>1000 mg/day).[42] Enteric-coated preparations or the concurrent use of medications that protect the stomach (ie, histamine antagonists or antacids) lessen the risk of gastric side effects.

Aspirin is recommended for lowering the risk of stroke for most high-risk patients with arterial disease[1] (Class I Recommendation, Level of Evidence A). It is the usual choice for the medical prevention of thromboembolism in patients with ischemic symptoms in either the carotid or vertebrobasilar circulation. It is used for treatment of patients with either intracranial or extracranial atherosclerosis. Aspirin is effective in a broad range of doses.

While early trials tested daily doses >1000 mg, more recent trials established the usefulness of lower doses.[43-45] A trial compared four different doses of aspirin in preventing stroke, MI, and vascular death among patients undergoing CEA.[46] Daily doses of 81 mg to 325 mg were found to be superior to higher doses. Current data support the use of aspirin in a daily dose of 81–325 mg for prevention of stroke in high-risk patients, including those with a recent stroke[1,47,48] (Class I Recommendation, Level of Evidence A). If a low dose is used, prompt inhibition of platelet aggregation may be achieved with an initial "loading" dose of 325 mg, although this is unproven. Thereafter, a daily dose of 81 mg aspirin will maintain suppression of platelet function. If the patient has problems with compliance and misses multiple doses, the 325-mg

11

dose may be superior to the 81-mg regimen because the larger dose will be more effective in reestablishing impaired platelet aggregation. There are no data to support increasing the dose of aspirin if a patient has an ischemic event (aspirin failure) despite treatment with low-dose aspirin.

While some patients may develop laboratory evidence of "resistance" to aspirin, the clinical correlates of this laboratory finding are lacking.[49,50] Currently, testing for aspirin sensitivity is complex and secondary adjustment (increase) in aspirin dose is not recommended. Aspirin, in a daily dose of 325 mg, is effective in preventing embolization among patients with AF. Still, in this setting, aspirin is inferior to warfarin and it should be used only when a patient cannot tolerate oral anticoagulants[1] (Class I Recommendation, Level of Evidence A). Aspirin has been used in conjunction with warfarin for treatment of patients who have recurrent symptoms despite "therapeutic" levels of anticoagulation[1] (Class I Recommendation, Level of Evidence A). The major concern here is the potential increase in hemorrhagic complications with the combination.

■ Dipyridamole and Aspirin/Dipyridamole

Dipyridamole has reversible effects on platelet aggregation through its inhibition of phosphodiesterase-5. The medication also produces vasodilation. Dipyridamole may be given as an adjunct to warfarin to treat patients with high-risk cardiac lesions, including those with mitral valve disease. Dipyridamole has few side effects; headaches are the most common complaint. In particular, headaches are a problem in patients with a past history of migraine. In addition, some patients with unstable angina may not tolerate the medication. Because of potential effects on coronary artery blood flow, dipyridamole may not be administered to a patient with a recent MI. Bleeding complications are few.

A European trial found that a combination of extended-release dipyridamole (400 mg/day) with aspirin (50 mg/day) was superior to aspirin (50 mg/day) alone in prevention of stroke.[51-53] Because the agents affect platelet aggregation by different mechanisms, there appears to be an increased effect when they are administered together. The same trial found that the combination was superior to dipyridamole alone and the risk of bleeding with the combination was not increased. A panel of the American College of Chest Physicians concluded that the combination of aspirin (50 mg/day) and extended-release dipyridamole (400 mg/day) was superior to aspirin in prevention of stroke among high-risk patients.[2] Currently, no data are available comparing the efficacy of aspirin and dipyridamole to that of clopidogrel in preventing ischemic events. Based on indirect evidence, Albers and associates[2] concluded that the combination of aspirin and dipyridamole might be superior to clopidogrel. A trial currently is testing the usefulness of clopidogrel or aspirin/dipyridamole in prevention of stroke. The combination of low-dose aspirin and extended-release dipyridamole is an important medical option for prevention of stroke among patients with TIA or stroke[1] (Class I Recommendation, Level of Evidence A).

11

■ Ticlopidine

Ticlopidine is a potent antiplatelet agent that blocks adenosine diphosphate (ADP)–induced platelet aggregation.[54] Clinical trials demonstrate the efficacy of ticlopidine in preventing ischemic events in high-risk patients.[55,56] In one trial, ticlopidine reduced the risk of stroke and other ischemic events by approximately 15% in comparison to aspirin. A study that tested the utility of aspirin or ticlopidine in prevention of recurrent among a group of high-risk African American patients found no benefit from treatment with ticlopidine.[57] Unfortunately, ticlopidine is associated with a relatively high rate of serious adverse experiences that limit its usefulness (**Table 11.5**). Approximately 0.5% of patients develop severe neutropenia (agranulocytosis).[58] Thrombotic thrombocytopenia purpura/hemolytic uremic syndrome is a potentially life-threatening complication that apparently is due to an antibody to von Willebrand metalloproteinase that is induced by the medication.[59-61] The hematologic abnormalities of ticlopidine generally happen during the first 3 to 4 months after starting the medication. As a result, regular hematologic assessments should be performed during this time period. While ticlopidine is an effective antiplatelet agent, the associated hematologic problems greatly limit its use. In general, clopidogrel now is used instead of ticlopidine.

■ Clopidogrel

Clopidogrel is a member of the same class of antiplatelet agents as ticlopidine. The usual daily dose is 75 mg. A "loading dose" of approximately 300 mg may be administered to initiate therapy in order to rapidly achieve maximal effects on platelet aggregation. This tactic is used when treating patients with acute myocardial ischemia or to achieve maximal effects on platelet function during endovascular procedures.[62,63] The need for this approach in the setting of general stroke prevention is not clear. Many of the side effects of clopidogrel are similar to those found with ticlopidine. A relatively low risk of thrombotic thrombocytopenic purpura (TTP) is reported.[64] Although the risk is less than that associated with ticlopidine, some patients with the complication have needed plasma exchanges or have had recurrent symptoms despite treatment for the hematological disorder. Most cases of TTP associated with clopidogrel are discovered within 2 weeks of starting treatment.

The agent was tested in a large clinical trial that enrolled patients with ischemic cerebrovascular dis-

296

ease as well as those with coronary artery disease and peripheral vascular disease.[65] The assumption was that the presence of ischemic symptoms in one vascular territory would denote a high risk of ischemic events in other parts of the body. This hypothesis makes considerable sense. However, there may be differences in the pathophysiology of ischemia in the lower extremities, myocardium, or brain. The symptoms of angina pectoris or intermittent claudication of the legs may be secondary to hypoperfusion aggravated by a temporary increase in metabolic demands. Acute MI is most commonly due to a local arterial thrombosis occurring at the site of a fractured plaque in a coronary artery. Many strokes are due to thromboembolism. Thus responses to a medication may not be identical in these three populations. The trial of clopidogrel found a modest reduction in ischemic events in comparison to aspirin, but the difference was noted primarily among patients who presented with symptomatic peripheral vascular disease. No significant difference between aspirin and clopidogrel was noted among patients who had a TIA or stroke as the qualifying event.

Because clopidogrel affects the P2Y12 receptor on platelets and aspirin affects cyclooxygenase, the combination of the two medications could have additive effects on preventing thrombosis. However, this combination of antiplatelet agents is associated with an increased risk of bleeding complications over monotherapy. Clopidogrel, in combination with aspirin, is prescribed to many patients with coronary artery disease, including those who undergo endovascular procedures. It also may be useful as an adjunctive therapy for treatment of acute myocardial ischemia. Patients who undergo cerebrovascular angioplasty or stenting often are prescribed clopidogrel in addition to aspirin for a period that usually lasts 6 to 12 weeks after the procedure.

Recently, a large trial tested the safety and efficacy of aspirin and clopidogrel vs clopidogrel alone for prevention of recurrent ischemic events among patients with TIA or stroke.[66,67] No difference in the frequency of ischemic events was noted between treatment groups, but the combination of medications was accompanied by an increase is serious bleeding complications. Another trial testing the utility of aspirin and clopidogrel demonstrated that adding clopidogrel to aspirin did not prevent ischemic events but was associated with an increased risk of bleeding.[68] The combination of aspirin and clopidogrel is not recommended for treatment of most patients with ischemic stroke[1] (Class I Recommendation, Level of Evidence A). Clopidogrel may be considered as a treatment alternative for a patient who has recurrent symptoms despite the use of aspirin or when treatment with aspirin is contraindicated[1] (Class I Recommendation, Level of Evidence A).

■ Other Antiplatelet Aggregating Agents

Sulfinpyrazone was tested in comparison with aspirin in a large clinical trial but it was found to be inferior.[69] As a result, sulfinpyrazone is not used for stroke prophylaxis. Several trials tested the utility of the glycoprotein (GP) IIb/IIIa inhibitors alone or in combination with aspirin. While the trials recruited patients with coronary artery disease, stroke was an important secondary outcome measure. In general, these trials found that the GP IIb/IIIa inhibitors were not more effective than aspirin, but they were associated with an increased risk of serious bleeding complications. As a result of these negative studies, these agents likely will not become a useful medical therapy to prevent ischemic stroke.

Combinations of Medications

Because antiplatelet agents and anticoagulants affect thrombosis by different mechanisms, the combination of medications might be more effective than the use of either class of agents alone. Similarly, because the several antiplatelet agents affect different aspects of platelet function, combinations also may be useful. However, the use of a combination of medications may be associated with an increased risk of bleeding complications. In particular, the combination of an antiplatelet agent and an anticoagulant may be associated with a high chance of serious hemorrhage.

Already, the combination of low-dose aspirin and extended-release dipyridamole is being used for stroke prophylaxis.[2] The combination of aspirin and clopidogrel is being used widely in cardiology and as an adjunct to endovascular procedures. The combination of aspirin and clopidogrel does have more effect on platelets than a single agent.[70] However, one recent trial that enrolled patients with ischemic cerebrovascular disease did not demonstrate an increase in efficacy with the combination of aspirin and clopidogrel when compared with clopidogrel alone.[66] In addition, the combination was dangerous, with an increase in the risk of serious bleeding. This finding gives pause to the use of aspirin and clopidogrel for treatment of patients with TIA or stroke. Aspirin (81 mg/day) or dipyridamole may be added to warfarin for prevention of thromboembolism among patients with very high-risk cardiac lesions, especially those persons who have had embolic events despite adequate levels of anticoagulation.[71,72] The combination of fixed-dose warfarin and aspirin is not as effective as adjusted-dose warfarin in preventing thromboembolic events among patients with AF.[73] There are no data about the usefulness of clopidogrel in combination with warfarin.

Surgical Procedures

Several surgical procedures are available to treat patients with intracranial or extracranial vascular disease. The goals of these operations are to either remove a source for thromboembolism or to improve flow to a vulnerable area of the brain. Carotid endarterectomy (CEA) is the most widely performed operation for prevention of stroke.[74] With advances in techniques and technology, the role of endovascular interventions is growing rapidly.

■ Carotid Endarterectomy

CEA is of proven utility for prevention of stroke among patients with symptomatic stenosis >50% at the origin of the internal carotid artery.[75-78] In the past, the role of the operation for prevention of stroke among patients with an asymptomatic stenosis >60% was controversial.[72-80] However, recent evidence suggests that CEA is effective for this indication, too.[81] This trial demonstrated that surgery reduced the 5-year risk of ipsilateral stroke from approximately 12% to approximately 6%. The data demonstrate that CEA is an important surgical intervention to prevent stroke among patients with advanced atherosclerotic disease at the origin of the internal carotid artery[1] (Class I Recommendation, Level of Evidence A). In general CEA is recommended to be performed within the first 2 weeks following a TIA or minor stroke[1] (Class IIa Recommendation, Level of Evidence B). Several factors influence the decision to recommend CEA (**Table 11.6**).

The advantage of surgical treatment increases among patients with the more severe narrowing (>70%) of the carotid artery. The operation is effective among both symptomatic men and women who have had high-grade narrowing.[82] The benefit of operation among patients with the most severe narrowing (preocclusive stenosis >99%) is clear.[83] The presence of ulceration in addition to a high-grade stenosis increases the potential benefit from CEA.[84] Patients with an occlusion do not benefit from surgery unless the arterial occlusion is known to be acute because restoration of

TABLE 11.6 — Factors That Predict an Increased Risk of Perioperative Complications or Contraindications for Carotid Endarterectomy

Contraindications for Carotid Endarterectomy
- Recent (<6 weeks) major ischemic stroke:
  – Major neurologic impairments
  – Major infarction found on brain imaging
- Recent (<6 weeks) myocardial infarction
- Unstable angina pectoris

Neurological Factors Associated With Increased Risk
- Unstable neurologically:
  – Crescendo TIA
  – Stroke in evolution
- Recent ischemic symptoms (greater than asymptomatic patients)

Epidemiological Factors Associated With Increased Risk
- Women (may be related to smaller caliber of artery)
- Age (advanced age is not a contraindication)

Medical Factors Associated With Increased Risk
- Past history of myocardial infarction of angina pectoris
- Obstructive lung disease
- Diabetes mellitus
- Hypertension
- Obesity

Arteriographic (Vascular) Factors Associated With Increased Risk
- Occlusion of the contralateral internal carotid artery
- Severe stenosis of the contralateral internal carotid artery
- Presence of an intraluminal thrombus
- Presence of intracranial arterial disease
- Absence of major collateral vessels in the circle of Willis
- Severe disease of the vertebrobasilar arteries

11

flow generally is unsuccessful. Those patients with an intraluminal thrombus usually are not initially treated with CEA; they often receive anticoagulants as a preoperative therapy with the goal of having the thrombus resolve prior to surgery.[85] There is insufficient evidence to recommend CEA as a prophylactic procedure to treat an asymptomatic stenosis prior to general surgical procedures.[86] Stroke is an important noncardiac complication of major cardiovascular operations, including coronary artery bypass graft (CABG) procedures.[87,88] The morbidity and mortality from combined CEA and CABG surgery is unacceptably high.

CEA may be recommended if the following criteria are met:

- The patient is a reasonable operative risk.
- The vascular lesion is appropriate for surgical management.
- A skilled surgeon is available.

If the above criteria cannot be met, a patient should either forego CEA or be referred to another medical institution where the operation may be performed safely. Overall, the surgeon should report that <2% to 3% of symptomatic and 1% to 2% of asymptomatic patients experience serious morbidity after CEA.[74,89,90] A systematic review has demonstrated that the operative risks of CEA are increased among women and persons older than 75 years.[91]

The operation may be associated with a number of medical and neurologic complications (**Table 11.7**). In general, patients with recent neurologic symptoms are at higher risk for serious complications than are those who are asymptomatic. Neurologically unstable patients are at highest risk. Surgery often is delayed for several weeks following a major hemispheric infarction. However, a patient with a mild stroke (minimal neurologic impairments and no major lesion found on brain imaging) probably can be treated immedi-

TABLE 11.7 — Leading Complications of Carotid Endarterectomy

- Ischemic stroke:
  - Hypoperfusion
  - Postoperative carotid occlusion
  - Artery-to-artery embolism
- Hemorrhagic stroke:
  - Hyperperfusion syndrome
  - Related to antithrombotic medications
- Seizures
- Cranial nerve palsies:
  - Vagal/recurrent laryngeal nerve
  - Hypoglossal nerve
- Local hematoma or infection
- Myocardial infarction

ately.[92,93] There is some evidence that CEA is associated with more adverse experiences among women than among men.[82] The leading causes of death following CEA are stroke and MI.[94] Intracerebral hemorrhage and hyperperfusion syndromes are potential complications of CEA for treatment of high-grade stenosis.[95,96]

Several techniques are used to lessen the risk of complications. Local anesthesia may be associated with a lower risk of cardiovascular complications than operations performed with general anesthesia. In addition, the neurologic status of an alert patient may be monitored during the operation. If general anesthesia is used, electroencephalographic or evoked potential monitoring may be used to screen for changes reflecting brain dysfunction during surgery. Placement of a shunt may be used to maintain flow during the operation. Patients scheduled for CEA usually receive antiplatelet agents (aspirin) before surgery. A trial showed that low doses of aspirin (81 mg to 325 mg) are superior to larger doses in preventing stroke, MI, or death in the first months after CEA.[46] Postoperative management usually includes antiplatelet agents.

■ Other Revascularization Operations

Superficial temporal artery to middle cerebral artery anastomosis (extracranial–intracranial [EC/IC] bypass) was tested in a large clinical trial that enrolled patients with occlusion of the internal carotid artery and stenosis of the middle cerebral artery.[97] Although the patients undergoing surgery did very well, their outcomes were not superior to those patients who were treated medically. As a result, EC/IC bypass was abandoned other than for treatment of exceptional cases, such as moyamoya. EC/IC bypass outside the setting of a clinical trial is not recommended[1] (Class III Recommendation, Level of Evidence A). However, there may be a group of patients with internal carotid artery occlusion who are at very high risk for recurrent stroke and who might benefit from EC/IC bypass.[98,99] Patients with borderline perfusion and high oxygen extraction appear to be at very high risk for new ischemic events and EC/IC bypass may be beneficial. This situation is being tested in a clinical trial.[100] With the advent of interventional techniques, such as angioplasty and stenting, the role of EC/IC bypass likely will be limited to treatment of a subset of patients with symptomatic occlusion of the internal carotid artery. Other revascularization procedures have been used to improve blood flow among patients with moyamoya syndrome.[101,102]

Occasionally, patients with severe atherosclerotic disease of major cervical arteries (subclavian, common carotid, or vertebral) are treated with vascular reconstructive operations. Endarterectomy of the external carotid artery may be done if the patient has an occlusion of the ipsilateral internal carotid artery. If the stump of an occluded internal carotid artery serves as the nidus for thrombus formation, it may be plicated.[103] Occlusion of the proximal subclavian artery with a symptomatic subclavian steal syndrome is a potential indication for surgery, but the value of operative repair is not known.[104]

Endovascular Interventions

With advances in technology and physician expertise, the role of angioplasty, with or without stenting, in treatment of patients with cerebrovascular disease is expanding. Among the technical advances is the use of distal protective devices that collect emboli that are released at the time of the angioplasty.[105] A stent often is inserted to maintain patency. The use of the device is reported in select series to reduce the risk of thromboembolic complications in the brain.[106,107] Negative experiences are generally not reported. Atherosclerotic lesions of both intracranial and extracranial vessels in the carotid and vertebrobasilar circulations are being treated. While the origin of the internal carotid artery is the most common site for endovascular treatment, the vertebral artery and intracranial vessels also may be treated[108-110] (**Table 11.8**). In general, the goal is to improve or restore flow. This procedure does not

---

TABLE 11.8 — Endovascular Procedures

Potential Settings
- Atherosclerotic disease – stenosis
- Fibromuscular dysplasia
- Recurrent stenosis (postoperative)
- Radiation-induced arterial stenosis
- Arterial dissection
- Vasculitis

Locations
- Internal carotid artery:
  - Origin
  - Base of skull
  - Cavernous segment
- Middle cerebral artery
- Basilar artery
- Vertebral artery:
  - Origin
  - Distal segment

remove an atherosclerotic lesion that is the source of emboli. Most patients receive aspirin and clopidogrel in preoperative and postoperative management in an effort to reduce thromboembolism. GP IIb/IIIa receptor blockers also have been used as an adjunctive medical intervention.[111] But these reports are anecdotal.

Angioplasty without stenting can be associated with a relatively high rate of moderate to severe recurrent stenosis.[112] Besides embolic stroke, endovascular treatment of a high-grade arterial stenosis may be complicated with a hyperperfusion syndrome or hemorrhage following treatment.[113,114] Other complications include arterial dissection or vasospasm. Arterial rupture during an intracranial procedure may be complicated by subarachnoid hemorrhage. Overall, the frequency of serious complications varies considerably among institutions.[115-118] Generally, the safety of endovascular therapy appears to be equal to that of CEA.[119]

Carotid angioplasty and stenting are also being recommended for treatment of patients considered at high risk for complications following CEA[1,120] (Class IIa Recommendation, Level of Evidence B). Among the potential indications for the procedures are treatment of recurrent stenosis following a prior CEA, fibromuscular dysplasia, arterial dissection, and radiation-induced stenosis.[121,122] A European trial compared angioplasty with CEA in treatment of carotid artery disease.[117] The rates of complications generally were similar but the trial found a higher rate of recurrent stenosis among the patients undergoing angioplasty. However, most patients having endovascular treatment did not have a stent placed. A subsequent trial that enrolled asymptomatic or symptomatic patients with carotid stenosis found that CEA or angioplasty and stenting generally had similar profiles in safety and efficacy.[123] Another trial compared angioplasty and stenting with the use of distal protective device to CEA in treatment of patients with either symptomatic or asymptomatic carotid stenosis.[118] Overall, the trial found that endovascular treatment was not inferior to CEA.

Currently, the utility of endovascular therapies to prevent ischemic stroke is in a state of flux. Already, they are being used to treat some patients with severe, symptomatic atherosclerotic disease of the posterior circulation and intracranial arteries[1] (Class IIb Recommendation, Level of Evidence C). Whether endovascular treatment could replace CEA for management of many patients with severe atherosclerotic disease of the extracranial segment of the internal carotid artery remains to be tested.

REFERENCES

1. Sacco RL, Adams R, Albers G, et al; American Heart Association; American Stroke Association Council on Stroke; Council on Cardiovascular Radiology and Intervention; American Academy of Neurology. Guidelines for prevention of stroke in patients with ischemic stroke or transient ischemic attack. A statement for healthcare professionals from the American Heart Association/American Stroke Association Council on Stroke: co-sponsored by the Council on Cardiovascular Radiology and Intervention: the American Academy of Neurology affirms the value of this guideline. *Stroke*. 2006;37:577-617.

2. Albers GW, Amarenco P, Easton JD, Sacco RL, Teal P. Antithrombotic and thrombolytic therapy for ischemic stroke: the Seventh ACCP Conference on Antithrombotic and Thombolytic Therapy. *Chest*. 2004;126:483S-512S.

3. Gorelick PB, Sacco RL, Smith DB, et al. Prevention of a first stroke: a review of guidelines and a multidisciplinary consensus statement from the National Stroke Association. *JAMA*. 1999;281:1112-1120.

4. Albers GW. Choice of antithrombotic therapy for stroke prevention in atrial fibrillation: warfarin, aspirin, or both? *Arch Intern Med*. 1998;158:1487-1491.

5. Hirsh J, Dalen J, Anderson DR, et al. Oral anticoagulants: mechanism of action, clinical effectiveness, and optimal therapeutic range. *Chest*. 2001;119:8S-21S.

6. Hart RG. Atrial fibrillation and stroke prevention. *N Engl J Med*. 2003;349:1015-1016.

7. Go AS, Hylek EM, Chang Y, et al. Anticoagulation therapy for stroke prevention in atrial fibrillation. How well do randomized trials translate into clinical practice? *JAMA*. 2003;290:2685-2692.

8. Homma S, Di Tullio MR, Sciacca RR, Sacco RL, Mohr JP; PICSS Investigators. Effect of aspirin and warfarin therapy in stroke patients with valvular strands. *Stroke*. 2004;35:1436-1442.

9. Hart RG, Halperin JL. Atrial fibrillation and thromboembolism: a decade of progress in stroke prevention. *Ann Intern Med*. 1999;131:688-695.

11

10. Hart RG, Palacio S, Pearce LA. Atrial fibrillation, stroke, and acute antithrombotic therapy: analysis of randomzied clinical trials. *Stroke*. 2002;33:2722-2727.

11. Salem DN, Levine HJ, Pauker SG, Eckman MH, Daudelin DH. Antithrombotic therapy in valvular heart disease. *Chest*. 1998;114(suppl 5):590S-601S.

12. Pullicino PM, Halperin JL, Thompson JL. Stroke in patients with heart failure and reduced left ventricular ejection fraction. *Neurology*. 2000;54:288-294.

13. Hurlen M, Abdelnoor M, Smith P, Erikssen J, Arnesen H. Warfarin, aspirin, or both after myocardial infarction. *N Engl J Med*. 2002;347:969-974.

14. Ezekowitz MD. Anticoagulation management of valve replacement patients. *J Heart Valve Dis*. 2002;11(suppl 1):S56-S60.

15. Khamashta MA, Cuadrado MJ, Mujic F, Taub NA, Hunt BJ, Hughes GR. The management of thrombosis in the antiphospholipid-antibody syndrome. *N Engl J Med*. 1995;332:993-997.

16. Bauer KA. Management of thrombophilia. *J Thromb Haemost*. 2003;1:1429-1434.

17. Crowther MA, Kelton JG. Congenital thrombophilic states associated with venous thrombosis: a qualitative overview and proposed classification system. *Ann Intern Med*. 2003;138:128-134.

18. Levine SR, Brey RL, Tilley BC, et al; APASS Investigators. Antiphospholipid antibodies and subsequent thrombo-occlusive events in patients with ischemic stroke. *JAMA*. 2004;291:576-584.

19. A randomized trial of anticoagulants versus aspirin after cerebral ischemia of presumed arterial origin. The Stroke Prevention in Reversible Ischemia Trial (SPIRIT) Study Group. *Ann Neurol*. 1997;42:857-865.

20. Mohr JP, Thompson JL, Lazar RM, et al; Warfarin-Aspirin Recurrent Stroke Study Group. A comparison of warfarin and aspirin for the prevention of recurrent ischemic stroke. *N Engl J Med*. 2001;345:1444-1451.

21. Chimowitz MI, Lynn MJ, Howlett-Smith H, et al; Warfarin-Aspirin Symptomatic Intracranial Disease Trial Investigators. Comparison of warfarin and aspirin for symptomatic intracranial arterial stenosis. *N Engl J Med*. 2005;352:1305-1316.

22. Leys D, Kwiecinski H, Bogousslavsky J, et al; EUSI Executive Committee; EUSI Writing Committee. Prevention. European Stroke Initiative. *Cerebrovasc Dis*. 2004;17(suppl 2):15-29.

23. Lyrer P, Engelter S. Antithrombotic drugs for carotid artery dissection. *Stroke*. 2004;35:613-614.

24. Hirsh J, Poller L. The international normalized ratio. A guide to understanding and correcting its problems. *Arch Intern Med*. 1994;154:282-288.

25. Weser JK, Sellers E. Drug interactions with coumarin anticoagulants. 2. *N Engl J Med*. 1971;285:547-558.

26. Sato Y, Kuno H, Kaji M, Ohshima Y, Asoh T, Oizumi K. Increased bone resorption during the first year after stroke. *Stroke*. 1998;29:1373-1377.

27. Sato Y, Metoki N, Iwamoto J, Satoh K. Amelioration of osteoporosis and hypovitaminosis D by sunlight exposure in stroke patients. *Neurology*. 2003;61:338-342.

28. Ginsberg JS, Greer I, Hirsh J. Use of antithrombotic agents during pregnancy. *Chest*. 2001;119(suppl 1):122S-131S.

29. Cotrufo M, De Feo M, De Santo LS, et al. Risk of warfarin during pregnancy with mechanical valve protheses. *Obstet Gynecol*. 2002;99:35-40.

30. Yasaka M, Minematsu K, Naritomi H, Sakata T, Yamaguchi T. Predisposing factors for enlargement of intracerebral hemorrhage in patients treated with warfarin. *Thromb Haemost*. 2003;89:278-283.

31. Oates A, Jackson PR, Austin CA, Channer KS. A new regimen for starting warfarin therapy in out-patients. *Br J Clin Pharmacol*. 1998;46:157-161.

32. Shine D, Patel J, Kumar J, et al. A randomized trial of initial warfarin dosing based on simple clinical criteria. *Thromb Haemost*. 2003;89:297-304.

33. Olsson SB; Executive Steering Committee on behalf of the SPORTIF III Investigators. Stroke prevention with the oral direct thrombin inhibitor ximelagatran compared with warfarin in patients with non-valvular atrial fibrillation (SPORTIF III): randomised controlled trial. *Lancet*. 2003;362:1691-1698.

34. Albers GW, Diener HC, Frison L, et al; SPORTIF Executive Steering Committee for the SPORTIF V Investigators. Ximelagatran vs warfarin for stroke prevention in patients with nonvalvular atrial fibrillation: a randomized trial. *JAMA*. 2005;293:690-698.

35. Antithrombotic Trialists' Collaboration. Collaborative meta-analysis of randomised trials of antiplatelet therapy for prevention of death, myocardial infarction, and stroke in high risk patients. *BMJ*. 2002;324:71-86.

36. Patrono C, Coller B, Dalen JE, et al. Platelet-active drugs: the relationships among dose, effectiveness, and side effects. *Chest*. 1998;114:470S-488S.

37. Patients with nonvalvular atrial fibrillation at low risk of stroke during treatment with aspirin: Stroke Prevention in Atrial Fibrillation III Study. The SPAF III Writing Committee for the Stroke Prevention in Atrial Fibrillation Investigators. *JAMA*. 1998;279:1273-1277.

38. Hart RG, Sherman DG, Easton JD, Cairns JA. Prevention of stroke in patients with nonvalvular atrial fibrillation. *Neurology*. 1998;51:674-681.

39. The International Stroke Trial (IST): a randomised trial of aspirin, subcutaneous heparin, both, or neither among 19435 patients with acute ischaemic stroke. International Stroke Trial Collaborative Group. *Lancet*. 1997;349:1569-1581.

40. CAST: randomised placebo-controlled trial of early aspirin use in 20,000 patients with acute ischaemic stroke. CAST (Chinese Acute Stroke Trial) Collaborative Group. *Lancet*. 1997;349:1641-1649.

41. Gorelick PB, Weisman SM. Risk of hemorrhagic stroke with aspirin use: an update. *Stroke*. 2005;36:1801-1807.

42. Isles C, Norrie J, Paterson J, Ritchie L. Risk of major gastrointestinal bleeding with aspirin. *Lancet*. 1999;353:148-150.

43. United Kingdom transient ischaemic attack (UK-TIA) aspirin trial: interim results. UK-TIA Study Group. *Br Med J*. 1988;296:316-320.

44. The Dutch TIA Trial: protective effects of low-dose aspirin and atenolol in patients with transient ischemic attacks or nondisabling stroke. The Dutch TIA Study Group. *Stroke*. 1988;19:512-517.

45. Swedish Aspirin Low-Dose Trial (SALT) of 75 mg aspirin as secondary prophylaxis after cerebrovascular ischaemic events. The SALT Collaborative Group. *Lancet*. 1991;338:1345-1349.

46. Taylor DW, Barnett HJ, Haynes RB, et al. Low-dose and high-dose acetylsalicylic acid for patients undergoing carotid endarterectomy: a randomized controlled trial. ASA and Carotid Endarterectomy (ACE) Trial Collaborators. *Lancet*. 1999;353:2179-2184.

47. Algra A, van Gijn J. Aspirin at any dose above 30 mg offers only modest protection after cerebral ischaemia. *J Neurol Neurosurg Psychiatry*. 1996;60:197-199.

48. Adams HP Jr, Bendixen BH. Low- versus high-dose aspirin in prevention of ischemic stroke. *Clin Neuropharmacol*. 1993;16:485-500.

49. Alberts MJ, Bergman DL, Molner E, Jovanovic BD, Ushiwata I, Teruya J. Antiplatelet effect of aspirin in patients with cerebrovascular disease. *Stroke*. 2004;35:175-178.

50. Grundmann K, Jaschonek K, Kleine B, Dichgans J, Topka H. Aspirin non-responder status in patients with recurrent cerebral ischemic attacks. *J Neurol*. 2003;250:63-66.

51. Diener HC, Cunha L, Forbes C, Sivenius J, Smets P, Lowenthal A. European Stroke Prevention Study. 2. Dipyridamole and acetylsalicylic acid in the secondary prevention of stroke. *J Neurol Sci*. 1996;143:1-13.

52. Sivenius J, Cunha L, Diener HC, et al. Second European Stroke Prevention Study: antiplatelet therapy is effective regardless of age. ESPS2 Working Group. *Acta Neurol Scand*. 1999;99:54-60.

53. Wilterdink JL, Easton JD. Dipyridamole plus aspirin in cerebrovascular disease. *Arch Neurol*. 1999;56:1087-1092.

54. Sharis PJ, Cannon CP, Loscalzo J. The antiplatelet effects of ticlopidine and clopidogrel. *Ann Intern Med*. 1998;129:394-405.

55. Hass WK, Easton JD, Adams HP Jr, et al. A randomized trial comparing ticlopidine hydrochloride with aspirin for the prevention of stroke in high-risk patients. Ticlopidine Aspirin Stroke Study Group. *N Engl J Med*. 1989;321:501-507.

56. Gent M, Blakely JA, Easton JD, et al. The Canadian American Ticlopidine Study (CATS) in thromboembolic stroke. *Lancet*. 1989;1:1215-1220.

57. Gorelick PB, Richardson D, Kelly M, et al; African American Antiplatelet Stroke Prevention Study Investigators. Aspirin and ticlopidine for prevention of recurrent stroke in black patients: a randomized trial. *JAMA*. 2003;289:2947-2957.

58. Love BB, Biller J, Gent M. Adverse haematological effects of ticlopidine. Prevention, recognition and management. *Drug Saf*. 1998;19:89-98.

59. Bennett CL, Weinberg PD, Rozenberg-Ben-Dror K, Yarnold PR, Kwaan HC, Green D. Thrombotic thrombocytopenic purpura associated with ticlopidine. A review of 60 cases. *Ann Intern Med*. 1998;128:541-544.

60. Steinhubl SR, Tan WA, Foody JM, Topol EJ. Incidence and clinical course of thrombotic thrombocytopenic purpura due to ticlopidine following coronary stenting. EPISTENT Investigators. Evaluation of Platelet IIb/IIIa Inhibitor for Stenting. *JAMA*. 1999;281:806-810.

61. Tsai HM, Rice L, Sarode R, Chow TW, Moake JL. Antibody inhibitors to von Willebrand factor metalloprotease and increased binding of von Willebrand factor to platelets in ticlopidine-associated thrombotic thrombocytopenic purpura. *Ann Intern Med*. 2000;132:794-799.

62. Yusuf S, Zhao F, Mehta SR, Chrolavicius S, Tognoni G, Fox KK; Clopidogrel in Unstable Angina to Prevent Recurrent Events Trial Investigators. Effects of clopidogrel in addition to aspirin in patients with acute coronary syndromes without ST-segment elevation. *N Engl J Med*. 2001;345:494-502.

63. Yusuf S, Mehta SR, Zhao F, et al; Clopidogrel in Unstable angina to prevent Recurrent Events Trial Investigators. Early and late effects of clopidogrel in patients with acute coronary syndromes. *Circulation*. 2003;107:966-972.

64. Bennett CL, Connors JM, Carwile MJ, et al. Thrombotic thrombocytopenic purpura associated with clopidogrel. *N Engl J Med*. 2000;342:1773-1777.

65. A randomised, blinded, trial of clopidogrel versus aspirin in patients at risk of ischaemic events (CAPRIE). CAPRIE Steering Committee. *Lancet*. 1996;348:1329-1339.

66. Diener HC, Bogousslavsky J, Brass LM, et al; MATCH investigators. Aspirin and clopidogrel compared with clopidogrel alone after recent ischaemic stroke or transient ischaemic attack in high-risk patients (MATCH): randomised, double-blind, placebo-controlled trial. *Lancet*. 2004;364:331-337.

67. Diener HC, Bogousslavsky J, Brass LM, et al. Management of atherothrombosis with clopidogrel in high-risk patients with recent transient ischaemic attack or ischaemic stroke (MATCH): study design and baseline data. *Cerebrovasc Dis*. 2004;17:253-261.

68. Bhatt DL, Fox KA, Hacke W, et al; for the CHARISMA Investigators. Clopidogrel and aspirin versus aspirin alone for the prevention of atherothrombotic events. *N Engl J Med*. 2006;354:1706-1717.

69. A randomized trial of aspirin and sulfinpyrazone in threatened stroke. The Canadian Cooperative Study Group. *N Engl J Med*. 1978;299:53-59.

70. Serebruany VL, Malinin AI, Ziai W, et al. Effects of clopidogrel and aspirin in combination versus aspirin alone on platelet activation and major receptor expression in patients after recent ischemic stroke: for the Plavix Use for Treatment of Stroke (PLUTO-Stroke) trial. *Stroke*. 2005;36:2289-2292.

71. Hurlen M, Erikssen J, Smith P, Arnesen H, Rollag A. Comparison of bleeding complications of warfarin and warfarin plus acetylsalicylic acid: a study in 3166 outpatients. *J Intern Med*. 1994;236:299-304.

72. Fagan SC, Kertland HR, Tietjen GE. Safety of combination aspirin and anticoagulation in acute ischemic stroke. *Ann Pharmacother*. 1994;28:441-443.

73. Thrombosis prevention trial: randomised trial of low-intensity oral anticoagulation with warfarin and low-dose aspirin in the primary prevention of ischaemic heart disease in men at increased risk. The Medical Research Council's General Practice Research Framework. *Lancet*. 1998;351:233-241.

74. Biller J, Feinberg WM, Castaldo JE, et al. Guidelines for carotid endarterectomy: a statement for healthcare professionals from a Special Writing Group of the Stroke Council, American Heart Association. *Circulation*. 1998;97:501-509.

75. Barnett HJ, Taylor DW, Eliasziw M, et al. Benefit of carotid endarterectomy in patients with symptomatic moderate or severe stenosis. North American Symptomatic Carotid Endarterectomy Trial Collaborators. *N Engl J Med*. 1998;339:1415-1425.

76. Randomised trial of endarterectomy for recently symptomatic carotid stenosis: final results of the MRC European Carotid Surgery Trial (ECST). *Lancet*. 1998;351:1379-1387.

77. Rothwell PM, Eliasziw M, Gutnikov SA, Warlow CP, Barnett HJ; Carotid Endarterectomy Trialists' Collaboration. Endarterectomy for symptomatic carotid stenosis in relation to clinical subgroups and timing of surgery. *Lancet*. 2004;363:915-924.

78. Rothwell PM, Mehta Z, Howard SC, Gutnikov SA, Warlow CP. Treating individuals 3: from subgroups to individuals: general principles and the example of carotid endarterectomy. *Lancet*. 2005;365:256-265.

79. Endarterectomy for asymptomatic carotid artery stenosis. Executive Committee for the Asymptomatic Carotid Atherosclerosis Study. *JAMA*. 1995;273:1421-1428.

80. Rothwell PM, Goldstein LB. Carotid endarterectomy for asymptomatic carotid stenosis: asymptomatic carotid surgery trial. *Stroke*. 2004;35:2425-2427.

81. Halliday A, Mansfield A, Marro J, et al; MRC Asymptomatic Carotid Surgery Trial (ACST) Collaborative Group. Prevention of disabling and fatal strokes by successful carotid endarterectomy in patients without recent neurological symptoms: randomised controlled trial. *Lancet*. 2004;363:1491-1502.

82. Alamowitch S, Eliasziw M, Barnett HJ; North American Symptomatic Carotid Endarterectomy Trial (NASCET); ASA Trial Group; Carotid Endarterectomy (ACE) Trial Group. The risk and benefit of endarterectomy in women with symptomatic internal carotid artery disease. *Stroke*. 2005;36:27-31.

83. Morgenstern LB, Fox AJ, Sharpe BL, Eliasziw M, Barnett HJ, Grotta JC. The risks and benefits of carotid endarterectomy in patients with near occlusion of the carotid artery. North American Symptomatic Carotid Endarterectomy Trial (NASCET) Group. *Neurology*. 1997;48:911-915.

84. Eliasziw M, Streifler JY, Fox AJ, Hachinski VC, Ferguson GG, Barnett HJ. Significance of plaque ulceration in symptomatic patients with high-grade carotid stenosis. North American Symptomatic Carotid Endarterectomy Trial. *Stroke*. 1994;25:304-308.

85. Buchan A, Gates P, Pelz D, Barnett HJ. Intraluminal thrombus in the cerebral circulation. Implications for surgical management. *Stroke*. 1988;19:681-687.

86. Paciaroni M, Caso V, Acciarresi M, Baumgartner RW, Agnelli G. Management of asymptomatic carotid stenosis in patients undergoing general and vascular surgical procedures. *J Neurol Neurosurg Psychiatry*. 2005;76:1332-1336.

87. Brown KR. Treatment of concomitant carotid and coronary artery disease. Decision-making regarding surgical options. *J Cardiovasc Surg*. 2003;44:395-399.

88. Naylor AR, Cuffe RL, Rothwell PM, Bell PR. A systematic review of outcomes following staged and synchronous carotid endarterectomy and coronary artery bypass. *Eur J Vasc Endovasc Surg*. 2003;25:380-389.

89. Cowan JA Jr, Dimick JB, Thompson BG, Stanley JC, Upchurch GR Jr. Surgeon volume as an indicator of outcomes after carotid endarterectomy: an effect independent of specialty practice and hospital volume. *J Am Coll Surg*. 2002;195:814-821.

90. Kresowik TF, Hemann RA, Grund SL, et al. Improving the outcomes of carotid endarterectomy: results of a statewide quality improvement project. *J Vasc Surg*. 2000;31:918-926.

91. Bond R, Rerkasem K, Cuffe R, Rothwell PM. A systematic review of the associations between age and sex and the operative risks of carotid endarteretomy. *Cerebrovasc Dis*. 2005;20:69-77.

92. Eckstein HH, Ringleb P, Dorfler A, et al. The Carotid Surgery for Ischemic Stroke trial: a prospective observational study on carotid endarterectomy in the early period after ischemic stroke. *J Vasc Surg*. 2002;36:997-1004.

93. Eckstein HH, Schumacher H, Laubach H, et al. Early carotid endarterectomy after non-disabling ischaemic stroke: adequate therapeutical option in selected patients. *Eur J Vasc Endovasc Surg*. 1998;15:423-428.

94. Lanska DJ, Kryscio RJ. In-hospital mortality following carotid endarterectomy. *Neurology*. 1998;51:440-447.

95. Cheung RT, Eliasziw M, Meldrum HE, Fox AJ, Barnett HJ; North American Symptomatic Carotid Endarterectomy Trial Group. Risk, types, and severity of intracranial hemorrhage in patients with symptomatic carotid artery stenosis. *Stroke*. 2003;34:1847-1851.

96. Naylor AR, Evans J, Thompson MM, et al. Seizures after carotid endarterectomy: hyperperfusion, dysautoregulation or hypertensive encephalopathy? *Eur J Vasc Endovasc Surg*. 2003;26:39-44.

97. Failure of extracranial-intracranial arterial bypass to reduce the risk of ischemic stroke. Results of an international randomized trial. The EC/IC Bypass Study Group. *N Engl J Med*. 1985;313:1191-1200.

98. Grubb RL Jr. Extracranial-intracranial arterial bypass for treatment of occlusion of the internal carotid artery. *Curr Neurol Neurosci Rep*. 2004;4:23-30.

99. Klijn CJ, van Gijn J. Extracranial to intracranial bypass. *Adv Neurol*. 2003;92:329-333.

100. Adams HP Jr. Occlusion of the internal carotid artery: reopening a closed door? *JAMA*. 1998;280:1093-1094.

101. Iwama T, Hashimoto N, Miyake H, Yonekawa Y. Direct revascularization to the anterior cerebral artery territory in patients with moyamoya disease: report of five cases. *Neurosurgery*. 1998;42:1157-1161.

102. Golby AJ, Marks MP, Thompson RC, Steinberg GK. Direct and combined revascularization in pediatric moyamoya disease. *Neurosurgery*. 1999;45:50-58.

103. Ryan PG, Day AL. Stump embolization from an occluded internal carotid artery. Case report. *J Neurosurg*. 1987;67:609-611.

104. Molnar RG, Naslund TC. Vertebral artery surgery. *Surg Clin North Am*. 1998;78:901-913.

105. Cosottini M, Michelassi MC, Puglioli M, et al. Silent cerebral ischemia detected with diffusion-weighted imaging in patients treated with protected and unprotected carotid artery stenting. *Stroke*. 2005;36:2389-2393.

106. Cremonesi A, Manetti R, Setacci F, Setacci C, Castriota F. Protected carotid stenting: clinical advantages and complications of embolic protection devices in 442 consecutive patients. *Stroke*. 2003;34:1936-1941.

107. McKevitt FM, Macdonald S, Venables GS, Cleveland TJ,Gaines PA. Complications following carotid angioplasty and carotid stenting in patients with symptomatic carotid artery disease. *Cerebrovasc Dis*. 2004;17:28-34.

108. Cloud GC, Crawley F, Clifton A, McCabe DJ, Brown MM, Markus HS. Vertebral artery origin angioplasty and primary stenting: safety and restenosis rates in a prospective series. *J Neurol Neurosurg Psychiatry*. 2003;74:586-590.

109. Mori T, Mori K, Fukuoka M, Honda S. Percutaneous transluminal angioplasty for total occlusion of middle cerebral arteries. *Neuroradiology*. 1997;39:71-74.

110. Higashida RT. Intracranial stenting: which patients and when? *Cleve Clin J Med*. 2004;71(suppl 1):S50-S51.

111. Wholey MH, Eles G, Toursakissian B, Bailey S, Jarmolowski C, Tan WA. Evaluation of glycoprotein IIb/IIIa inhibitors in carotid angioplasty and stenting. *J Endovasc Ther*. 2003;10:33-41.

112. Albuquerque FC, Fiorella D, Han P, Spetzler RF, McDougall CG. A reappraisal of angioplasty and stenting for the treatment of vertebral origin stenosis. *Neurosurgery*. 2003;53:607-614.

11

113. Schoser BG, Heesen C, Eckert B, Thie A. Cerebral hyperperfusion injury after percutaneous transluminal angioplasty of extracranial arteries. *J Neurol*. 1997;244:101-104.

114. Mori T, Fukuoka M, Kazita K, Mima T, Mori K. Intraventricular hemorrhage after carotid stenting. *J Endovasc Surg*. 1999;6:337-341.

115. Kastrup A, Groschel K, Krapf H, Brehm BR, Dichgans J, Schulz JB. Early outcome of carotid angioplasty and stenting with and without cerebral protection devices: a systematic review of the literature. *Stroke*. 2003;34:813-819.

116. Kastrup A, Skalej M, Krapf H, Nagele T, Dichgans J, Schulz JB. Early outcome of carotid angioplasty and stenting versus carotid endarterectomy in a single academic center. *Cerebrovasc Dis*. 2003;15:84-89.

117. Endovascular versus surgical treatment in patients with carotid stenosis in the Carotid and Vertebral Artery Transluminal Angioplasty Study (CAVATAS): a randomised trial. *Lancet*. 2001;357:1729-1737.

118. Yadav JS, Wholey MH, Kuntz RE, et al; Stenting and Angioplasty with Protection in Patients at High Risk for Endarterectomy Investigators. Protected carotid-artery stenting versus endarterectomy in high-risk patients. *N Engl J Med*. 2004;351:1493-1501.

119. Coward LJ, Featherstone RL, Brown MM. Safety and efficacy of endovascular treatment of carotid artery stenosis compared with carotid endarterectomy: a Cochrane systematic review of the randomized evidence. *Stroke*. 2005;36:905-911.

120. Fox DJ Jr, Moran CJ, Cross DT 3rd, et al. Long-term outcome after angioplasty for symptomatic extracranial carotid stenosis in poor surgical candidates. *Stroke*. 2002;33:2877-2880.

121. Ahuja A, Blatt GL, Guterman LR, Hopkins LN. Angioplasty for symptomatic radiation-induced extracranial carotid artery stenosis: case report. *Neurosurgery*. 1995;36:399-403.

122. Lanzino G, Mericle RA, Lopes DK, Wakhloo AK, Guterman LR, Hopkins LN. Percutaneous transluminal angioplasty and stent placement for recurrent carotid artery stenosis. *J Neurosurg*. 1999;90:688-694.

123. CaRESS Steering Committee. Carotid Revascularization Using Endarterectomy or Stenting Systems (CaRESS) phase I clinical trial: 1-year results. *J Vasc Surg*. 2005;42:213-219.

12   Rehabilitation After Stroke

Rehabilitation is an integral component of management of patients with stroke. A key to successful rehabilitation is a coordinated team approach that involves the active participation of several rehabilitation specialists.[1,2] Rehabilitation should begin as soon as the patient is medically stable. Education of the patient and family about stroke and its consequences is an important step in rehabilitation. For example, family members should be informed about the nature of the neurologic impairments. In particular, prominent cognitive or emotional impairments, including language disorders, sleep disturbances, and depression, should be discussed. Patients with stroke in the nondominant hemisphere may not exhibit much emotionality and may not recognize the emotions of others.

Rehabilitation Specialists

Several different rehabilitation specialists may provide services to patients selected on a case-by-case basis. The most commonly involved rehabilitation services are occupational therapy, physical therapy, and speech pathology. In some cases, vocational rehabilitation specialists, recreation therapists, or neuropsychologists/cognitive rehabilitation specialists are needed. In addition, it is important to enlist the assistance of a social service specialist/discharge planner and a dietitian. The involvement of the nursing service also is critical. These professionals should assess the patient and tailor a treatment plan for the patient's individual needs. Plans should respect the wishes of the patient and family. Each rehabilitation service specializes in different aspects of the patient's recovery.

Physical therapy concentrates on the following activities:

- Mobilization
- Walking
- Addressing major motor or sensory impairments of the limbs
- Prescribing devices, such as a cane or walker.

Speech pathologists address the following activities:

- Improving recovery from language impairments
- Improving recovery of articulation (speech)
- Improving recovery of swallowing.

In an effort to help the patient function independently, occupational therapy focuses on the following issues:

- Facilitating fine movements of the hand
- Improving arm function
- Utilizing tools, such as dinnerware
- Prescribing assistive devices, such as splints.

While the preliminary steps in rehabilitation begin in an acute-care setting, a plan should be developed for subsequent outpatient or inpatient treatment.[3-7] In the United States, patients are eligible for intensive inpatient rehabilitation in an acute-care or stand-alone rehabilitation facility if they need at least two rehabilitation services (occupational, speech, or physical) and if they can tolerate at least 3 hours of treatment daily.[7] Skilled nursing facilities can provide inpatient rehabilitation for those patients who cannot tolerate more intensive patient care. Patients with minimal impairments often may be treated as outpatients.[8,9] Aggressive outpatient rehabilitation has important attributes, including the patient living at home, which improves morale and allows the patient to use the training in an actual real-life setting.

New interventions to help motor recovery after stroke include constraint-induced movement therapy and medications to treat spasticity.[10-12] In particular, local injections of botulinum toxin are effective in reducing the effects of spasticity.[13-16] There has been interest in the use of amphetamines as an adjunct to speed motor recovery after stroke, but data are not sufficient to recommend this intervention.[17-20]

Other promising therapies include robot training, electrical stimulation, intermittent compression, and intensive physical therapy.[21-26] Some of these interventions are being tested in clinical trials and results are confirming which therapies are most helpful.[27] Aggressive treatment of aphasia also is a component of rehabilitation.[28-30]

Patients should be assessed at regular intervals during their recovery from the stroke. The types and settings of rehabilitation are adjusted in response to the patient's recovery. The goal will be for the patient to be as independent as possible. Subsequently, issues such as sexuality or driving an automobile should be addressed. Another important subject is the ability of the patient to return to work.

The patient's living quarters may need to be modified to permit a return to home. In order to accommodate the patient's impairments, alterations should be made to facilities, such as the following:

- Toilet
- Bath/shower
- Rugs
- Stairs
- Kitchen
- Trip hazards (eg, electric cords).

Depression is common following stroke.[31-35] The mood disorder may be an emotional response to the sudden and devastating change in a patient's life and independence. Depression after stroke also is an organic consequence of the brain injury. Less commonly, stroke may cause mania. Emotional disturbances may hamper recovery from the stroke and limit the efficacy of rehabilitation. Often, counseling and the use of antidepressant medications are needed.

Discharge Planning

In an era of constrained health care budgets and short lengths of stay in acute-care settings, plans for management after discharge from the hospital should begin as soon as the patient is medically stable.[36] Many hospitals have a care-management/discharge planner who may provide assistance in arranging for continued treatment after hospitalization. The goal should be to provide continued long-term medical treatment and rehabilitation to meet the patient's and family's wishes and needs.

REFERENCES

1. Ronning OM, Guldvog B. Outcome of subacute stroke rehabilitation: a randomized controlled trial. *Stroke*. 1998;29:779-784.
2. Dombovy ML. Understanding stroke recovery and rehabilitation: current and emerging approaches. *Curr Neurol Neurosci Rep*. 2004;4:31-35.
3. Alexander MP. Stroke rehabilitation outcome. A potential use of predictive variables to establish levels of care. *Stroke*. 1994;25:128-134.
4. Cifu DX, Stewart DG. Factors affecting functional outcome after stroke: a critical review of rehabilitation interventions. *Arch Phys Med Rehabil*. 1999;80:S35-S39.
5. Lofgren B, Nyberg L, Osterlind P, Mattsson M, Gustafson Y. Stroke rehabilitation - discharge predictors. *Cerebrovasc Dis*. 1997;7:168-174.
6. Harvey RL, Roth EJ, Heinemann AW, Lovell LL, McGuire JR, Diaz S. Stroke rehabilitation: clinical predictors of resource utilization. *Arch Phys Med Rehabil*. 1998;79:1349-1355.
7. Gresham GE, Duncan PW, Stason WB, et al. Post-Stroke Rehabilitation. U.S. Department of Health and Human Services, 1995.
8. Werner RA, Kessler S. Effectiveness of an intensive outpatient rehabilitation program for postacute stroke patients. *Am J Phys Med Rehabil*. 1996;75:114-120.
9. Legg L, Langhorne P; Outpatient Service Trialists. Rehabilitation therapy services for stroke patients living at home: systematic review of randomised trials. *Lancet*. 2004;363:352-356.

10. Miltner WH, Bauder H, Sommer M, Dettmers C, Taub E. Effects of constraint-induced movement therapy on patients with chronic motor deficits after stroke: a replication. *Stroke*. 1999;30:586-592.

11. Liepert J, Bauder H, Wolfgang HR, Miltner WH, Taub E, Weiller C. Treatment-induced cortical reorganization after stroke in humans. *Stroke*. 2000;31:1210-1216.

12. Page SJ, Sisto S, Johnston MV, Levine P. Modified constraint-induced therapy after subacute stroke: a preliminary study. *Neurorehabil Neural Repair*. 2002;16:290-295.

13. Brashear A, Gordon MF, Elovic E, et al; Botox Post-Stroke Spasticity Study Group. Intramuscular injection of botulinum toxin for the treatment of wrist and finger spasticity after a stroke. *N Engl J Med*. 2002;347:395-400.

14. Brashear A, McAfee AL, Kuhn ER, Fyffe J. Botulinum toxin type B in upper-limb poststroke spasticity: a double-blind, placebo-controlled trial. *Arch Phys Med Rehabil*. 2004;85:705-709.

15. Pittock SJ, Moore AP, Hardiman O, et al. A double-blind randomised placebo-controlled evaluation of three doses of botulinum toxin type A (Dysport) in the treatment of spastic equinovarus deformity after stroke. *Cerebrovasc Dis*. 2003;15:289-300.

16. Johnson CA, Burridge JH, Strike PW, Wood DE, Swain ID. The effect of combined use of botulinum toxin type A and functional electric stimulation in the treatment of spastic drop foot after stroke: a preliminary investigation. *Arch Phys Med Rehabil*. 2004;85:902-909.

17. Martinsson L, Eksborg S, Wahlgren NG. Intensive early physiotherapy combined with dexamphetamine treatment in severe stroke: a randomized, controlled pilot study. *Cerebrovasc Dis*. 2003;16:338-345.

18. Martinsson L, Hardemark HG, Wahlgren NG. Amphetamines for improving stroke recovery: a systematic cochrane review. *Stroke*. 2003;34:2766.

19. Martinsson L, Wahlgren NG. Safety of dexamphetamine in acute ischemic stroke: a randomized, double-blind, controlled dose-escalation trial. *Stroke*. 2003;34:475-481.

20. Treig T, Werner C, Sachse M, Hesse S. No benefit from D-amphetamine when added to physiotherapy after stroke: a randomized, placebo-controlled study. *Clin Rehabil*. 2003;17:590-599.

21. Fasoli SE, Krebs HI, Stein J, Frontera WR, Hogan N. Effects of robotic therapy on motor impairment and recovery in chronic stroke. *Arch Phys Med Rehabil*. 2003;84:477-482.

22. Moreland JD, Goldsmith CH, Huijbregts MP, et al. Progressive resistance strengthening exercises after stroke: a single-blind randomized controlled trial. *Arch Phys Med Rehabil*. 2003;84:1433-1440.

23. Cambier DC, De Corte E, Danneels LA, Witvrouw EE. Treating sensory impairments in the post-stroke upper limb with intermittent pneumatic compression. Results of a preliminary trial. *Clin Rehabil*. 2003;17:14-20.

24. Pollock A, Baer G, Pomeroy V, Langhorne P. Physiotherapy treatment approaches for the recovery of postural control and lower limb function following stroke. *Cochrane Database Syst Rev*. 2003;CD001920.

25. da Cunha IT Jr, Lim PA, Qureshy H, Henson H, Monga T, Protas EJ. Gait outcomes after acute stroke rehabilitation with supported treadmill ambulation training: a randomized controlled pilot study. *Arch Phys Med Rehabil*. 2002;83:1258-1265.

12

26. Ada L, Dean CM, Hall JM, Bampton J, Crompton S. A treadmill and overground walking program improves walking in persons residing in the community after stroke: a placebo-controlled, randomized trial. *Arch Phys Med Rehabil*. 2003;84:1486-1491.

27. Duncan P, Studenski S, Richards L, et al. Randomized clinical trial of therapeutic exercise in subacute stroke. *Stroke*. 2003;34:2173-2180.

28. Ferro JM, Mariano G, Madureira S. Recovery from aphasia and neglect. *Cerebrovasc Dis*. 1999;9(suppl 5):6-22.

29. Selnes OA. Recovery from aphasia: activating the "right" hemisphere. *Ann Neurol*. 1999;45:419-420.

30. Greener J, Enderby P, Whurr R. Pharmacological treatment for aphasia following stroke. *Cochrane Database Syst Rev*. 2001;CD000424.

31. Astrom M, Adolfsson R, Asplund K. Major depression in stroke patients. A 3-year longitudinal study. *Stroke*. 1993;24:976-982.

32. Palomaki H, Kaste M, Berg A, et al. Prevention of poststroke depression: 1 year randomised placebo controlled double blind trial of mianserin with 6 month follow up after therapy. *J Neurol Neurosurg Psychiatry*. 1999;66:490-494.

33. Robinson RG. Poststroke depression: prevalence, diagnosis, treatment, and disease progression. *Biol Psychiatry*. 2003;54:376-387.

34. Hackett ML, Yapa C, Parag V, Anderson CS. Frequency of depression after stroke: a systematic review of observational studies. *Stroke*. 2005;36:1330-1340.

35. Hackett ML, Anderson CS. Predictors of depression after stroke: a systematic review of observational studies. *Stroke*. 2005;36:2296-2301.

36. Wentworth DA, Atkinson RP. Implementation of an acute stroke program decreases hospitalization costs and length of stay. *Stroke*. 1996;27:1040-1043.

INDEX

Note: Entries followed by "f" indicate figures; "t" tables.

Symbols and Numbers

α-3-Hydroxy-5-methyl-4-isooxazoloproprionic acid/kainate antagonists. *See* AMPA (alpha-3-hydroxy-5-methyl-4-isooxazoloproprionic acid)/kainate antagonists.

α-Blockers, 44

β-Blockers, 44, 45t, 153-154

3-Hydroxy-3-methyglutaryl coenzyme A reductase inhibitors. *See* HMG-CoA (3-hydroxy-3-methyglutaryl coenzyme A reductase) inhibitors.

4a-Phemamthrenamine derivatives, 270

4-S (Scandinavian Simvastatin Stroke Study), 49t

Abciximab, 252

Abdominal aortic aneurysm, 35

ACAPS (Asymptomatic Carotid Artery Progression Study), 49t

ACE (angiotensin-converting enzyme) inhibitors, 44-46, 45t, 153-154

Acetaminophen, 150, 184

Activity levels, 179-181, 180t-181t

Acute stroke management (prevention, evaluation, and treatment) topics. *See also under individual topics.*

  clinical trials and research studies. *See* Clinical trials and research studies.

  diagnoses and evaluations, 69-101

  drug therapies and drug-related considerations. *See* Drug therapies and drug-related considerations.

  emergency medical management, 147-173

  fundamental concepts, 13-19

  hemorrhagic stroke management, 189-219

  hospital admissions and general management, 175-188

  imaging techniques (brain and blood vessels), 103-145

  ischemic stroke acute management, 221-314

    brain blood supply, 221-264

    neuroprotection, 265-278

    prevention measures and therapies, 279-314

  overviews and summaries. *See* Overviews and summaries.

  post-stroke rehabilitation, 315-320

  prevention measures and therapies, 33-68, 279-314

    general measures, 33-68

    for ischemic and recurrent ischemic stroke, 279-314

  reference resources. *See* Reference resources.

  services organization, 21-32

Acute stroke-care teams, 24-27, 26t

13

Adenosine receptor agonists, 268

Admissions, 175-188. *See also* Hospital admissions and general management.

Age-related risk factors, 34t

Airway and breathing support, 147-149

Akinetic segments, 36t

Albers, et al study, 231t

Alcohol consumption, excessive, 51-52, 193t, 287-290, 289t

Algorithms, 90f-95f, 282f-283f. *See also under individual topics.*
  for diagnoses and evaluations, 90f-95f
  for recurrent ischemic and ischemic stroke (prevention measures and therapies), 282f-283f

Alpha-3-hydroxy-5-methyl-4-isooxazoloproprionic acid/kainate antagonists. *See* AMPA (alpha-3-hydroxy-5-methyl-4-isooxazoloproprionic acid)/kainate antagonists.

Alpha-blockers, 44

Altepase Thrombolysis for Acute Noninterventional Therapy in Ischemic Stroke study. *See* ATLANTIS (Altepase Thrombolysis for Acute Noninterventional Therapy in Ischemic Stroke) study.

Alzheimer's disease, 13

Amaurosis fugax, 56-57

Amlyloid angiopathy, 42t

AMPA (alpha-3-hydroxy-5-methyl-4-isooxazoloproprionic acid)/kainate antagonists, 269-270

Amphetamines, 43t, 198

Amyloid angioplasty, central, 199

Analgesics, 184, 205t

Ancrod, 222t

Aneurysms, 35, 36t-37t, 42t, 203-211, 205t-206t, 208f-209f, 273-274
  abdominal aortic, 35
  aneurysmal rupture, 273-274
  atrial septal, 36t
  descriptions of, 36t-37t, 42t
  fusiform (dolichoectatic), 37t
  nonsaccular, 203-204
  risk factors and, 36t-37t, 42t
  saccular, 203-211, 205t-206t, 208f-209f
  ventricular, 36t

Angina pectoris, 35

Angiotensin receptor blockers. *See* ARBs (angiotensin receptor blockers).

Angiotensin-converting enzyme inhibitors. *See* ACE (angiotensin-converting enzyme) inhibitors.

Antacids, 184-185, 293

Antibiotics, 183, 288, 289t

Anticoagulants, 25t, 43t, 81, 178t, 185-186, 190, 193-195, 193t, 196t, 221, 222t, 232, 241-250, 242t-243t, 246t-247t, 249t, 298-299

Anticoagulants, long-term, 280-281, 280t
Anticoagulants, oral, 194-195, 196t, 250, 281-291, 282f-283f,
    284t-285t, 292
Anticonvulsants, 160, 205t
Antiemetic agents, 184, 205t
Antifibrinolytic agents, 205t, 207
Antihypertensive agents, 46, 155, 184, 205t-206t
Antiplatelet aggregate agents, 43t, 193-195, 196t, 221-223, 222t,
    232, 250-252, 280-281, 280t, 291-298, 292t, 298-299
Antipyretics, 150
Antithrombotic agents, 154-155, 221-223
Aortic atherosclerosis, 37t
Apnea, sleep, 51-52
Aptiganel, 269270
ARBs (angiotensin receptor blockers), 44, 45t, 46
Argatroban, 222t
Arrhythmias, 150-151, 151t
Arterial hypertension, 151-158, 156t-157t
  descriptions of, 151-152
  long-term treatment initiation for, 155-158
  treatment of, 153-155, 153t. 156t-157t
Arterial hypotension, 158
Aspirin, 150, 205t, 222t, 242t-243t, 246t-247t, 250-252, 280-281,
    280t, 282f-283f, 287, 291-294, 292t
Aspirin, low dose, 282f-283f, 293-295, 298-299
Aspirin/clopidogrel, 195, 297-298, 298-299
Aspirin/dipyridamole, 194, 252, 280-281, 280t, 282f-283f, 294-295,
    298-299
Asymptomatic Carotid Artery Progression Study. See ACAPS
    (Asymptomatic Carotid Artery Progression Study).
Asymptomatic cervical (carotid) stenosis or bruit, 54-56
Atherosclerotic causes, 35-43, 37t
ATLANTIS (Altepase Thrombolysis for Acute Noninterventional
    Therapy in Ischemic Stroke) study, 227-232
Atrial appendage thrombus, 36t
Atrial fibrillation, 36t, 53-54
Atrial lesions, 36t
Atrial septal aneurysm, 36t
Atrial septic defect, 36t
Atrial thrombus, 36t
Atrial turbulence, 36t
Atropine, 206t

Background perspectives, 13-14
Barbiturates, 272
Barthel Index, 225t-226t

13

Basic concepts. *See* Fundamental concepts; Overviews and summaries.
Basic FGF (basic fibroblastic growth factor), 270-271
Beta-blockers, 44, 45t, 153-154
Bezodiazepines, short-acting, 160
Bladder care, 183
Bleeding diatheses, 42t, 193-197, 193t, 197t
Brain attack (stroke)-heart attack (myocardial infarction) difference summaries, 22t
Brain blood supply, 221-264. *See also* Ischemic stroke acute management.
  anticoagulants, 241-250
  antiplatelet agents, 250-252
  embolectomy, 257
  endovascular extraction of thrombus, 255-257
  intervention summaries, 222t
  nonpharmacologic surgical measures, 255-257
  novel pharmacologic therapies, 254
  overviews and summaries of, 221-223, 222t
  pharmacologic thrombolysis, 223-240
  reference resources for, 258-264
Brain edema, 160-166, 163t
Brain imaging techniques, 103-145. *See also* Imaging techniques (brain and blood vessels).
Brain stem signs, 75t-76t
Breathing and airway support, 147-149
Bupropion, 51

Calcium channel blockers, 44, 45t, 153-154, 266-268, 274
Calcium channel blockers, L-type, 267-268
Camerlingo, et al study, 242t-243t, 246t-247t
Candesartan, 153
Cardiac causes, 36t
Cardiac complications, 150-151, 151t
Cardioembolism, 35-40
Cardiomyopathy, dilated, 36t
Cardioversion, pharmacologic, 54
CARE (Cholesterol and Recurrent Events) study, 49t
Carotid circulation territories, 73t
Carotid duplex scanning, 130-132, 133f
Carotid endarterectomy, 300-303, 301t, 303t
Centers of excellence, 23-24
Central amyloid angioplasty, 199
Cerebellum signs, 75t-76t
Cerebral hemisphere infarction signs, 78t-79t
Cerebral ischemia, secondary, 207-211
Cerebrobasilar circulation territories, 73t

Cerebrovascular accidents. *See* CVAs (cerebrovascular accidents).

Cerebrovascular disease, 13

Certoparin, 242t-243t, 246t-247t

CGP-40116, 270

CGS 19755, 270

CHARISMA (Clopidogrel for High Atherothrombotic Risk and Ischemic Stabilization, Management, and Avoidance) trial, 251

Chemotherapy, 200

Cholesterol and Recurrent Events study. *See* CARE (Cholesterol and Recurrent Events) study.

Choline, 270

Cimetidine, 184-185

Citicholine, 270

Classes of Recommendations, 16t, 27, 44-52, 148-166, 198, 232, 284-304

  Class I, 16t, 27, 44-52, 148-159, 198, 232, 284-304

  Class II, 16t

  Class IIa, 16t, 51, 154-155, 159, 163-166, 285-286, 300-304

  Class IIb, 16t, 47, 51-52, 285-286

  Class III, 16t, 148-151, 154-155, 160, 162-166, 287

  overviews and summaries of, 16t

Claudication, 35

Clinical features, 70-75, 71t-75t. *See also* Diagnoses and evaluations.

Clinical trials and research studies. *See also under individual topics.*

  4-S, 49t

  ACAPS, 49t

  Albers, et al study, 231t

  ATLANTIS study, 227-232

  Camerlingo, et al study, 242t-243t, 246t-247t

  CARE study, 49t

  CHARISMA trial, 251

  ECASS-1, 227-232, 228t

  ECASS-2, 227-232

  Eckert, et al study, 252

  Egan, et al study, 231t

  FISS, 242t-243t, 244-248, 246t-247t

  FISS-bis, 242t-243t, 246t-247t

  Grond, et al study, 231t

  HAEST, 242t-243t, 246t-247t

  IST, 241-244, 242t-243t, 246t-247t

  KAPS, 49t

  Katzan, et al study, 231t

  LIPID trial, 49t

  MERCI trial, 255-257

  NINDS studies, 224-236, 225t-226t, 229t

  PROACT study, 237-240, 248-250

13

Clinical trials and research studies *(continued)*
  PROACT-II study, 238-240
  RAPID study, 242t-243t, 246t-247t
  STAT parallel studies, 252
  TAIST, 242t-243t, 246t-247t
  Tanne, et al study, 231t
  TOAST, 242t-243t, 246t-247t
  TOPAS study, 242t-243t, 246t-247t
  Wang, et al study, 231t
  WARCEF trial, 286
  WARSS trial, 248
  WOSCOPS, 49t
Clomethiazole, 268, 273
Clopidogrel, 251-252, 280-281, 280t, 282f-283f, 292t, 296-298
Clopidogrel for High Atherothrombotic Risk and Ischemic
    Stabilization, Management, and Avoidance trial. *See*
    CHARISMA (Clopidogrel for High Atherothrombotic Risk and
    Ischemic Stabilization, Management, and Avoidance) trial.
Clopidogrel/aspirin, 195, 297-299
Clumsy hand syndrome, 76t
CNS 5161A, 270
Coagulation disorders, 35
Cocaine, 43t, 198
Collaboration considerations, 21
Common misconceptions, 14-15
Common symptoms summaries, 22t
Complications, 180t-181t, 184-185
  summaries of, 180t-181t
  treatment of, 184-185
Computed tomography. *See* CT (computed tomography).
Computed tomography angiography. *See* CTA (computed
    tomography angiography).
Concomitant diseases, 184-185
Contraceptives, oral, 34t, 51
Corticosteroids, 162
Coumarins, 250, 282f-283f, 284t-285t
Crural paresis, 76t
Crystalloids, 253-254
CT (computed tomography), 103-118, 104t-107t, 108f, 110f-115f,
    116t
CTA (computed tomography angiography), 133-136, 135f-136f
CVAs (cerebrovascular accidents), 14
Cytidine, 270
Cytidine diphosphocholine, 270

Dalteparin, 242t-243t, 246t-247t
Danaparoid, 222t, 242t-243t, 245-248, 246t-247t

Deep vein thrombosis prevention, 185-186
Dementia, 13, 193t, 289t
Dementia, degenerative, 13
Desmoteplase, 222t, 240
Dextran, low molecular weight, 222t, 253-254
Dextrorphan, 269-270
Diabetes mellitus, insulin resistance, and metabolic syndrome, 46-47
Diagnoses and evaluations, 69-101
  algorithm for, 90f-95f
  brain stem signs, 75t-76t
  carotid circulation territories, 73t
  cerebellum signs, 75t-76t
  cerebral hemisphere signs, 76t
  cerebrobasilar circulation territories, 73t
  clinical features, 70-75, 71t-75t
  diagnosis and treatment summaries, 17
  diagnostic testing, 83-85, 84t-88t, 90f-95f
  differential diagnoses, 69-70, 70t
  emergency diagnostic studies summaries, 88t
  general examinations, 75-80, 76t-80t
  Glasgow Coma Scale, 87t
  historical features, 71t
  Hunt and Hess Scale, 86t
  immediate evaluations, 80-83, 82t-83t
  infarction signs, cerebral hemisphere, 78t-79t
  ischemic vs hemorrhagic stroke features, 80t, 82t-83t
  lacunar syndromes, 76t
  localizing signs, 78t-79t
  neurologic worsening causes, 72t
  NIHSS, 85t
  overview and summaries of, 69
  reference resources for, 95-101
  SAH signs, 84t, 86t
Diatheses, bleeding, 42t, 193-197, 193t, 197t
Digital substraction angiography. *See* DSA (digital substraction angiography).
Dipyridamole, 292t
Dipyridamole, extended-release, 298-299
Dipyridamole/aspirin, 194, 252, 280-281, 280t, 282f-283f, 294-295, 298-299
Direct thrombin inhibitors, 222t, 250, 290-291
Diuretics and diuretic agents, 44, 45t, 46, 153-154, 182-183
Dopamine, 158, 206t
Drug abuse, 51-52, 193t, 198, 289t
Drug therapies and drug-related considerations, 252, 298. *See also under individual drug classes and names.*
  α-blockers, 44

13

Drug therapies and drug-related considerations *(continued)*
β-blockers, 44, 45t, 153-154
4a-phemamthrenamine derivatives, 270
abciximab, 252
ACE inhibitors, 44, 45t, 46, 153-154
acetaminophen, 150, 184
adenosine receptor agonists, 268
AMPA/kainate antagonists, 269-270
amphetamines, 43t, 198
analgesics, 184, 205t
ancrod, 222t
antacids, 184-185, 293
antibiotics, 183, 288, 289t
anticoagulants, 25t, 43t, 81, 178t, 185-186, 190, 193-195, 193t,
    196t, 221, 222t, 232, 241-250, 242t-243t, 246t-247t, 249t,
    298-299
anticoagulants, long-term, 280-281, 280t
anticoagulants, oral, 194-195, 196t, 250, 281-291, 282f-283f,
    284t-285t, 292
anticonvulsants, 160, 205t
antiemetic agents, 184, 205t
antifibrinolytic agents, 205t, 207
antihypertensive agents, 46, 155, 184, 205t-206t
antiplatelet aggregate agents, 43t, 193-195, 196t, 221-223, 222t,
    232, 250-252, 280-281, 280t, 291-298, 292t, 298-299
antipyretics, 150
antithrombotic agents, 154-155, 221-223
aptiganel, 269270
ARBs, 44, 45t, 46
argatroban, 222t
aspirin, 150, 205t, 222t, 242t-243t, 246t-247t, 250-252, 280-281,
    280t, 282f-283f, 287, 291-294, 292t
aspirin, low dose, 282f-283f, 293-295, 298-299
aspirin/clopidogrel, 195, 297-299
aspirin/dipyridamole, 194, 252, 280-281, 280t, 282f-283f, 294-295,
    298-299
atropine, 206t
barbiturates, 272
basic FGF, 270-271
bezodiazepines, short-acting, 160
bupropion, 51
calcium channel blockers, 44, 45t, 153-154, 266-268, 274
calcium channel blockers, L-type, 267-268
candesartan, 153
cardioversion, pharmacologic, 54
certoparin, 242t-243t, 246t-247t
CGP-40116, 270

Drug therapies and drug-related considerations *(continued)*
  CGS 19755, 270
  chemotherapy, 200
  choline, 270
  cimetidine, 184-185
  citicholine, 270
  clomethiazole, 268, 273
  clopidogrel, 251-252, 280-281, 280t, 282f-283f, 292t, 296-298
  CNS 5161A, 270
  cocaine, 43t, 198
  contraceptives, oral, 34t, 51
  corticosteroids, 162
  coumarins, 250, 282f-283f, 284t-285t
  crystalloids, 253-254
  cytidine, 270
  cytidine diphosphocholine, 270
  dalteparin, 242t-243t, 246t-247t
  danaparoid, 222t, 242t-243t, 245-248, 246t-247t
  desmoteplase, 222t, 240
  dextran, low molecular weight, 222t, 253-254
  dextrorphan, 269-270
  dipyridamole, 292t
  dipyridamole, extended-release, 298-299
  direct thrombin inhibitors, 222t, 250, 290-291
  diuretics and diuretic agents, 44, 45t, 46, 153-154, 182-183
  dopamine, 158, 206t
  eliprodil, 269-270
  fibrinogen-depleting agents, 222t, 252
  fibrinolytic agents, 221-223
  fosphenytoin, 160
  fraxiparin, 242t-243t, 244-248
  free-radical scavengers, 273
  furosemide, 163t, 164
  GABA agonists, 268
  gemfibrozil, 50
  glutamate receptor antagonists, 266
  glutamate release inhibitors, 268
  glycerol, 164
  GM1, 272
  GP IIa/IIb inhibitors, 252, 298
  GP IIa/IIb receptor blockers, 222t
  GPI 3000, 270, 298
  hemostatic medications, 191
  heparin, 40t, 185-186, 196t, 222t, 238-244, 239t, 242t-243t,
    246t-247t, 248-250, 249t
  heparin, low molecular weight (LMWH), 222t, 244-248, 246t-247t,
    289-290

13

Drug therapies and drug-related considerations *(continued)*
  histamine antagonists, 184-185, 293
  HMG-CoA inhibitors, 48, 49t
  hydroxyethyl starch, 253-254
  hypertonic saline, 163t, 164
  ibuprofin, 150
  insulin, 46-47, 69-70
  labetalol, 155, 156t-157t
  laxitives, 182-183
  leukocyte-endothelial cell adhesion receptor inhibitors, 222t
  licostinel, 269-270
  lovastatin, 49t
  lubeluzole, 268, 273
  magnesium sulfate, 270
  mannitol, 163t, 164
  memantine, 270
  membrane-active agents, 270
  nadroparin, 242t-243t, 246t-247t
  naloxone, 272
  neuroprotectants-reperfusion combinations, 273
  neuroprotective agents, 266
  neurotrophic factors, 270-271
  nicardipine, 155, 156t-157t
  nicotine products (smoking cessation), 51
  nifedipine, sublingual, 155
  nimodipine, 206t, 211, 267-268, 273-274
  nitrites, 44, 45t, 153-154
  nitroglycerin, topical, 155
  nitropaste, 156t-157t
  nitroprusside. *See* Sodium nitroprusside.
  NMDA antagonists, 269-270, 274
  NO modulators, 271
  nonagonist opiate receptor antagonists, 272
  nonsteroidal anti-inflammatory agents, 205t
  normal saline, 148t, 182-183
  novel pharmacologic therapies, 254
  NXY-059, 273
  ondansetron, 184
  opiates, 205t, 272
  ORG 10172, 242t-243t
  PAs, 221-237, 225t-226t, 228t-229t, 231t, 234f-235f, 240, 248-250,
    249t, 255
  phenylpropanolamine, 43t
  phenytoin, 160
  pioglitazone, 47
  pravastatin, 49t
  prourokinase, 222t, 237-240, 239t

Drug therapies and drug-related considerations *(continued)*
remacemide, 269-270
reteplase, 222t
r-Factor VIIa, 191
as risk factors, 42. *See also* Risk factors.
rt-PA/alteplase, 26t, 27-28, 91f, 154-155, 191, 222t, 223-238,
    225t-226t, 228t-229t, 231t, 234f-235f, 240, 248-252, 249t,
    255, 268, 273
saline, 254
saline, hypertonic, 163t, 164
saline, normal, 148t, 182-183
scu-PA, 222t
sedatives, 205t
selfotel, 269-270
S-emopamil, 267-268
simuvastin, 49t
sodium channel blockers, 268
sodium nitroprusside, 155, 156t-157t
statins, 48, 49t, 50
stimulants, 198
stool softeners, 182-183, 205t
streptokinase, 222t, 224
sulfinpyrazone, 298
TGF-β, 270-271
thrombolytic agents, 43t, 81, 154-155, 190, 193t, 194-195, 196t,
    201, 222t, 223-236, 225t-226t, 228t-229t, 231t, 234f-235f,
    252, 274
thrombolytic agents, intra-arterial, 236-240, 239t
ticlopidine, 280-281, 280t, 282f-283f, 292t, 295-296
tinzaparin, 242t-243t, 246t-247t
tirilazad mesylate, 272
TNK, 222t, 240
tranquilizers, major, 184
triple-H therapy, 211
urokinase, 222t
vasoconstrictors, 222t, 254
vasodilators, 222t
vasopressors, 158, 206t, 222t, 254
VSCC antagonists, 266
VSCC blockers, N-type and T-type, 267-268
warfarin, 89, 280-281, 280t, 282f-283f, 284t-285t, 286, 292, 299
white cell receptor blockers, 254
ximelagatran, 290-291
ZK200775, 269-270
DSA (digital substraction angiography), 136-140, 137f, 141t
Duplex scanning, carotid, 130-132, 133f
Dysarthria, 76t

13

ECASS-1 (European Cooperative Acute Stroke Study-1), 227-232, 228t

ECASS-2 (European Cooperative Acute Stroke Study-2), 227-232

EC/IC (extracranial-intracranial) bypass, 304

Eckert, et al study, 252

Edema, brain, 160-166, 163t

Egan, et al study, 231t

Electrocardiographic abnormalities, 150-151t

Eliprodil, 269-270

Embolectomy, 257

Emergency medical management, 147-173
  arterial hypertension, 151-158, 156t-157t
    descriptions of, 151-152
    long-term treatment initiation for, 155-158
    treatment of, 153-155, 153t, 156t-157t
  arterial hypotension, 158
  brain edema, 160-166, 163t
  emergency diagnostic studies summaries, 88t
  emergency evaluation component summaries, 25-27
  emergency life-support, 147-151, 148t, 151t
    airway and breathing support, 147-149
    arrhythmias, 150-151, 151t
    cardiac complications, 150-151, 151t
    components of, 148t
    electrocardiographic abnormalities and, 150-151t
    fever, 149-150
    hyperbaric oxygen, 149
  emergency medical services and. *See* EMSs (emergency medical services).
  for hemorrhagic stroke management, 190-191. *See also* Hemorrhagic stroke management.
  hyperglycemia vs hypoglycemia and, 158-159
  ICP, 160-166, 163t
  overviews and summaries of, 147
  palliative care and, 166
  papilledema, 161-162
  reference resources for, 167-173
  SAH, 159-160
  seizures, 159-160

EMSs (emergency medical services), 22t, 23-27, 25t-26t. *See also* Services organization.
  acute stroke-care teams, 24-27, 26t
  common symptoms summaries and, 22t
  emergency evaluation component summaries and, 25-27
  governmental support and, 23
  HMOs and, 24

EMSs (emergency medical services) *(continued)*
  Joint Commission on Accreditation Healthcare Organizations and, 23
  required field information summaries, 24-26, 25t
  stroke centers of excellence and, 23-24
  stroke (brain attack)-myocardial infarction (heart attack) difference summaries and, 22t
Endarterectomy, carotid, 300-303, 301t, 303t
Endovascular extraction of thrombus, 255-257
Endovascular interventions, 305-307, 305t
Epidemiology and etiology, 13-14, 33-42, 34t
  epidemiologic risk factors, 33-35, 34t. *See also* Risk factors.
    age, 34t
    descriptions of, 33-35, 34t
    family histories, 34t, 40-42
    geography, 34t
    race, 34t
  fundamental concepts, 13-14
Ethnic- and race-related risk factors, 34t
Etiology and epidemiology, 13-14. *See also* Epidemiology and etiology.
European Cooperative Acute Stroke Study-1. *See* ECASS-1 (European Cooperative Acute Stroke Study-1).
European Cooperative Acute Stroke Study-2. *See* ECASS-2 (European Cooperative Acute Stroke Study-2).
Evaluations and diagnoses, 69-101
  algorithm for, 90f-95f
  carotid circulation territories, 73t
  cerebellum signs, 75t-76t
  cerebral hemisphere infarction signs, 78t-79t
  cerebrobasilar circulation territories, 73t
  clinical features, 70-75, 71t-75t
  diagnosis and treatment summaries, 17
  emergency diagnostic studies summaries, 88t
  evaluation component summaries, 25-27
  general examinations, 75-80, 76t-80t
  Glasgow Coma Scale, 87t
  historical features, 71t
  Hunt and Hess Scale, 86t
  immediate evaluations, 80-83, 82t-83t
  ischemic vs hemorrhagic stroke features, 80t, 82t-83t
  lacunar syndromes, 76t
  localizing signs, 78t-79t
  neurologic worsening causes, 72t
  NIHSS, 85t
  overview and summaries of, 69
  reference resources for, 95-101
  SAH signs, 84t, 86t

13

Evidence levels. *See* Levels of Evidence.

Examinations, general, 75-80, 76t-80t. *See also* Diagnoses and evaluations.

Excessive alcohol consumption, 51-52

Exercise, lack of, 51-52

Extended-release dipyridamole, 298-299

Extracranial large-artery atherosclerosis, 37t

Extracranial-intracranial bypass. *See* EC/IC (extracranial-intracranial) bypass.

Extraction of thrombus, endovascular, 255-257

Family histories, 34t, 40-42

Features, clinical, 70-75, 71t-75t. *See also* Diagnoses and evaluations.

Female vs male risk factors, 34t, 40-42

Fever, 149-150

FGF, basic. *See* Basic FGF (basic fibroblastic growth factor).

Fibrinogen-depleting agents, 222t, 252

Fibrinolytic agents, 221-223

Field information summaries, 24-26, 25t

FISS (Fraxiparine Ischemic Stroke Study), 242t-243t, 244-248, 246t-247t

FISS-bis (second Fraxiparine Ischemic Stroke Study), 242t-243t, 246t-247t

Fosphenytoin, 160

Four-S (Scandinavian Simvastatin Stroke Study), 49t

Fraxiparin, 242t-243t, 244-248

Fraxiparine Ischemic Stroke Study. *See* FISS (Fraxiparine Ischemic Stroke Study).

Fraxiparine Ischemic Stroke Study (second). *See* FISS-bis (second Fraxiparine Ischemic Stroke Study).

Free-radical scavengers, 273

Fundamental concepts, 13-19. *See also* Overviews and summaries.
  common misconceptions, 14-15
  diagnosis and treatment summaries, 17
  etiology and epidemiology, 13-14
  historical perspectives, 13-14
  Levels of Evidence and Classes of Recommendations, 16-17, 16t.
See also Classes of Recommendations; Levels of Evidence.
  management options summaries, 14-17, 16t
  overviews and summaries of, 13
  prevention summaries, 14-15
  reference resources for, 18-19

Fusiform (dolichoectatic) aneurysm, 37t

GABA (gamma-aminobutyric acid) agonists, 268

Gemfibrozil, 50

General examinations, 75-80, 76t-80t. *See also* Diagnoses and evaluations.

General management, 175-188. *See also* Hospital admissions and general management.

General observations and vital signs, 181

General prevention measures, 33-68. *See also* Prevention measures and therapies.

  overviews and summaries of, 33-35

  primary vs secondary prevention and, 33-35

  reference resources for, 59-68

  risk factors and, 33-52, 34t, 36t-40t, 42t-43t, 45t, 49-50t. *See also* Risk factors.

Geography-related risk factors, 34t

Glasgow Coma Scale, 25t, 87t

Glasgow Outcome Scale, 225t-226t

Glutamate receptor antagonists, 266

Glutamate release inhibitors, 268

Glycerol, 164

Glycoprotein (GP) IIa/IIb inhibitors, 252, 298

Glycoprotein (GP) IIa/IIb receptor blockers, 222t

GM1 (monosialoganglioside), 272

Governmental support, 23

GP (glycoprotein) IIa/IIb inhibitors, 252, 298

GP (glycoprotein) IIa/IIb receptor blockers, 222t

GPI 3000, 270, 298

Grond, et al study, 231t

HAEST (Heparin Aspirin Ischemic Stroke Trial), 242t-243t, 246t-247t

Heart attack (myocardial infarction)-brain attack (stroke) difference summaries, 22t

Hematologic risk factors, 40t

Hemorrhagic infection, secondary, 199-201

Hemorrhagic stroke management, 189-219

  causation management and prevention, 192-211. *See also* Prevention measures and therapies.

  bleeding diatheses, 193-197, 193t, 197t

  central amyloid angioplasty, 199

  drug abuse, 198

  hypertensive hemorrhage, 192-193

  nonsaccular aneurysms, 203-204

  rebleeding prevention, 205-207

  saccular aneurysms, 203-211, 205t-206t, 208f-209f

  SAH, 203-211, 205t-206t, 208f-209f

  secondary cerebral ischemia, 207-211

  tumors, 197

  vascular malformations, 201-203

  vasculitis, 197-198

  vasospasm prevention, 206t, 207-211

  venous thrombosis with secondary hemorrhagic infection, 199-201

13

Hemorrhagic stroke management *(continued)*
emergency management, 190-191. *See also* Emergency medical
management.
descriptions of, 190
hemostatic medications, 190
surgical management, hematomas, 190
hemorrhagic vs ischemic stroke features, 80t, 82t-83t
overviews and summaries of, 189-190
reference resources for, 212-219
Hemorrhagic transformation of infarction, 42t
Hemostatic medications, 190, 191
Heparin, 40t, 185-186, 196t, 222t, 238-244, 239t, 242t-243t,
246t-247t, 248-250, 249t
Heparin Aspirin Ischemic Stroke Trial *See* HAEST (Heparin
Aspirin Ischemic Stroke Trial).
Heparin, low molecular weight (LMWH), 222t, 244-248, 246t-247t,
289-290
Highest risk factors, 53-59, 58t-63t. *See also* Risk factors.
amaurosis fugax, 56-57
asymptomatic cervical (carotid) stenosis or bruit, 54-56
atrial fibrillation, 53-54
descriptions of, 53
TIA, 56-57, 58t-61t
warning leak, 57-59, 62t-63t
Histamine antagonists, 184-185, 293
Historical features, 71t. *See also* Diagnoses and evaluations.
Historical perspectives, 13-14
HMG-CoA (3-hydroxy-3-methyglutaryl coenzyme A reductase)
inhibitors, 48, 49t
HMOs (health maintenance organizations), 24
Homolateral ataxia, 76t
Hospital admissions and general management, 175-188
activity levels, 179-181, 180t-181t
bladder care, 183
complications, 180t-181t, 184-185
summaries of, 180t-181t
treatment of, 184-185
concomitant diseases, 184-185
deep vein thrombosis prevention, 185-186
general management, 176-179, 178t-179t
hypovolemia and, 182-183
multidisciplinary management, 178t-179t
neurologic worsening causes, 176t
nutrition and hydration, 182-183
overviews and summaries of, 175-176, 176t
pulmonary embolism prevention, 185-186
reference resources for, 187-188

Hospital admissions and general management *(continued)*
  rehabilitation, 186
  SIADH and, 182-183
  symptomatic management, 184
  vital signs and general observations, 181
Hunt and Hess Scale, 86t
Hydration and nutrition, 182-183
Hydroxyethyl starch, 253-254
Hyperbaric oxygen, 149
Hypercholesterolemia, 47-50, 49t
Hyperglycemia vs hypoglycemia, 158-159
Hyperhomocysteinemia, 51-52
Hypertension, arterial, 151-158, 156t-157t
Hypertensive hemorrhage, 192-193
Hypertonic saline, 163t, 164. *See also* Saline.
Hypoglycemia vs hyperglycemia, 158-159
Hypotension, arterial, 158
Hypothermia, 271-273
Hypovolemia, 182-183

Ibuprofin, 150
ICP (increased intracranial pressure), 160-166, 163t
Imaging techniques (brain and blood vessels), 103-145
  brain imaging, 103-129
  carotid duplex scanning, 130-132, 133f
  CT, 103-118, 104t-107t, 108f, 110f-115f, 116t
  CTA, 133-136, 135f-136f
  DSA, 136-140, 137f, 141t
  MRA, 133-134, 134f
  MRI, 118-129, 120f, 122t-123t, 124f-127f, 128t, 129t
  MRV, 133-134, 134f
  overviews and summaries of, 103, 104t-105t
  PC sequences, 132-133
  PI, 140
  reference resources for, 142-145
  TCD ultrasonography, 130-132, 133f
  TOF sequences, 132-133
  vascular imaging, 129-140
Immediate evaluations, 80-83, 82t-83t. *See also* Diagnoses and
  evaluations.
Increased intracranial pressure. *See* ICP (increased intracranial
  pressure).
Insulin, 46-47, 69-70
Insulin resistance. *See* Diabetes mellitus, insulin resistance, and
  metabolic syndrome.
Interarterial lesions, 36t
International Stroke Trial *See* IST (International Stroke Trial).

13

Intervention summaries, 222t

Intra-arterial thrombolytic agents, 236-240, 239t. *See also* Thrombolytic agents.

Intraatrial lesions, 36t

Intracranial causes, 42t

Intraventricular lesions, 36t

Intraventricular thrombus, 36t

Introductory concepts. *See* Fundamental concepts; Overviews and summaries.

Ischemic stroke acute management, 221-314. *See also under individual topics.*

  brain blood supply, 221-264

    anticoagulants, 241-250

    antiplatelet agents, 250-252

    embolectomy, 257

    endovascular extraction of thrombus, 255-257

    intervention summaries, 222t

    nonpharmacologic surgical measures, 255-257

    novel pharmacologic therapies, 254

    overviews and summaries of, 221-223, 222t

    pharmacologic thrombolysis, 223-240

    reference resources for, 258-264

  neuroprotection, 265-278

    AMPA antagonists, 269-270

    aneurysmal rupture, 273-274

    calcium channel blockers, 267-268

    free-radical scavengers, 273

    glutamate release inhibitors, 268

    hypothermia, 271-273

    membrane-active agents, 270

    neurotrophic factors, 270-271

    NMDA antagonists, 269-270

    NO modulation, 271

    novel interventions, 272-273

    overviews and summaries of, 256-267

    reference resources for, 275-278

    SAH, 273-274

    window of treatment, 274-275

  prevention measures and therapies, 279-314

    endovascular interventions, 305-307, 305t

    general measures for, 279-280

    medications for, 280-298

    overviews and summaries of, 279

    reference resources for, 307-314

    surgical procedures for, 299-304

Isolated sensory/motor stroke, 76t

IST (International Stroke Trial), 241-244, 242t-243t, 246t-247t

Joint Commission on Accreditation Healthcare Organizations, 23-24

KAPS (Kuopio Atherosclerosis Prevention Study), 49t
Katzan, et al study, 231t
Kuopio Atherosclerosis Prevention Study. *See* KAPS (Kuopio
   Atherosclerosis Prevention Study).

Labetalol, 155, 156t-157t
Lack of exercise, 51-52
Lacunar syndromes, 76t
Lacunes, 35
Large-artery atherosclerosis, 35
Laxitives, 182-183
Left atrial lesions, 36t
Left ventricular lesions, 36t
Leukocyte-endothelial cell adhesion receptor inhibitors, 222t
Levels of Evidence, 16t, 27-52, 148-166, 198, 232, 284-304
  Level A, 16t, 27-29, 44-52, 158-159, 232, 284-304
  Level B, 16t, 51-52, 148-151, 154-155, 159, 162-166, 198,
    285-286, 300-304
  Level C, 16t, 47, 51, 148-151, 154-155, 160
  overviews and summaries of, 16-17, 16t
Libman-Sacks endocarditis, 36t
Licostinel, 269-270
Life-support, emergency, 147-151, 148t, 151t. *See also* Emergency
   medical management.
  airway and breathing support, 147-149
  arrhythmias, 150-151, 151t
  cardiac complications, 150-151, 151t
  components of, 148t
  electrocardiographic abnormalities and, 150-151t
  fever, 149-150
  hyperbaric oxygen, 149
LIPID (Long-term Intervention With Pravastatin in Ischemic
   Disease) trial, 49t
Lipophyalinosis, 37t
LMW (low molecular weight) dextran, 222t, 253-254
LMWH (low molecular weight heparin), 222t, 244-248, 246t-247t,
   289-290. *See also* Heparin.
Localizing signs, 78t-79t. *See also* Diagnoses and evaluations.
Long-term anticoagulants, 280-281, 280t. *See also* Anticoagulants.
Long-term Intervention With Pravastatin in Ischemic Disease.
   See LIPID (Long-term Intervention With Pravastatin in
   Ischemic Disease) trial
Long-term treatment initiation, 155-158
Lovastatin, 49t
Low dose aspirin, 282f-283f, 293-295, 298-299. *See also* Aspirin.

13

Low molecular weight dextran, 222t, 253-254

Low molecular weight heparin (LMWH), 222t, 244-248, 246t-247t, 289-290

L-type calcium channel blockers, 267-268

Lubeluzole, 268, 273

Magnesium sulfate, 270

Magnetic resonance angiography. *See* MRA (magnetic resonance angiography).

Magnetic resonance imaging. *See* MRI (magnetic resonance imaging).

Magnetic resonance veonography. *See* MRV (magnetic resonance venography).

Major tranquilizers, 184

Malabsorption cautions, 289t

Male vs female risk factors, 34t, 40-42

Malformations, vascular, 201-203

Management of stroke (prevention, evaluation, and treatment) topics. *See also under individual topics.*

  brain and blood vessel imaging techniques, 103-145

  clinical trials and research studies. *See* Clinical trials and research studies.

  diagnoses and evaluations, 69-101

  drug therapies and drug-related considerations. *See* Drug therapies and drug-related considerations.

  emergency medical management, 147-173

  fundamental concepts, 13-19

  hemorrhagic stroke management, 189-219

  hospital admissions and general management, 175-188

  ischemic stroke acute management, 221-314

    brain blood supply, 221-264

    neuroprotection, 265-278

    prevention measures and therapies, 279-314

  overviews and summaries. *See* Overviews and summaries.

  post-stroke rehabilitation, 315-320

  prevention measures and therapies, 33-68, 279-314

    general measures, 33-68

    for ischemic and recurrent ischemic stroke, 279-314

  reference resources. *See* Reference resources.

  services organization, 21-32

Mannitol, 163t, 164

Mechanical Embolus Removal in Cerebral Ischemia. *See* MERCI (Mechanical Embolus Removal in Cerebral Ischemia) trial.

Medications. *See* Drug therapies and drug-related considerations.

Memantine, 270

Membrane-active agents, 270

MERCI (Mechanical Embolus Removal in Cerebral Ischemia) trial, 255-257

Metabolic syndrome. *See* Diabetes mellitus, insulin resistance, and metabolic syndrome.

Microatheroma, 37t

Migraine, 51-52

Mineral supplementation. *See* Supplements (vitamins, minerals, etc).

Misconceptions, common, 14-15

Mitrial annulus calcification, 36t

Modifiable risk factors, 34t, 43-52, 45t, 49t-50t. *See also* Risk factors.
  alcohol consumption, excessive, 51-52
  apnea, sleep, 51-52
  descriptions of, 34t, 43
  drug abuse, 51-52
  exercise, lack of, 51-52
  hypercholesterolemia, 47-50, 49t
  hyperhomocysteinemia, 51-52
  hypertension, 43-46, 45t
  migraine, 51-52
  obesity, 51-52
  oral contraceptive use, 51-52
  sleep disorders, 51-52

Modified Rankin Scale, 225t-226t

Monocular blindless, transient, 56-57

Monosialoganglioside (GM1), 272

MRA (magnetic resonance angiography), 133-134, 134f

MRI (magnetic resonance imaging), 118-129, 120f, 122t-123t, 124f-127f, 128t, 129t

MRV (magnetic resonance venography), 133-134, 134f

Multidisciplinary management, 178t-179t

Mural thrombus, 36t

Myocardial infarction (heart attack)-stroke (brain attack) difference summaries, 22t, 34t, 35, 40-42

Myxoma, 36t

Nadroparin, 242t-243t, 246t-247t

Naloxone, 272

National Institutes of Health Stroke Scale. *See* NIHSS (National Institutes of Health Stroke Scale).

National Institutes of Neurological Disorders and Stroke. *See* NINDS (National Institutes of Neurological Disorders and Stroke) studies.

Neoplasm, 42t. *See also* Tumors.

Neurologic worsening causes, 72t, 176t

Neuroprotectants-reperfusion combinations, 273

13

Neuroprotection, 265-278. *See also* Ischemic stroke acute management.
  AMPA antagonists, 269-270
  aneurysmal rupture, 273-274
  calcium channel blockers, 267-268
  free-radical scavengers, 273
  glutamate release inhibitors, 268
  hypothermia, 271-273
  membrane-active agents, 270
  neurotrophic factors, 270-271
  NMDA antagonists, 269-270
  NO modulation, 271
  novel interventions, 272-273
  overviews and summaries of, 256-267
  reference resources for, 275-278
  SAH, 273-274
  window of treatment, 274-275
Neuroprotective agents, 266
Neurotrophic factors, 270-271
Nicardipine, 155, 156t-157t
Nicotine products (smoking cesession), 51
Nifedipine, sublingual, 155
NIHSS (National Institutes of Health Stroke Scale), 26t, 85t, 225t-226t, 238-240, 249t
Nimodipine, 206t, 211, 267-268, 273-274
NINDS (National Institutes of Neurological Disorders and Stroke) studies, 224-236, 225t-226t, 229t
Nitric oxide modulators. *See* NO (nitric oxide) modulators.
Nitrites, 44, 45t, 153-154
Nitroglycerin, topical, 155
Nitropaste, 156t-157t
Nitroprusside. *See* Sodium nitroprusside.
NMDA (N-methyl-D-aspartate) antagonists, 269-270, 274
NO (nitric oxide) modulators, 271
Nonagonist opiate receptor antagonists, 272
Nonatherosclerotic vasculopathies, 35
Nonpharmacologic surgical measures, 255-257
Nonsaccular aneurysms, 203-204
Nonsteroidal anti-inflammatory agents, 205t
Normal saline, 148t, 182-183. *See also* Saline.
Novel pharmacologic therapies, 254
N-type and T-type VSCC (voltage-sensitive calcium channel) blockers, 267-268
Nutrition and hydration, 182-183
NXY-059, 273

Obesity, 51-52

Observations, general, 181

Ondansetron, 184

Opiates, 205t, 272

Oral anticoagulants, 194-195, 196t, 250, 281-291, 282f-283f, 284t-285t, 292. *See also* Anticoagulants.

Oral contraceptives, 34t, 51-52

ORG 10172, 242t-243t

Organization of services, 21-32
  collaboration considertations for, 21
  EMSs, 22t, 23-27, 25t-26t
    acute stroke-care teams, 24-27, 26t
    common symptoms summaries and, 22t
    emergency evaluation component summaries and, 25-27
    governmental support and, 23
    HMOs and, 24
    Joint Commission on Accreditation Healthcare Organizations and, 23
    required field information summaries, 24-26, 25t
    stroke centers of excellence and, 23-24
    stroke (brain attack)-myocardial infarction (heart attack) difference summaries and, 22t

Overviews and summaries. *See also under individual topics.*
  of diagnoses and evaluations, 69
  of emergency medical management, 147
  of fundamental concepts, 13
  of hemorrhagic stroke management, 189-190
  of hospital admissions and general management, 175-176, 176t
  of imaging techniques (brain and blood vessels), 103, 104t-105t, 221-223, 222t
  of ischemic stroke acute management, 221-223, 222t, 256-267, 279
    neuroprotection, 256-267
    prevention measures and therapies, 279
  of prevention measures and therapies, 33-35, 279
    general measures, 33-35
    ischemic and recurrent ischemic stroke, 279
  of services organization, 21

Oxygen, hyperbaric, 149

Palliative care, 166

Papilledema, 161-162

PAs (plasminogen activators), 221-237, 225t-226t, 228t-229t, 231t, 234f-235f, 240, 248-250, 249t, 255

Patent foramen ovale, 36t

PC (phase contrast) sequences, 132-133

Perfusion imaging. *See* PI (perfusion imaging).

Pharmacologic therapies. *See* Drug therapies and drug-related considerations.

13

Phase contrast sequences. *See* PC (phase contrast) sequences.
Phenylpropanolamine, 43t
Phenytoin, 160
PI (perfusion imaging), 140
Pioglitazone, 47
Plasminogen activators. *See* PAs (plasminogen activators).
Post-stroke rehabilitation, 315-320
  discharge planning and, 315, 318
  overviews and summaries of, 315
  patient education and, 315
  reference resources for, 318-320
  rehabilitation specialists, 315-318
    acute care setting-outpatient/inpatient setting transitions, 316-317
    constraint-induced movement therapy and, 317
    occupational therapists, 316
    physical therapists, 316
    roles of, 315-318
    speech pathologists, 316
  rehabilitation specialists roles in, 315-318
Pravastatin, 49t
Prevention measures and therapies, 33-68, 279-314. *See also under
    individual topics.*
  for deep vein thrombosis prevention, 185-186
  fundamental concepts of, 14-15
  general measures, 33-68
    overviews and summaries of, 33-35
    primary vs secondary prevention and, 33-35
    reference resources for, 59-68
    risk factors and, 33-52, 34t, 36t-40t, 42t-43t, 45t, 49-50t. *See
        also* Risk factors.
  for hemorrhagic stroke management, 192-211. *See also*
      Hemorrhagic stroke management.
  for ischemic and recurrent ischemic stroke, 279-314
    endovascular interventions, 305-307, 305t
    general measures for, 279-280
    medications for, 280-298
    overviews and summaries of, 279
    reference resources for, 307-314
    surgical procedures for, 299-304
  for pulmonary embolism, 185-186
  for vasospasm, 206t, 207-211
Primary vs secondary prevention, 33-35. *See also* Prevention
    measures and therapies.
PROACT (Prolyse in Acute Cerebral Thromboembolism) study,
    237-240, 248-250
PROACT-II (Prolyse in Acute Cerebral Thromboembolism-II)
    study, 238-240

Prolyse in Acute Cerebral Thromboembolism. *See* PROACT
(Prolyse in Acute Cerebral Thromboembolism) study.
Prolyse in Acute Cerebral Thromboembolism-II study. *See*
PROACT-II (Prolyse in Acute Cerebral Thromboembolism-II)
study.
Prourokinase, 222t, 237-240, 239t
Pulmonary embolism prevention, 185-186
Pure motor hemiparesis, 76t
Pure sensory stroke, 76t

Race- and ethnic-related risk factors, 34t
Rankin Scale, Modified, 225t-226t
RAPID (Rapid Anticoagulation Prevents Ischemic Damage) study,
242t-243t, 246t-247t
Rebleeding prevention, 205-207
Recombinant activated Factor VII. *See* r-Factor VIIa (recombinant
activated Factor VII).
Recombinant tissue plasminogen activator. *See* rt-PA/alteplase
(recombinant tissue plasminogen activator).
Recommendation classes. *See* Classes of Recommendations.
Recurrent ischemic and ischemic stroke (prevention measures and
therapies), 279-314. *See also* Prevention measures and therapies.
algorithm for, 282f-283f
general measures for, 279-280
medications for, 280-298. *See also* Drug therapies and drug-
related considerations.
anticoagulants, oral, 281-285, 285t
antiplatelet agents, 291-298, 292t
arterial diseases and, 287
aspirin, 291-294
cardioembolic stroke and, 284-286, 284t
coagulation disorders and, 286
clopidogrel, 296-298
descriptions of, 280-281, 280t
dipyridamole and aspirin/dipyridamole, 294-295
direct thrombin inhibitors, 290-291
GP IIa/IIb inhibitors, 298-299
poentital complications of, 287-290, 289t
sulfinpyrazone, 298-299
ticlopidine, 295-296
overviews and summaries of, 279
reference resources for, 307-314
surgical procedures for, 300-305, 301t, 303t, 305t
carotid endarterectomy, 300-303, 301t, 303t
descriptions of, 299-300
endovascular interventions, 305-307, 305t
revasculatization operations, 304

13

Recurrent ischemic and ischemic stroke (prevention measures and therapies), surgical procedures for *(continued)*
    superficial temporal artery to middle cerebral artery anastomosis (extracranial-intracranial [EC/IC] bypass), 304

Reference resources. *See also under individual topics.*
  for diagnoses and evaluations, 95-101
  for emergency medical management, 167-173
  for fundamental concepts, 18-19
  for hemorrhagic stroke management, 212-219
  for hospital admissions and general management, 187-188
  for imaging techniques (brain and blood vessels), 142-145
  for ischemic stroke acute management, 258-264, 275-278, 307-314
    brain blood supply, 258-264
    neuroprotection, 275-278
    prevention measures and therapies, 307-314
  for prevention measures and therapies, 59-68, 307-314
    general measures, 59-68
    ischemic and recurrent ischemic stroke, 307-314
  for services organization, 29-32

Rehabilitation, 186

Remacemide, 269-270

Reperfusion-neuroprotectants combinations, 273

Required field information summaries, 24-26, 25t

Research studies. *See* Clinical trials and research studies.

Reteplase, 222t

Revasculatization operations, 304

r-Factor VIIa (recombinant activated Factor VII), 191

Risk factors, 33-52, 34t, 36t-40t, 42t-43t, 45t, 49-50t. *See also* Prevention measures and therapies.
  amlyloid angiopathy, 42t
  aneurysm, 36t-37t, 42t
  atherosclerotic causes, 35-43, 37t
  bleeding diatheses, 42t
  cardiac causes, 36t
  cardioembolism, 35-40
  coagulation disorders, 35, 40t
  drugs and pharmacologic agents, 42
  epidemiologic, 33-35, 34t
    age, 34t
    descriptions of, 33-35, 34t
    family histories, 34t, 40-42
    geography, 34t
    race, 34t
    sex, 34t, 40-42
  hematologic, 40t
  hemorrhagic transformation of infarction, 42t

Risk factors (continued)
  highest, 53-59, 58t-63t
    amaurosis fugax, 56-57
    asymptomatic cervical (carotid) stenosis or bruit, 54-56
    atrial fibrillation, 53-54
    descriptions of, 53
    TIA, 56-57, 58t-61t
    warning leak, 57-59, 62t-63t
  intracranial causes, 42t
  large-artery atherosclerosis, 35
  modifiable, 34t, 43-52, 45t, 49t-50t
    alcohol consumption, excessive, 51-52
    apnea, sleep, 51-52
    descriptions of, 34t, 43
    diabetes mellitus, insulin resistance, and metabolic syndrome,
      46-47
    drug abuse, 51-52
    exercise, lack of, 51-52
    hypercholesterolemia, 47-50, 49t
    hyperhomocysteinemia, 51-52
    hypertension, 43-46, 45t
    migraine, 51-52
    obesity, 51-52
    oral contraceptive use, 51-52
    sleep disorders, 51-52
    smoking, 50-51
  neoplasm, 42t
  nonatherosclerotic vasculopathies, 35, 38t-39t
  overviews and summaries of, 33-35, 34t
  primary vs secondary prevention and, 33-35. See also Prevention
    measures and therapies.
  small-artery occlusive diseases (lacunes), 35
  trauma, 42t
  vascular malformation, 42t
  vasculitis, 42t
  venous thrombosis, 42t
rt-PA/alteplase (recombinant tissue plasminogen activator), 26t,
    27-28, 91f, 154-155, 191, 222t, 223-238, 225t-226t, 228t-229t,
    231t, 234f-235f, 240, 248-252, 249t, 255, 268, 273
Rupture, aneurysmal, 273-274

Saccular aneurysms, 203-211, 205t-206t, 208f-209f
SAH (subarachnoid hemorrhage), 84t, 86t, 159-160, 203-211,
    205t-206t, 208f-209f, 273-274
Saline, 254
Saline, hypertonic, 163t, 164
Saline, normal, 148t, 182-183

13

Scandinavian Simvastatin Stroke Study. *See* 4-S (Scandinavian Simvastatin Stroke Study).

Scavengers, free-radical, 273

scu-PA (single-chain urokinase plasminogen activator), 222t. *See also* PAs (plasminogen activators).

Second Fraxiparine Ischemic Stroke Study. *See* FISS-bis (second Fraxiparine Ischemic Stroke Study).

Secondary cerebral ischemia, 207-211

Secondary hemorrhagic infection, 199-201

Secondary prevention vs primary prevention, 33-35. *See also* Prevention measures and therapies.

Sedatives, 205t

Segments, akinetic, 36t

Seizures, 159-160

Selected readings. *See* Reference resources.

Selfotel, 269-270

S-emopamil, 267-268

Services organization, 21-32

  collaboration considerations for, 21

  EMSs, 22t, 23-27, 25t-26t

    acute stroke-care teams, 24-27, 26t

    common symptoms summaries and, 22t

    emergency evaluation component summaries and, 25-27

    governmental support and, 23

    HMOs and, 24

    Joint Commission on Accreditation Healthcare Organizations and, 23

    required field information summaries, 24-26, 25t

    stroke centers of excellence and, 23-24

    stroke (brain attack)-myocardial infarction (heart attack) difference summaries and, 22t

    third-party payers support and, 23

  overviews and summaries of, 21

  public education and responses, 21-23, 22t

    common symptoms awareness and recognition, 21-23, 22t

    correct responses, 21-23

    EDs and, 21-23

  reference resources for, 29-32

  stroke units, 26t, 27-29, 28t

    benefits of, 27

    components of, 28t

    definitions of, 27-28

    ICUs and, 28-29

    NIHSS score determinations and, 26t

    step-down unit concept of, 28-29

    success of, 27-29

Sex-related risk factors, 34t, 40-42

Shagbark aorta, 37t

Short-acting bezodiazepines, 160

SIADH (syndrome of inappropriate secretion of antidiruetic hormone), 182-183

Sign descriptions and summaries. *See* Diagnoses and evaluations.

Simuvastin, 49t

Single-chain urokinase plasminogen activator. *See* scu-PA (single-chain urokinase plasminogen activator).

Sleep apnea and other sleep disorders, 51-52

Small-artery disease, 37t

Small-artery occlusive diseases (lacunes), 35

Smoking, 50-51

Sodium channel blockers, 268

Sodium nitroprusside, 155, 156t-157t

STAT parallel studies (North American and European), 252

Statins, 48, 49t, 50. *See also under individual drug names.*

Stimulants, 198

Stool softeners, 182-183, 205t

Streptokinase, 222t, 224

Stroke centers of excellence, 23-24

Stroke management (prevention, evaluation, and treatment) topics. *See also under individual topics.*

  brain and blood vessel imaging techniques, 103-145

  clinical trials and research studies. *See* Clinical trials and research studies.

  diagnoses and evaluations, 69-101

  drug therapies and drug-related considerations. *See* Drug therapies and drug-related considerations.

  emergency medical management, 147-173

  fundamental concepts, 13-19

  hemorrhagic stroke management, 189-219

  hospital admissions and general management, 175-188

  imaging techniques (brain and blood vessels), 103-145

  ischemic stroke acute management, 221-314

    brain blood supply, 221-264

    neuroprotection, 265-278

    prevention measures and therapies, 279-314

  overviews and summaries. *See* Overviews and summaries.

  post-stroke rehabilitation, 315-320

  prevention measures and therapies, 33-68, 279-314

    general measures, 33-68

    for ischemic stroke, 279-314

  reference resources. *See* Reference resources.

  services organization, 21-32

Stroke (brain attack)-myocardial infarction (heart attack) difference summaries, 22t

Stroke services organization, 21-32. *See also* Services organization.

13

Studies, research. *See* Clinical trials and research studies.

Subarachnoid hemorrhage. *See* SAH (subarachnoid hemorrhage).

Sublingual nifedipine, 155

Suggested readings. *See* Reference resources.

Sulfinpyrazone, 298-299

Summary topics. *See* Overviews and summaries.

Superficial temporal artery to middle cerebral artery anastomosis, 304

Supplements (vitamins, minerals, etc). *See also under individual*
   supplement names.
  calcium, 45t
  folic acid, 51-52
  magnesium, 45t
  niacin, 50
  potassium, 45t, 182-183
  pyridoxine, 51-52
  vitamin B$_{12}$, 51-52
  vitamin K, 281, 288, 289t

Surgical procedures, 255-257, 300-305, 301t, 303t, 305t
  carotid endarterectomy, 300-303, 301t, 303t
  descriptions of, 299-300
  endovascular interventions, 305-307, 305t
  nonpharmacologic surgical measures, 255-257
  revasculatization operations, 304
  superficial temporal artery to middle cerebral artery anastomosis
    (extracranial-intracranial [EC/IC] bypass), 304

Symptoms summaries, 22t

Syndrome of inappropriate secretion of antidiuretic hormone. *See*
  SIADH (syndrome of inappropriate secretion of antidiuretic
  hormone).

TAIST (Tinzaparin in Acute Ischemic Stroke Trial), 242t-243t,
  246t-247t

Tanne, et al study, 231t

TCD (transcranial Doppler) ultrasonography, 130-132, 133f

Teams, acute stroke-care, 24-27, 26t

TEEs (transesophageal echocardiograms), 88-89

Tenecteplase. *See* TNK (tenecteplase).

TGF-β (transforming growth factor-β), 270-271

Therapy of Patients With Acute Stroke. *See* TOPAS (Therapy of
  Patients With Acute Stroke) study.

Thrombin inhibitors, direct, 222t, 250, 290-291

Thrombolysis, pharmacologic, 223-240

Thrombolytic agents, 43t, 81, 154-155, 190, 193t, 194-195, 196t, 201,
  222t, 223-236, 225t-226t, 228t-229t, 231t, 234f-235f, 252, 274

Thrombolytic agents, intra-arterial, 236-240, 239t

Thrombus extraction, endovascular, 255-257

TIA (transient ischemic attack), 56-57, 58t-61t

Ticlopidine, 280-281, 280t, 282f-283f, 292t, 295-296

Time-of-flight sequences. *See* TOF (time-of-flight) sequences.

Tinzaparin, 242t-243t, 246t-247t

Tinzaparin in Acute Ischemic Stroke Trial *See* TAIST (Tinzaparin in Acute Ischemic Stroke Trial).

Tirilazad mesylate, 272

TNK (tenecteplase), 222t, 240

TOAST (Trial of ORG 10172 in Acute Stroke Treatment), 242t-243t, 246t-247t

Tobacco use, 50-51

TOF (time-of-flight) sequences, 132-133

TOPAS (Therapy of Patients With Acute Stroke) study, 242t-243t, 246t-247t

Topical nitroglycerin, 155

Tranquilizers, major, 184

Transcranial Doppler ultrasonography. *See* TCD (transcranial Doppler) ultrasonography.

Transesophageal echocardiograms. *See* TEEs (transesophageal echocardiograms).

Transforming growth factor-β. *See* TGF-β (transforming growth factor-β).

Transient ischemic attack. *See* TIA (transient ischemic attack).

Transient monocular blindness. *See* Amaurosis fugax.

Transthoracic echocardiograms. *See* TTEs (transthoracic echocardiograms).

Trauma-related risk factors, 42t

Treatment windows, 274-275

Trial of ORG 10172 in Acute Stroke Treatment. *See* TOAST (Trial of ORG 10172 in Acute Stroke Treatment).

Trials, clinical *See* Clinical trials and research studies.

Triple-H therapy, 211

TTEs (transthoracic echocardiograms), 88-89

T-type and N-type VSCC (voltage-sensitive calcium channel) blockers, 267-268

Tumors, 197. *See also* Neoplasm.

13

Ultrasonography, transcranial Doppler. *See* TCD (transcranial Doppler) ultrasonography.

Unilateral ocular (III) nerve palsy, 160

Urokinase, 222t

Vascular imaging, 129-140. *See also* Imaging techniques (brain and blood vessels).

Vascular lesions, 36t

Vascular malformations, 42t, 201-203

Vasculitis, 42t, 197-198

Vasoconstrictors, 222t, 254

Vasodilators, 222t

Vasopressors, 158, 206t, 222t, 254

Vasospasm prevention, 206t, 207-211

Venous thrombosis, 42t

Venous thrombosis with secondary hemorrhagic infection, 199-201

Ventricular aneurysm, 36t

Vital signs and general observations, 181

Vitamins supplementation. *See* Supplements (vitamins, minerals, etc).

VSCC (voltage-sensitive calcium channel) antagonists, 266

VSCC (voltage-sensitive calcium channel) blockers, N-type and
  T-type, 267-268

Wang, et al study, 231t

WARCEF (Warfarin versus Aspirin in patients with Reduced
  Cardiac Ejection Fraction) trial, 286

Warfarin, 89, 280-281, 280t, 282f-283f, 284t-285t, 286, 292, 299

Warfarin versus Aspirin in patients with Reduced Cardiac Ejection
  Fraction trial. *See* WARCEF (Warfarin versus Aspirin in patients
  with Reduced Cardiac Ejection Fraction) trial.

Warning leak, 57-59, 62t-63t

WARSS trial, 248

West of Scotland Coronary Prevention Study. *See* WOSCOPS
  (West of Scotland Coronary Prevention Study).

White cell receptor blockers, 254

Window of treatment, 274-275

Worsening, neurologic, 72t, 176t

WOSCOPS (West of Scotland Coronary Prevention Study), 49t

Ximelagatran, 290-291

ZK200775, 269-270